PESTILENCE AND THE BODY POLITIC IN LATIN LITERATURE

Pestilence and the Body Politic in Latin Literature

HUNTER H. GARDNER

OXFORD
UNIVERSITY PRESS

OXFORD
UNIVERSITY PRESS

Great Clarendon Street, Oxford, OX2 6DP,
United Kingdom

Oxford University Press is a department of the University of Oxford.
It furthers the University's objective of excellence in research, scholarship,
and education by publishing worldwide. Oxford is a registered trade mark of
Oxford University Press in the UK and in certain other countries

First Edition published in 2019

Published in the United States of America by Oxford University Press
198 Madison Avenue, New York, NY 10016, United States of America

British Library Cataloguing in Publication Data
Data available

Library of Congress Control Number: 2019931473

ISBN 978–0–19–879642–8

For Syda, *filiae carissimae*

Acknowledgments

It is the twentieth-century zombie film that first afforded me the unique combination of thrills and moral discomfort inspired by the contagion narrative. For that reason, I must first give thanks to George Romero, and then to my older brother, Jamin, who introduced me to the genre and endured many late-night VHS screenings with me. Without him, I surely would have run across what is now an oversaturated market, but perhaps not at such an impressionable age.

Many friends and colleagues have helped me clarify and strengthen the arguments put forth in this book: Paul Allen Miller, Jim O'Hara, Alison Keith, Dominic Machado, Ted Gellar-Goad, Christine Perkell, Megan Drinkwater, and John Muckelbauer all read sections of this project in various stages of its development. The anonymous readers for the Press provided invaluable feedback on earlier chapter drafts. Christine Boeckl was gracious enough to help me, through a good deal of written correspondence and telephone conversation, with my ideas concerning the engraving by Raimondi that appears on the cover of this volume. I am of course solely responsible for any errors of content or argumentation that remain.

Grants from the Loeb Classical Library Foundation and the University of South Carolina's Provost's Office allowed me the time and mental space needed to complete the project. Funds from a Peter and Bonnie McCausland Fellowship assisted my travel to various sites in France and Italy, where I was able to view a good number of Renaissance and Baroque plague paintings. I owe a special *grazie mille* to the clergy at San Bartolomeo all' Isola in Rome, where I was allowed an unscheduled viewing of the interior plague painting by Carracci as well as the preserved foundations of the temple of Asclepius that once stood on the site. Charlotte Loveridge and Tom Perridge at Oxford University Press offered invaluable support as this manuscript developed over the past few years. Georgina Leighton showed remarkable patience and guidance (and a consistently cheerful disposition) in response to the myriad emails I sent her in the final stages of the book.

Students in my classes, especially Olivia Semler, and impressive audiences at the University of North Carolina, Hampden-Sydney

College, and Wake Forest University also provided useful feedback to my presentations on epidemic disease in Latin literature and its resonance of civil war.

Others have provided help in less direct but no less essential ways: Sharon James, Sarah Spence, my wonderful colleagues in USC's department of Languages, Literatures, and Cultures, Andrea Hebert, Susan Scoven, and Hartley Barber. I could not have managed this without the encouragement of my parents (Jackie and Ben) and my daughter, Svda, who is just beginning her own study of Latin and to whom this volume is dedicated.

Translations throughout are mine unless otherwise noted.

Sections of Chapters 4 and 5 were excerpted from an article originally published in *Vergilius* (2014, "Bees, Ants, and the Body Politic: Vergil's Noric Plague and Ovid's Origin of the Myrmidons." *Vergilius* 60: 3–31) and are reproduced with kind permission of the editor.

Contents

List of Illustrations

Introduction

Experiments in Plague Discourse

In his second-century CE treatise, *How to Write History*, Lucian comments on the pernicious spread of a certain disease among the Abderites:

> They say, my dear Philo, that during the reign of King Lysimachus, a sickness (νόσημα) fell up the people of Abdera. These were the symptoms: first everyone of them fell ill with fever, violent and obstinate; around the seventh day, after the fever broke, a lot of blood flowed from the nose, or they experienced heavy sweating; but the illness left their minds in a ridiculous state—they all went mad reciting tragedy!
> (*Hist. Conscr.*1, translation modified from Kilburn 1913)

The epidemic Lucian refers to in the passage, a disease spread by exposure to the theater, prompts all Abderites to quote tragedy until a change in the weather at last causes the νόσημα to abate. The literary critic then turns from tragedy to an account of a similar epidemic among writers of history, and the contagion that has infected a population of fledgling historians with pretensions of rivaling Thucydides, Herodotus, and Xenophon. The "Abderite" complaint thus offers Lucian the opportunity to "draw a comparison" (ἕν . . . ἐνὶ παραβαλεῖν, 2), and the νόσημα provides a more general metaphor for the rapid transmission of conventions, trends, and topoi among writers staking their claim within a given literary genre.

By using disease as a figure for generic (re-) production, Lucian anticipates by 2000 years those theoretical models that apply the metaphor of contagion to the infective power of literary discourses.[1]

[1] See Cooke (2009, 5–6), who focuses on the cross-contamination of terms in metaphor generally speaking (a discussion owing much to Derrida's *Dissemination*

Within its immediate context of precepts for composing history, however, Lucian's polemic against banal transmission of conventions cannot but evoke one of the most imitated passages in all of historiography, Thucydides' description of the Athenian plague. In Lucian we sense the same weariness with authors who narrate pestilence that Jürgen Grimm suggests in his mid-twentieth century survey of ancient plague discourse: after Vergil's rendering of plague in Noricum and beginning somewhere around the histories of Livy, pestilence narratives became overwrought with conventions, and stripped of emotive capacity (1965, 63).[2]

While I disagree with Grimm's disparaging evaluation and Lucian's implicit jab, their assessments raise the question of why the plague narrative morphed from purported eye-witness account into a literary topos, and why, of the many historiographic trends Lucian might have cited, he brings plague to the fore. While we may concede that certain conventions of narrating plague became trite from overuse, a more productive approach to their excesses is to ask why pestilence has proven such an irresistible discursive experiment: what ideological work do accounts of plague perform for the cultures that produce them? As various recent studies on contagion discourse have illustrated, the allure of writing pestilence lies partly in its representational capacity and, more specifically, in the way that infection and the social proximity it assumes allow writers to define communities and the norms that govern them.[3] Despite his attention to fever, sweating, and bloody noses, Lucian's account of the "Abderite disease" says as much about the values of the Abderites, flocking to convene in a

[2004]), and of terms in the plague metaphor in particular. See also Steel (1981, 106–7) on the "odd affinity between literature and contagious disease."

[2] Quintilian also implies the familiarity of the topos in his advice to orators concerning arguments about conjectural causes (*Inst. Orat.* 7.2.3), where he reviews commonly cited causes of pestilence in plague narratives; see further, Chapter 6, pp. 187–8.

[3] Two especially rich treatments of the topic are those of Cooke (2009) and Wald (2008), though both deal primarily with twentieth- and twenty-first-century discourses. Gomel's article length study (2000) also offers useful insights, while focusing primarily on the late twentieth-century novel. For earlier representations of plague (beginning with Boccaccio) and their metaphoric import, see Leavy (1992); these studies, along with the more explicitly theoretical approaches I outline in Chapter 1, have played important roles in allowing me to formulate my ideas about Roman pestilence.

theater dominated by productions of Euripidean tragedy (*Hist. Concrs.* 1), as it does about the nature of the disease that afflicts them.

As social pathologies of a community evolve over time and space, so too do those conventions of writing pestilence best suited to address them. Thus, although Lucretius purports to describe the same calamity that afflicted Athens in 430 BCE, included in Thucydides' history of the Peloponnesian war, he imagines a very different epidemic: in his account, victims of disease suffer in a way that addresses the chaotic world of Rome in the 50s BCE and promotes his Epicurean agenda as a means of achieving equanimity in the face of such chaos. While certain features of Thucydides' description of the Athenian plague—the ubiquity of death, contamination of the sacred with the profane, the neglect of the ill—reassert themselves in Latin treatments of epidemic disease, the Romans introduced unique physical, moral, and social symptoms as characteristics of Latin pestilence, symptoms that would better address the pathologies defining the social and cultural context in which such accounts were generated. This book explores the constitution of distinctively Roman features of contagion, initially as they evolved within three epic treatments of plague, those of Lucretius, Vergil, and Ovid, produced during the late Republic and early Empire.

When scholars turn to antiquity for representations linking plague to the disruption of the social bond, they largely confine discussion to Greek models, especially those offered in Sophocles' *Oedipus Rex* and Thucydides' history (Grimm 1965; Girard 1974; Cooke 2009).[4] Alternatively, a resurgence of interest in the first known outbreak of bubonic plague (541–750 CE) has shed light on the histories of Procopius and his Greek models (Little 2007; Rosen 2007). While these trends have left the bookends of the classical pestilence tradition well documented, they have neglected what the Romans were doing with that tradition in between.[5] In turning attention to Latin

[4] As will become clearer in my discussion of Seneca's *Oedipus*, references to the plague (λοιμός, 38) that befalls Thebes in Sophocles' tragedy are highly symbolic of (*inter alia*) Oedipus' polluted status, but the Greek text contains only the barest outline of a plague narrative and lacks detailed attention to symptomatology and epidemiology.

[5] Important exceptions include Grimm's monograph, cited above, and the initial chapters of Raymond Crawfurd's *Plague and Pestilence in Literature and Art* (1914). The only recent monograph on plague's representational capacity in the ancient world is that of Robin Mitchell-Boyask (2008), whose work, an exploration of the resonance

innovations in discourses of contagion, I have identified a revival of plague narratives during the late Republic and early Empire (*c.*55 BCE–8 CE), offered as self-conscious representations, rather than purported eyewitness accounts, of outbreaks of pestilence. I argue that Lucretius, Vergil, and Ovid, relying on the metaphoric relationship between the human body and the body politic, use representations of epidemics to address the collapse of the social order due to recurrent episodes of civil discord and to evaluate various remedies for recovery. Plague as such functions frequently in Roman texts to enact a drama in which the concerns of the individual must be weighed against those of the collective. As ancient and modern chronicles of the period have demonstrated, an individual's striving for political advancement, frequently termed *ambitio* and mobilized by popular support, often conflicted with familial devotion and the *res publica*'s well-being, and was diagnosed as a primary cause of civil strife.[6] Pestilence narratives, in which efforts for self-preservation must compete with bonds of kinship and *amicitia*, allow writers to reflect on the choices and sacrifices made in the event of a communally experienced crisis. In the context of a Republic brought down by intense competition for limited *honores*, the homogenizing force of contagious disease, in which all

of plague in fifth-century Athenian discourse, I invoke in my comments on Sophocles' *Oedipus* (Chapter 6). In the area of Latin representations of plague, there have been important article contributions, especially on the pestilences described in Lucretius and Vergil, but no monograph treatment. Vallillee's (1960) dissertation is a useful starting point in so far as it tracks certain topoi and literary echoes in the tradition of Latin plague narratives, but it does not attempt to account for those traditions either in terms of social and historical context or in terms of the range of theories emerging in the twentieth century used to explain contagion discourse. Julia Hawkins' (2019) monograph promises to add much to the discussion of metaphors of illness and healing in the Augustan period. She locates the origins of communal health and its management in the Hellenistic period under Ptolemaic rule and argues that Vergil and Ovid appropriate authority over communal health in their development of the imagery of poet and statesman as healers of a war-weary civic body. While my overall interpretation of the power assigned to the Princeps by the Augustan poets to manage community health is ultimately more cynical, and problematizes rather than confirms the efficacy of state-sponsored approaches to communal health (see Gardner 2014), we concur on a number of significant points discussed in Chapters 4 and 5.

6 Of course, *ambitio* was not uniformly cast in a negative light (e.g., Quint. *Inst.* 1.2.22). For *ambitio* as a cause of ill will (*invidia*) and hostile rivalry, cf. Cic. *Sul.*1; as a source of political instability, cf. Tac. *Ann.* 16.23; at *AUC* 3.35.1 Livy uses the term in its narrower sense of canvassing for votes, though the process takes on a decidedly negative valence through its association with the Decemvir Appius Claudius. Lintott (1990) discusses ancient views that the corrupt practices linked to the pursuit of public office were a source of the Republic's demise.

succumb equally to death, enacts a dissolution of conflict—catastrophic for sure, but also a preliminary step towards reconstructing a populace less at odds with itself.

While recognition of verbal allusions and terminology that intersects with contemporary discourses of civil war has shaped my understanding of how plague narratives function during the period, this analysis is also informed by twentieth-century approaches to representations of epidemic disease, those of Antonin Artaud, René Girard, Susan Sontag, and Michel Foucault, in particular. The work of these theorists regularly underscores the symbolic cleansing, renewal, and reordering of society that frequently operate within plague narratives. At the same time, as Elana Gomel's more recent approach to contagious disease reminds us, plague narratives, frequently posited as precursors to apocalyptic and post-apocalyptic scenarios, often leave us with remainders, discursively dwelling on the suffering of survivors left in the aftermath of a (not entirely) clean sweep (2000, 408; cf. Berger 1999). Such theoretical perspectives, weighing the expurgating power of plague against its ultimate resistance to a clean break from the past, allow us to better understand Roman fictions of disease and the ideological work they perform.

Lucretius' rendering of Athenian plague at the end of *De Rerum Natura*, Vergil's accounts of plague among cattle and apian communities in *Georgics* 3 and 4, and Ovid's account of pestilence in Aegina in *Metamorphoses* 7 combine the mythic dimensions of the Homeric νόσος that opens the *Iliad* with Thucydides' sustained interest in the impact of plague on the social order. Such a combination, articulated through the epic meter often, if problematically, associated with *reges et proelia* (Verg. *E*.6.3), results in narratives that call attention to their fictive status as often as they invoke ancient clinical accounts of disease in historians and medical writers. Epic accounts of pestilence in Latin generate meaning through exaggeration and inversion of tropes, shifts of perspective, vivid pathos, and structural experimentation, qualities not altogether absent from historical and medical accounts, but which operate under fewer constraints when projected within the realms of myth and legend, or even the relatively "ancient" history of fifth-century Athens.

Four features frequently define imaginative treatments of plague in Latin: 1) Roman pestilence confuses prelasparian or "Golden-Age" motifs with apocalyptic imagery; plague restores some aspects of the relationship between humans and a beneficent earth, but only after the eradication (or serious modification) of human civilization. 2) Such a return to primitive conditions, as it collapses social hierarchies and strife between species, is articulated as a consequence of the methods and symptoms of the disease pathogen, which works by dissolving barriers of the body, often resulting in liquefaction of flesh. 3) The liquefaction and resultant homogeneity of the body anticipates the dissolution of the individual subject and signals a similar dissolution in the body politic. 4) The collapse of discrete human subjects is often met with resistance,[7] a resistance dramatized through recognition of familial ties between parents, children, and siblings, usually in the moment of succumbing to disease or death. While I argue that these features emerge partly as a response to the civil discord of the late Republic and the gradual constitution of quasi-monarchical government under Augustus, they would have a lasting influence on literary successors writing in the genres of epic (Lucan and Silius Italicus) and tragedy (Seneca). Outbreaks of Roman plague also recur sporadically in the Western tradition, attesting to the capacity of Roman idioms of plague to address social dysfunction and offer a diseased foil against which a healthier social order might be imagined.

I have organized this book into three parts, the first of which ("*Tabula Rasa*: A New Kind of Plague Narrative") weighs the metaphoric potency of pestilence against its discursively constructed reality in Rome. Chapter 1, in considering evidence for the material conditions of Roman epidemics, examines how disease is documented, especially among medical writers and observers of Rome's cultural development. Such an examination allows us to isolate causes, symptoms, and demographic concerns associated with pestilence in the city (e.g., foul odors, liquefaction and putrefaction, contagious particles), which Latin poets manipulate in their fictionalized accounts. I then turn to contemporary theorists of disease discourse, particularly those who postulate the "clean slate" as one *telos* of the plague narrative, in effort to explain why the primarily physical features of epidemics isolated in the first part of the chapter might appeal to poets attempting to address dysfunction within the civic body. From different vantage points, Artaud, Foucault, Sontag, and Girard all observe the power of plague to purge a contaminated social

[7] Vergil's initial plague victims are of course not human, but are heavily anthropomorphized, a distinction I address in Chapter 4.

order and shed light on how symptomatologies and pathologies of epidemic disease frequently align with visions of a new order.

The expanding *scientia* of medicine and disease offers one source of common assumptions about epidemics informing the meaning of plague in the corpus of Latin epic. Alternatively, Rome's historical master narratives, as another source of evidence for the lived experience of Roman plague, offer a different set of assumptions about the shared Roman past that our poets draw from in upholding plague as a means of articulating political strife. In particular, Livy's *Ab Urbe Condita*, the subject of Chapter 2, frequently casts *pestilentia* as a collective crisis whose alleviation, abatement, or remedy must be sought through innovations in cultural and political institutions, innovations that in many cases prove salutary for the *res publica*'s developing stability and hegemony in Italy. Livy's narratives of contagion draw partly from the language of medical writers (Dutoit 1948) but equally from a historiographic tradition that correlated a diseased body with a diseased body politic (Woodman 2009). Close examination of Livy's language of epidemic disease and its contextualization within struggles between political classes reveals the historian's awareness of plague's metaphoric potential, in particular, its capacity to illustrate confusion within the social order and reflect on distinctions among members of different political *ordines*, especially the *patres/patricii* (highest class of citizens) and *plebs* (lowest class of citizens). While most episodes are relegated to the early Republican period, the historian invokes medical language programmatically in his history (*Praef.* 9–10) in ways that prompt us to apply the lessons learned from past outbreaks to the ailing body politic of the first century BCE.

Part II of this study consists of three chapters on "Experiments in Apocalyptic Thinking." Relying on the metaphor linking the human body to the body politic, accounts of plague in Lucretius, Vergil, and Ovid offer an evolution of responses to the breakdown of an aristocratically governed *res publica* in the mid-first century BCE and the eventual reconstitution of stabilized government under the Augustan Principate. Various discussions of plague texts have acknowledged how the discourse encourages a "drama of the self and other" to unfold (Stephanson 1987, 239; Leavy 1992, 7). While it would be anachronistic to equate the "self" postulated in many modern treatments of plague with the "self" of late-Republican Rome, Latin literature consistently demonstrates a notion of identity developed largely in relation to lineage, kinship networks, political alliances, and native *patria*.[8] In the context of civil war, these markers of identity are frequently rendered incompatible, as political rivalries often divided families against themselves (as, e.g., in the case of warring *fratres* who populate Lucretius' *De Rerum Natura*, 3.68–73, and Vergil's *Georgics*, cf. 2.510; 2.533).

Treatments of plague in Latin epic replicate confusion among traditional categories of self-identification by magnifying familial conflicts and confirmations in the face of disease: family members often neglect each other in a move for self-preservation, though *pietas* equally compels them to attend each other as they succumb to illness. More drastically, these treatments of pestilence invoke a link between human and civic *corpora* ("bodies"), and stage the dissolution of boundaries within and between *corpora* as the most explicit physical manifestation of the plague. Lucretius' treatment of the Athenian plague, the subject of Chapter 3, uses imagery of *corpora* to close his poem, in a move that, on the one hand, underscores the futility of Athenian citizens clinging to the material remnants of personal identity, as they struggle over the corpses of their kin (*rixantes potius quam corpora desererentur*, 6.1286; cf. Kelly 1980); on the other hand, the poet's sensitivity to blood relations within the community reconstitutes *corpora* as individuals whose humanity is expressed through their relationships as children and parents (6.1256–8).

Commager's (1957) analysis of the conclusion of *De Rerum Natura* has shown that the poet transfers the physical suffering brought about by plague not only to the moral condition of its victims but to the moral condition of the unenlightened human race, an opinion frequently echoed in attempts to find symbolic value in the episode since 1957.[9] While Commager does not emphasize civil war as a symptom

[8] A notion evident in the *sphragis* that concludes a number of poetry collections produced during the period (e.g., Prop. 1.22; Ov. *Am.* 3.15), as well as, e.g., Cicero's discussion of the family and *domus* in relation to the larger body politic (*De Off.* 1.53–4). I should stress that by "identity" I am referring above all to socially performed identity, in which family, *amicitiae*, and birthplace all play key roles (cf. Welch 2005, 8–9). Within the parameters of this project, I resist speculating on the interior lives of individual Romans, though social markers of identity indelibly impact an individual's self-awareness, as a number of psychoanalytic treatments of Latin poetry have demonstrated; see esp. Janan (2001) and Miller (2004).

[9] The episode's symbolic value is evident despite the poet's expressed antipathy toward metaphors: Lucretius rejects the use of musical harmony to describe the relationship between mind and body at *DRN* 3.124–35, cited in Sontag (1988, 95–6). She describes the passage as "the earliest attack I know on metaphoric thinking

of the unenlightened condition, recent analysis of the language of contemporary political struggles in the poem has dated its completion to 49 BCE, at the commencement of civil war between Pompey and Caesar (Hutchinson 2001).[10] As Pelling has emphasized (2010), Thucydides' account of the Peloponnesian war, as a war fought among Greek states, had heavily influenced Roman approaches to depicting Roman civil war. Lucretius' culling of the history for a prime example of human calamity would thus suggestively link his plague of Book 6 with recent incidents of civil strife, the Catilinarian conspiracy and the wars between Marius and Sulla, in particular. Reflecting on this larger context of contention among Rome's military and political elite, Lucretius describes the symptoms of the Athenian plague in language that echoes his earlier polemic against excessive desires for political *honores* (e.g., *DRN* 3.74–86). In doing so the poet primes *pestis* (or *pestilitas*) for application as a metaphor used to address destructive competition undertaken to augment individual *gloria*.[11]

Vergil's Noric cattle plague in *Georgics* 3, the subject of Chapter 4, develops a more direct correlation between contagious disease and civil discord. The initially conflicting symptoms (e.g., excessive heat and cold) effected by the disease soon collapse into liquefied homogeneity, and the open-ended spread of contagion that concludes Book 3 looks back to Lucretius' vision of the collapsing Athenian social order at the end of *De Rerum Natura*. Vergil, however, uses heavily anthropomorphized cattle to evoke a poignant image of the fraternal bond, a bond that is elsewhere in the poem depicted as bound to be severed through civil strife. Vergil's use of Golden-Age motifs, moreover, readies the Noric landscape for a fundamental shift in the order of things. All the same, the poet's resistance to identify a culprit of the disease and his failure to instruct readers of its remedy

about illness and health" (95). While Sontag's point concerning the particular metaphor she cites is valid, Lucretius necessarily employs metaphoric language throughout his poem, a tendency Kelly (1980, 96) has succinctly described as the use of *res apertae* to illuminate *res caecae*.

10 Hutchinson's argument, tentatively accepted by Schiesaro in 2007's *Cambridge Companion to Lucretius*, has been countered by Volk (2010), whose argument I address below, p. 98 n.31.

11 See Commager (1957, 112–13) for language in the plague that specifically echoes the poet's polemic against excessive political ambition.

indicate ambivalence toward prospects of recovery from contagion as civil war.

When disease strikes the apian community in the fourth *Georgic*, the competitive strivings of Orpheus and Aristaeus for Eurydice may be interpreted as a clearer source of the pestilence (*causa morbi*, 4.532); the slaughter of sacrificial animals, including four exceptional bulls, recommended by Cyrene is by some accounts a solution to the conflict between the two men, allowing Aristaeus to secure his position as master of his environment and restorer of a depleted population. Yet violence inherent in the remedy for the pestilence (institutionalized in the practice of the *bougonia*) as well as the homogenous, unflaggingly loyal offspring born from it fail to offer an adequate model for human existence: significantly, such a model cannot accommodate the interpersonal, often familial, connections that the poet privileges in other parts of the poem.

We can better understand Vergil's equivocation toward uniformity as an answer to the dilemmas of excessive *ambitio* by turning to Ovid's account of plague in *Metamorphoses* 7.490–660, the subject of Chapter 5. In Ovid's epic, the citizens of Aegina, nearly eradicated from a pestilence sent by Juno, are replaced by ant-born men, the Myrmidons, characterized in a manner reminiscent of the collective spirit and uniformity of the apian community in the *Georgics*. I argue that the episode should be read as a reflection of Ovid's cynical attitude toward Augustus' attempt to restore a war-depleted population by replacing it with a new generation of loyalists: the ant-born population of Myrmidons, bound to serve as soldiers in the war between Athens and Crete, constitute a new citizenry dreamt into existence by king Aeacus after he receives signs from Jupiter in the form of ants filing up a nearby oak tree. The privileges (grants of land) and functions (serving in war) awarded to this new population effectively sort out the confused heaps of those rotting *cadavera* of kin and acquaintances left in the wake of contagion, but hardly offer a sustainable model for the Roman citizenry. The poet's narrative of recovery thus broaches the political utility of pestilence, in such a way that not only reins in the uncontained post-apocalyptic visions of his predecessors in *DRN* 6 and *Georgics* 3, but also questions the rigorous mechanisms of recovery, often in the form of population controls, implemented by the Augustan Principate.

Part III of this study, "Transmitting Roman Plague," explores the early appropriation, by Imperial writers, of late-Republican and

Augustan treatments of pestilence, as well as the reception of Roman motifs of contagion in the Western tradition. In Chapter 6, I examine Seneca's version of Oedipus' tragedy: rather than turning to Sophocles for depiction of the Theban epidemic, Seneca relies heavily on Lucretius, Vergil, and Ovid to articulate the conditions of pestilence. This language reflects upon Oedipus' traditional role as *φαρμακός*, both infected "carrier" and savior to the Theban civic body, but also allows the dramatist to conjure the peculiar problems facing a Roman populace only recently pacified through the imperatives of the Julio-Claudian Principate.[12] Seneca's reception of those narratives preceding him brings into better focus how competing claims of individuality and collectivity have determined the pathology of earlier Augustan plagues. Characters throughout the play anticipate the conflict between Polyneices and Eteocles, establishing Thebes as a template for civil war (e.g., 738–50); and Oedipus' tentative status as unique or part of the collective is fervently negotiated in the plague passages (cf. *Oed.* 30, 76). Seneca's use of Golden-Age motifs in particular draws from his predecessors' narratives in order to conjure an atmosphere of epochal evolution amidst the epidemic, an atmosphere that both recognizes and questions the potential of a new order.

Two other instances of Imperial reception, the epics of Silius Italicus and Lucan, invoke the plagues of their predecessors in contexts of Roman civil discord, and both authors use the plague's power to enact the dissolution of individual identity as a way of illustrating the dangers of intense competition for political distinction. Lucan relies on the symptomatology of his predecessors in his account of the pestilence that afflicts Pompey's soldiers at Dyrrachium, but further emphasizes the link between contagion and internal conflict by casting both the disease and the fervor for civil war afflicting the armies of Caesar and Pompey as a *rabies* (*Bellum Civile* 6.63; 6.92). Moreover, Lucan's emphasis on unburied *corpora* in the context of a *pestis* echoes his constant attention to those corpses scattered on the battlefield as a result of strife and slaughter among *fratres*, signaling the dehumanizing effects of conflict within the Roman social order.

The civil discord of the *Punica* is less explicit, though recent scholarship has brought to light how war against a foreign foe allows Silius Italicus to comment on the internal discord of the year 69 CE that

12 On the uncertainties of dating the *Oedipus*, see Boyle (2011, xviii–xix), who tentatively suggests a Claudian date; see further below, Chapter 6, p. 208 n.31.

marked the end of the Julio-Claudian Principate.[13] Silius' pestilence in the context of the Roman attempt to besiege Syracuse during the Second Punic War brings about widespread, uniform destruction. In answer to the dehumanizing effects of those plagues that have preceded him, however, the poet recovers the distinction or "exemplarity" of the Roman general Marcellus within acceptable limits (Tipping 2010a). In so doing, he allows a kind of restrained individuality whose strivings will not fracture the collective efforts of the soldiery.[14] Such recuperative readings of plague, despite the tendency of the discourse to problematize hallmarks of individualism, also anticipate the possibility of renewal that follows in the wake of an epidemic.

The seventh and final chapter of this project demonstrates the persistent transmission of Roman plague in literary and visual arts, beginning with the early Christian period and proceeding up through the present day. Such a demonstration is necessarily selective rather than exhaustive and meant to indicate the range of interpretive possibilities available for readers who are sensitive to the conventions developed in the hexameter treatments of Lucretius, Vergil, and Ovid. Since their inception Roman plague topoi have emerged in a variety of media, from late-antique poetry and prose (e.g., Endelechius' fifth-century *Carmen de Mortibus Boum*; Paulus the Deacon's eighth-century *Historia Langobardorum*) to medical treatises and visual arts of the Italian Renaissance (e.g., Raphael's Vergilian *Plague of Phrygia* [1520's])[15] to contemporary films and novels. I concentrate on early Christian literary adaptations, paintings of the Italian Renaissance, and Anglo-American novels. These particular receptions crystallize the interplay between civil strife, familial discord, and epochal evolution evident in the pestilence narratives examined throughout this project, allowing further reflection on such dynamics as they are

[13] See, e.g., the articles of Marks and Fucecchi in the collection of essays edited by Augoustakis (2010).

[14] The poet's recognition of the positive impact of plague is not entirely anomalous; we observe it briefly in Grattius' late-Augustan poem, *Cynegetica*. The poem relies on Vergil's *Georgics* in its treatment of contagion among dogs, but instructs that pestilence is remediable with experience and devotion to the gods; see further, Chapter 4, p. 118 n.11.

[15] Raphael's drawing, a depiction of the Trojans beset by pestilence when they attempt to settle on Crete (*A.* 3.132–42), survives in the form of an engraving by Raimondi.

magnified or minimized in different dimensions.[16] In a concluding Epilogue, I address the post-millennial, and increasingly global, fixation on contagion evidenced in literature, television, and film.

Roman conventions of representing pestilence help us understand how visual and literary arts dramatize a tension between the ideals of autonomy and self-sufficiency and those that foster group cohesion and collectivity. As Roman plague texts demonstrate how the crisis of contagion offers an opportunity "to imagine as well as regulate" the ancient community, they also allow us to reflect on and better parse the discourse that governs contemporary outbreak narratives—both fiction and non-fiction.[17] Narratives of contagious disease show us not only how we are connected, but *with whom*, even as the threat of mortality, and the impulse to self-preservation, strain those relationships to the breaking point. Roman poets exploited that discursive power to the fullest in their attempt to track the pathologies that drove citizens toward a familially-inflected civil war. We too, as twenty-first-century *homo sapiens*, faced with equal drives to self-destruction and preservation, have indulged with aplomb, and occasional weariness, in the power of contagion to expose the frailties of those relationships that define us as a species.

[16] As will become evident in Chapters 6 and 7, my approach to reception and the power of later texts (broadly conceived) to provide insights into earlier texts is influenced by Martindale's "weak" thesis (1993, 7). His "strong" thesis—that any reading of ancient texts has already been conditioned by its various receptions—is also validated through my argument; the fact that we cannot get back to an originary meaning of any text should not prevent us from productively speculating on what plague might have meant to different Romans who encountered narratives about it in the late Republic and early Principate.

[17] See Wald 2008, 67. For non-fiction accounts relying on many tropes that define fictive plague narratives, cf. esp. *The Hot Zone* (Preston 1995) and *The Coming Plague* (Garrett 1994).

Part I

Tabula Rasa

A New Kind of Plague Narrative

1

Roman Pestilence

Tenor and Vehicle

Part of the potency of the plague metaphor is its function as an extension of the persistent analogy between human bodies and social units. As Turner (1984, 114) notes in *The Body and Society*:[1] the body is "the most potent metaphor of society . . . [and] disease is the most salient metaphor of a structural crisis. All disease is disorder—metaphorically, literally, socially, and politically." Ruth Padel has observed, similarly, of fifth-century Greek medical language used to explain social and moral transformation: "change in the body is an image for change in the body politic" (1992, 52–3; cf. Mitchell-Boyask 2008, 40–2). Such assertions of the body's role in political discourse have been confirmed less directly by Brooke Holmes, who investigates the ways in which the Hippocratic Corpus, by discursively mapping the human body, has expanded the representational capacity of the human form and its experience of disease (2010, esp. 13–18). In our post-structuralist world, representational thinking, and in particular the relative terms of a metaphor (the tenor and the vehicle) are of course rapidly destabilized.[2] How easily can parallels between human body and civic body or between "plague" as disease physically

[1] Cf. Woodman (2009, 59), citing Turner.

[2] Kennedy's (1993) study of the tropes and metaphors that populate Latin love elegy demonstrates the power struggles that determine primary and secondary fields of meaning: "All discourses seek by one means or another to control the potentiality for meaning that language has . . . The distinction between literal and metaphorical suggests that some uses of language are somehow more basic than others, that where the 'same' word can be used in two different contexts, for example, love and war, the one that gets called the 'literal' use, must be in some way prior or more important" (Kennedy 1993, 52). As K. goes on to argue, priority is always contested.

manifested and "plague" as a widespread disaster be confined within limited areas of signification, and carried efficiently and without ambiguity from one area to another?

Within the Latin literary tradition, that transference is particularly unstable. The Romans have various terms to indicate endemic and epidemic diseases:[3] *pestis, pestilentia, pestilitas, morbus, lues, contagium.* Despite its common appearance as an indicator of contagious disease in many of the narratives discussed in this book, the primary meaning of *pestis* is defined in the *Oxford Latin Dictionary* as a general term for "physical destruction" or "death," a usage attested as far back in the literary record as Ennius (*scen.* 168, Warmington's 1940 ed.); in the same author's *Annales* we find the word apparently referring to a contagious disease, and opposed to war, an alternate force of destruction (*hos pestis necuit, pars occidit illa duellis, Ann.* 476; Warmington's 1940 ed.). Apparent opposition, however, also forces a kind of elision, as *pestis* shares with war its role as a bane to human existence. Here Ennius may echo the coupling of war and disease (πόλεμος . . . λοιμός) first articulated by Achilles in his complaints to Agamemnon over the plague inflicted by Apollo at *Iliad* 1.61. As diachronic examination of the usage of *pestis* confirms, the word is frequently applied to the conditions of war, and it is likely that such military usage colors the term, even when its primary meaning refers to the conditions of disease.[4]

Moreover, by limiting the chronological range for our examination of *pestis* we observe a common invocation of the term in the context of the civil wars of the late Republic. Here too we can explain the

[3] These terms are used to describe the origins of diseases that afflict a population, whether repeatedly and arising from within a population (endemic) or sporadically and arising from outside a population (epidemic). While ancient writers do not apply these categories, the apparently "endemic" status of many of Rome's early diseases, observed by Crawfurd (1914, 42), is discussed further in Chapter 2. Unless using the adjectival forms (endemic and epidemic) to describe the origins of the disease, I apply the noun "epidemic" interchangeably with "pestilence" and "plague" to diseases afflicting a large portion of the population. The term "plague," while derived from a Latin word (*plaga*, "blow, wound"), originates in late Middle English.

[4] For a broader range of the metaphorical applications of *pestis* and *pestilentia,* see TLL esp. vol. 10.1, 1928.29–1930.58; see similar entries for *pestifer*, esp. 1921.37–51. I have emphasized usages of *pestis* here largely because the word and its cognates (*pestilentia, pestilitas*) recur with greater frequency in the literature under discussion. Other terms for contagious disease in poeticizing accounts of plague will be discussed further as they arise in subsequent chapters: e.g., *morbus* at *G.* 3.397, 504, 532 and *contagium* at *G.* 3.469 and *E.* 1.50.

association partly through Greek precedents, as Thucydides correlates the plague suffered by the Athenians in 430 BCE with the more general pathos of civil strife among Greek states (1.23; 2.59, 61; Parry 1969). *Pestis* and its compounds regularly appear in Cicero's orations and letters, with reference to Rome's internal discord:[5] the statesman describes Catiline's ascent as a *pestis* that has beset the body politic (Cic. *Sull.* 76), while he refers to the impending conflict (*bellum*) between Caesar and Pompey as "plague-bearing" (*pestifer*; *Att.* 8.14.2, 9.13.3). The later *Philippics* configure Antony as *pestis* to Rome's well-being (*Phil.* 8.15; cf. 5.43), and explicitly mark his return to the city from Brundisium in 41 BCE as "plague-bearing" (*pestiferum . . . M. Antoni reditum, Phil.* 3.2; 4.3), a threat to the state countered by the young Octavian's expedient levy of an army.

Addressing a wider swath of Roman history, but written only a few decades after Cicero's death, Livy's *Ab Urbe Condita* uses the terms in similar contexts of civil strife, for instance, in the case of Marcus Manlius, the single pestilent citizen (*unum pestiferum civem*, 6.19.6) whose attempt to instigate civil war in 384 BCE (*intestinum bellum*, 6.19.2) temporarily unites the patrician and plebeian orders. Similarly, in his account of the conflict between Marius and Sulla, Velleius Paterculus echoes Cicero's indictment of Antony by describing Marius' return to the city as a *pestifer reditus* (*Historiae Romanae*, 2.22). The anecdotes of Valerius Maximus, composed during the reign of Augustus' successor Tiberius, cast Quintus Varius as a "plague-bearing" tribune, and one of doubtful citizenship, in his own attempts to invoke civil war (*pestifer tribunus*, 8.6.4; cf. 5.4.1).

Perhaps the fullest flowering of the metaphor in roughly contemporary prose occurs in the *Controversiae* of Seneca the Elder (d. 30's CE?): in one series of rhetorical exercises, various arguments are offered from the perspective of a son whose poor father has given him up for adoption by a richer man, one who had already disinherited his own sons. The speaker Fabianus cites greed as the cause of similar infractions of familial piety, whose horrors have culminated on the battlefield in civil war: *quae tanta vos pestis, cum una stirps idemque sanguis sitis, quaeve furiae in mutuum sanguinem egere*? (2.1.10, "what monstrous

[5] For Cicero's figurative use of *pestis* to describe internal discord, see Schrijvers (1970, 320–1), who compares Lucretius' preference for *morbus* and suggests that the latter (as equivalent of the Greek νόσος) is more commonly applied to social and political movements.

disease, or what madness, drove you towards mutual bloodshed, though you are of a single stock and the same blood?"). The indictment against greed not only casts civil war as epidemic disease (*pestis*), but also observes a tendency, which we will examine more closely in subsequent chapters, to view civil war in distinctly familial terms. The trend in Roman political and historical discourses to some extent reflects a Greek tendency to characterize cities collectively as "sick" and to identify political strife (*stasis*) as one symptom of the sick city.[6] It is thus not surprising that Romans could consider the *Urbs* or *res publica* to be afflicted with illness. It is also worth considering, however, why a particular articulation of illness—a widespread epidemic, or *pestis*—would prove a suitable vehicle to convey the crisis of internal discord at Rome: what features of epidemic disease might discursively lend themselves to clarifying and reflecting on the experience of political strife?

1.1. EXPERIENCING AND OBSERVING EPIDEMIC DISEASE IN ANCIENT ROME

Cassius Dio informs us that an outbreak of pestilence during the early Augustan Principate (23–22 BCE) was considered by some a mandate for ceding to the Princeps consular authority, presumably to allow him to manage the disaster with more facility (cf. Gilliam 1961, 248):

> The pestilence (λοιμός) raged throughout all of Italy so that no one tilled the land, and I suppose the same was the case in foreign parts. The Romans therefore, reduced to dire straits by the diseases and by the consequent famine, believed that these woes had come upon them for no other reason than that they did not have Augustus for consul at this time as well. Accordingly, they wished to elect him dictator.
>
> (54.1.2–3, translation modified from Cary 1914)

Though Augustus refused this particular mandate (his powers already surpassed those of the office), its issuance aligned with his well-established identification with the premier god of healing, Apollo,

6 On the sick city (*polis nosousa*), see Kosak (2000).

who had been imported to Rome, with a temple built in his honor, in response to a plague of 433 BCE (cf. Livy 4.25).[7]

The incident stands as an illustration of the collision between real and representational notions of disease and the impact of such a collision in shoring up political authority. Augustus' powers to heal human bodies and heal the body politic became mutually reinforcing and nearly interchangeable. Apollo's association with bringing and alleviating contagious disease and his appropriation within what we can retroactively define as Augustan culture has been well documented (Galinsky 1996, 215–24; Zanker 1990, 44–71; Miller 2009). I offer this one evocation of the god's appropriation as an example of the potency of illness and its inverse, healing, as a metaphor used to inscribe a relationship between the statesman and the body politic.[8] Such a metaphor can only be effective in persuading concession to a new order within a context of a population familiar with the terms of real illness; that is, the tenor of the metaphor (ailing political institutions) can only make an impact on its audience if the vehicle (epidemic disease among human populations) is understood.

While bubonic plague did not befall Rome until the sixth century CE, the endemic conditions of certain pathogens in Rome compelled its citizens to experience pestilence as a matter of routine.[9] The role of plague in shaping the fate of the Roman Empire has been asserted, perhaps most famously by Niebuhr, though evidence for the actual impact of plague on Rome's population is less easily found.[10]

[7] This temple was later replaced by a temple to Apollo Medicus, the healer, three columns of which remain in Rome today. The more recent incarnation, while not as intimately connected with devotion to a relatively new god as a remedy against plague, may have had important political ramifications: its likely builder, the Antonian supporter Gaius Sosius, was perhaps contending with Augustus for proprietorship of the god and his healing properties during the aftermath of civil war; see Claridge (1998, 245–7). As such, some have interpreted the temple's erection as Antony's resistance to Octavian's appropriation of the god. See Williams (2009, 83), with further bibliography.

[8] On the statesman (and poet) as healer of the body politic, see Hawkins (2019).

[9] E.g., as was the case with malaria; see esp. Scheidel (2003, 158–76).

[10] Gilliam (1961, 225) cites Niebuhr's comment that during the reign of Marcus Aurelius plague "forms a turning point in so many things, and above all in literature and art, [and] I have no doubt that this crisis was brought about by the plague" (*Lectures on the History of Rome*, London 1849, p. 251). Gilliam goes on to assess evidence for the so-called Antonine plague more cautiously and implicitly reduce its impact on Rome's history. See also Littman and Littman (1973) who corroborate Gilliam's general assessment but suggest a higher mortality rate of around 10 percent. Harper (2017) credits the expansion of Rome's empire in combination with variously

Excellent recent edited collections have tackled the conditions of disease in the ancient city: the contributions in Bradley and Stow (2012) include plague as only one of many pollutants to afflict the *Urbs*, but usefully address the appropriation of a discourse of purity and pollution—or dirt as "matter out of place," using Mary Douglas' formulation—as a political weapon that has determined the physical development of Rome.[11] Scholarly surveys on the topic of disease have highlighted the resistance among many Romans to medical intervention and attempts to contain healing practices within the *paterfamilias*' realm of authority (Jackson 1988, 10–11; Keyser 2010, esp. 861–3). Despite this resistance there is also clear evidence of influence by Greek medical and philosophical texts upon Roman perceptions of the sick body,[12] and that influence is especially evident in Lucretius' discussions of disease, which establish a critical template for subsequent plague narratives in Latin poetry.[13]

By examining extra-poetic discourses about the causes and effects of epidemic disease we can better understand the efficacy of plague as

mobile populations as the driving forces behind disease in the later Empire, but evaluates the Antonine plague with some caution, calling it a "turning point" rather than a "fatal blow" (115).

[11] While many of the volume's insights apply to an era in which Christian doctrines determine the discourse of purity/pollution, its interest in "matter out of place" offers a useful way of conceptualizing the persistent problem survivors of disease faced in a crowded city, one where corpses of plague victims would pose a physical and psychological threat. See also Hope and Marshall's *Death and Disease in the Ancient City* (2000), where Bodel's contribution addresses the disposal of *cadavera* required during some of Rome's most devastating outbreaks of pestilence; discussion of epidemics in other contributions to this volume is confined mostly to the great plague of Athens, though Nutton's essay also addresses the prevalence of miasma theory, a tendency widespread throughout antiquity to attribute pestilence to an atmosphere corrupted by *miasmata* (in Hope and Marshall, 2000, 67–90); see further below, pp. 23–4. The collection edited by Little (2007) usefully introduces the perspectives of epidemiologists and forensic archaeologists, in addition to historical and literary perspectives, but its discussion is confined largely to the first recorded outbreak of bubonic plague in Constantinople under the reign of Justinian (541 CE). Of those essays in the collection that do address the spread of the pandemic into the Western Empire, Stoclet's (2007, 135, though still focusing on the 541 pandemic) is especially astute in using Livy's comments, cited in chapter two, pp. 67–8, on Roman responses to plague.

[12] Jackson (1988, 18–30). For this influence during the Augustan period in particular, see also Hawkins (2019).

[13] Nutton (1983, 9–10) makes this connection in his discussion of possible Epicurean contributions to the notion of seeds of disease and their illustration in Book 6 of *DRN*. Lucretius' articulation of diseased air as *semina* may have also had a reciprocal influence on medical writers, Galen in particular.

a metaphor—that is, the range of mental associations it might conjure in an audience with some experience (or at least historical awareness) of an epidemic. More specifically, we are able to gauge with better precision the degree to which epic poets exaggerated certain features of epidemic diseases as clinically described in medical writers, or manipulated recognizable developments of plague dramaturgy in historical anecdotes and cultural etiologies. The following comments are not intended as an exhaustive overview of what such writers have to say about epidemic disease, but instead survey a range of ancient writers attempting to understand, prevent, and predict the path of disease, in an effort to identify characteristics of and human responses to pestilence that may have informed treatments in Latin epic poetry.

As Hawkins observes in her work on "therapoetics" during the Augustan Principate, the Hippocratic Corpus and those medical texts influenced by it have little to say about plague, largely because the medical arts, which treated disease primarily through changes in human habits, were thought ineffective in combating it; pestilence appeared, at least by some accounts, to affect people regardless of diet and regimen.[14] Medical writers who operated within the Roman Empire, especially Celsus (*c.* 30 CE) and Galen (129–216 CE), the latter of whom may have fled the city during the outbreak of the so-called Antonine plague,[15] demonstrate a belief that epidemics were caused and transmitted by corrupt air, rather than being the result of lifestyle or direct physical contact with a sick individual, an explanation of disease known as miasma theory.[16] Influenced by the Hippocratic Corpus' emphasis on the role that weather patterns (or "constitutions," from *κατάστασις*, e.g., *Epidemics* 1.9) play in human diseases, doctors in Rome deemed places and the atmosphere surrounding them, more so than people, as sources of illness; illnesses, moreover, were manifested in the form of foul odors linked to putrefying materials and frequently considered to emanate from stagnant water supplies

[14] As evidence for this attitude, see especially the Hippocratic Corpus' *Nature of Man* 9.

[15] The initial outbreak occurred in 165/6 CE, though waves of the epidemic recurred periodically throughout the reign of Marcus Aurelius. Gilliam (1961, 227–8) compiles the relatively scarce evidence for the plague, including Galen's comments on it; cf. Jackson (1988, 174–5).

[16] Though some conditions, e.g., tuberculosis, psora (scabies), and lippitudo, were recognized as communicable, that communication was thought to occur through inhalation of exhaled diseased air; Jackson (1988, 172).

(cf. *Airs, Waters, Places* 8). That smells pervading the air were considered threatening in and of themselves is reflected in references to "cures" aimed at neutralizing bad odors.[17]

In addition to recognizing foul air as a cause of disease, ancient writers associate susceptibility to disease with proximity of place (e.g., Cels.1.10; Vitr. 1.2.7; Varro 1.4.5; Col. 1.5.6), and in turn recommend travel away from the site of an outbreak toward a healing spa or shrine. That certain geographic regions or topographic features were considered harmful develops a line of thinking that also extends to the Hippocratic Corpus, whose geographic indications, especially those examined in *Airs, Waters, Places*, mark certain regions as inherently unhealthy or salubrious. In his comments on the location of the temple of the healing god Aesculapius, brought to Rome from Epidaurus in 291 BCE after the Sibylline books were consulted during an outbreak of plague, Plutarch (*Roman Questions* 94) considers various alternatives to the site of the god's temple on the Insula Tiberina: he contrasts the location for the temple on a low-lying island with those Asclepieia built by many Greeks in clean and high places, and suggests that the Romans, in contrast, may have been following the model of the Epidaurians, who had their own temple to the god not within the city but just outside its walls. By many accounts the Romans were following the directive of the god, who had appeared and disappeared on the island in the form of a snake (Livy 10.47; cf. *Periocha* 11; Ovid *Met*.15.622–744). Plutarch's comments, however, underscore an implicit understanding that certain places were more conducive for healing (or sickness) and that decisions to promote good health in places deemed unhealthy needed additional justification.

At the same time, ancient medicine clearly did not restrict disease to single causes, but in general theorized a combination of weather patterns, places, and modes of life (δίαιτα) interacting with the humors of the body. The notion that the four humors (blood, phlegm, yellow bile, and black bile) constitute the human body and determine its health was developed by the Hippocratic authors as well as Aristotle and would be defended by Galen in particular (Hays 1998, 10). When writers shift the burden of explanation to that of the humors, they

[17] For instance, Diogenes Laertius notes that a plague in Selinus, cured by the philosopher Empedocles, was caused by a foul smell (D.L. 8.70; cited in Nutton 2000, 67).

acknowledge that particular constitutions are affected differently under certain atmospheric conditions, an acknowledgment that also implicitly establishes a degree of uniformity among the afflicted, in the event of a disease spreading rapidly and with similar symptoms throughout a population. While, as noted above, epidemic disease was thought to remain beyond the purview of medical arts because it did not appear to be affected by individual regimen, some diseases defined as "plague" were thought to be impacted by diet and lifestyle; thus "plague" in certain instances could presuppose both similar constitutions and habits.[18]

Such attitudes are reflected in anecdotes confirming a popular notion of shared constitutions and general receptivity to disease among certain groups (Nutton 1983, 16). In reporting a third-century epidemic experienced by Alexander Severus' troops encamped in northern Syria, and the subsequent abatement of disease once the men retreated to Antioch, the historian Herodian confirms a persistent understanding that similarly constituted bodies will respond somewhat uniformly when confronted with a change of environment (*Histories* 6.6.2; cf. Nutton 2000, 65). Humoral theory, at least in some cases, thus redoubles the homogenizing effects of pestilence: not only is the resulting population similarly stricken, but the same population, when healthy, must be similarly constituted—and share in certain habits of life—in order to be predisposed to the illness.

Since humors required agents to act on them in the event of illness, ancient medical writers broach the notion of contagion with some hesitation when considering agents beyond immediate atmospheric and geographic factors. Thucydides' influential account of Athenian plague indicates awareness, if not actual understanding, of contagion through physical contact between individuals (Longrigg 1992, 35–6; also Rusten 1989) and similar observations are detectible in an account of an epidemic in Thasos in the Hippocratic Corpus (*Epidemics* 1.1). Vivian Nutton's treatment of Galen's references to the seeds (σπέρματα)

[18] As with Livy's notation of *scabies* (a disease considered treatable) in the countryside that erupts as a *pestilentia* in the city (see Chapter 2, p. 57). Moreover, Galen's approach to treating a soldier stricken with the Antonine plague relies heavily on his understanding of the humors (*Methodus Medendi* 12; cf. Jackson 1988, 174). Part of the problem here is the frustratingly vague lexicography of disease; to assert a class of diseases that cannot be cured by rebalancing the humors, the Hippocratic *Nature of Man* (9) uses νοῦσος/νόσημα, which can refer to a range of epidemic and non-epidemic diseases (cf. the Latin *morbus*).

of disease suggests that the polymath and practicing doctor had some awareness of the transmissibility of disease-causing particles in the air, although the harmful potential of such particles was only actualized when they impinged on suitably receptive bodies (Nutton 1983, 7)—that is, bodies with the appropriate humoral balance:

> Suppose, for instance, that certain seeds of plague (τινα λοιμοῦ σπέρματα) are carried in the surrounding air, and of the bodies sharing it some are full of various residues already suitable to become putrefied (σήπεσθαι), while others are free of residues and clean. And let us add that in the former there is a blockage of pores, a so-called plethora and idle life given to gluttony, drink, sex and all the digestive disorders that necessarily come with them. The others, which are clean and lacking such residues, as well as being fine in and of themselves, all have a wholesome transpiration through pores neither blocked nor constricted; they take appropriate exercise and lead a temperate life. Assuming all this, which of these bodies is most likely to be affected by the inhalation of rotting air? (τῶν ἀναπνεομένων εἰς αὐτὰ σηπεδονωδῶν ἀέρων)
>
> (Galen, *On different types of fever* 1.6= vol. 7, pp. 289–91 in Kühn's text; translation modified from Nutton 1983)

Galen's remarks on the seeds of disease are embedded within a discussion of plague and putrid atmospheres, including swamps and the air surrounding unburied dead bodies on the battlefield. His use of σήπω and its cognates, equivalent to *tabeo* (cf. *tabes, tabum*) and *puteo* (cf. *puter, putris*) in Latin, reflects a perception that decaying organic matter, and the stench emanating from it, was a source of disease.[19] Galen's casual assignation of rotting flesh and properties of putrescence among a larger realm of disease-causing agents should perhaps come as no surprise, since the corpse is deemed universally taboo.[20] But in a passage that attempts to ground knowledge of disease-causing particles within a context of quasi-empirical observation, based on the flow and restriction of these particles throughout the body, decaying matter is curiously undertheorized. Moreover,

[19] *Epidemics* 3 of the Hippocratic Corpus, in describing the symptomatology of what may have been the Athenian plague, observes the presence of growths on pre-existing sores, which the author terms "rot" (σήψ; cf. Jones 1923, 143).

[20] For cultural provisions against decaying flesh and norms surrounding the corpse as abject substance, see Kristeva (1982, 2–6; 108–12), discussed further in Chapter 3. Practically speaking, as was demonstrated in the 2014 Ebola outbreak, corpses are highly contagious in the case of certain pathogens.

Galen casts a moral shadow over disease by explicitly judging certain lifestyles, those that accumulate "various residues," as more susceptible to putrescence; such rot emerges as a prominent source of disease in Latin epic and plays a key role in the process of its transmission.

The passage from Galen also recognizes, however dubiously, the possibility that noxious seeds (which, according to the terms of the metaphor, function as living entities with the potential for growth; Nutton 1983, 3) might be exhaled from one body and impinge on another. Thus even if Galen is more interested in the interaction of his seeds with the constitution of individual bodies, and wishes to argue against the notion that a disease pathogen could infect a person with a healthy humoral balance, he reflects an ancient awareness that illness might be spread through proximity and social contact: not only should places beset by corrupt air be avoided, but sick individuals as well. This point is worth emphasizing since it tacitly allows that disease might be communicable between kin and compatriots, and thus threaten the stability of relationships within the larger civic body.

Accounts of disease in Latin also imply an observation if not comprehension of contagion, and it is within Latin literature that there emerges a terminology of transmission through social proximity or "touch": Greek writers discussing disease in this period lack the equivalent to Latin *contagium*, which they might have used to indicate explicitly the transmission of disease through physical contact with sufferers (Nutton 1983, 5 n. 16). The *Thesaurus Linguae Latinae* cites multiple instances in which the writers discussed in this project, along with their contemporaries, use *contactus*, *contagio*, *contag (is)*, and *contagium* to indicate the spread of physical disease; the same writers apply identical terminology as they chart the spread of socially acquired habits, or *mores* (*TLL* vol. 4, 624.68–628.17)—to such an extent that the social network enabling physical corruption becomes hopelessly entangled with that enabling the spread of certain habits and the values that subtend them. Where Thucydides observes the "coming and going" (πρόσειμι; cf. 2.47, 51) of healthy patients among sick ones as a means of spreading disease,[21] it is with Lucretius and the Latin writers following him that "touch" explicitly

[21] He also uses the verb ἀναπίμπλημι (lit. "fulfill, fill up") to refer to infection, which suggests a rather different process of transmission than the Latin terms related to *contingo* ("touch").

signals transmission of physical maladies that are readily converted into spiritual ones.[22] Galen's morally inflected medical model linking corrupt habits of life with susceptibility to disease, combined with the power of social proximity as a vehicle for contagion, not only expands the figurative potential of disease in Roman thought, but also reflects on that potential in earlier discursive traditions.[23]

In sum, the experience of plague among the Roman population as documented in medical texts, historical anecdotes, and didactic treatises was defined by sensitivity to atmospheres and smells, awareness of a threat posed by organic decay, and the possibility of contagion through physical proximity, all features of epidemics exaggerated or sequentially varied in representations of plague in Latin epic. Moreover, while there is evidence that plague was considered beyond the purview of doctors who considered humoral balance the best means of determining the course and treatment of other illnesses, the susceptibility of certain populations to certain epidemics admits to a degree of similarity in humoral constitution among members of those populations. Evidence for a uniform response to a pathogen among a collectively defined group in a new region (e.g., Herodian's soldiers in Syria) suggests that the physical and moral homogeneity of a population might be conceptually strengthened through the shared experience of disease.

1.2. THEORIZING FICTIONS OF THE END

The perceived physical reality of pestilence in Rome, along with a nebulous but persistent notion of transmission through touch and

[22] In Book 3 of *DRN*, Lucretius uses *contagium* and its cognates without a negative valence, to describe the touching of atoms that comprise the *animus* with those that comprise the body (3.345, cf. 3.734, 740). In the same book, however, *contagium* marks the corruptive effects of the "contagion of disease" on the mind (*contagia morbi*, 3.471) as proof of the mind's mortality. His use of *contagia* in the plague episode of Book 6 introduces the explicitly destructive and demoralizing impact of disease (6.1236); discussed further in Chapter 3, p. 94.

[23] For the persistence of disease models that assign a degree of moral corruption to the sufferer, cf. Healy (2001, 22): "From classical times through the Renaissance and beyond, endogenous explanations of disease combined with exopathic ones to produce a model of infectious disease in which outer pollution could only corrupt a body suitably disordered and susceptible (physically and/or morally)."

social intercourse, allows us to understand better why the plague metaphor emerged so forcefully in poems produced during the period of intense civil strife that defined the late Republic. The remainder of this chapter extends my examination of figurative uses of plague into modern and contemporary theories of the discourse. My understanding of plague's development as a metaphor in the period of the late Republic and early Empire is indebted to moments in intellectual history when plague texts have been explicitly theorized; that is to say, to moments when thinkers such as Artaud, Foucault, Girard, and Sontag have observed the hermeneutic potential of plague and attempted to account for its proliferation as a metaphor. Such theoretical models recognize that certain features of plague discourse help us come to terms with how we envision ourselves as human beings who must function within a larger community: the theories outlined below recognize the appeal of narrating processes of decay and its resultant liquefaction, the desire for dissolution of identity, and the enjoyment of dwelling imaginatively within a post-apocalyptic landscape; they also explain, in light of those interests, how epidemic disease can be used to address intense rivalries over limited resources within a collectively defined group.

One of the earliest twentieth-century thinkers to make explicit plague's metaphoric potential is Antonin Artaud, who, in the opening essay of *The Theater and its Double*,[24] forges a link between the function of theatrical spectacle and the function of plague. The essay, first published independently as *The Theater and the Plague*, borrows from St. Augustine's comparison between *pestilentia* and the Roman theater (*ludi scaenici*) in order to lay the foundation of a more elaborate metaphoric relationship: for Artaud, plague and theater are both communicative and psychically transformative; both affect and upset collectivities in similar ways. Moreover, both phenomena have the potential to transgress the theoretical divide between body and mind, in so far as they physically instantiate psychic phenomena. According to Artaud, the psychic affectations of bubonic plague (e.g., lawlessness, impulsivity, drastic changes of character) reflected the physical, internal workings of the bacillus that caused it. The actor/playwright's unsettling observations on how plague operates within the individual

[24] The collection of essays and epistles was published as *Le Théâtre et son Double* by Gallimard in 1938 (reissued for the Folio/Essais collection in1964) and translated into English by Mary Richards for the 1958 Grove Press edition.

and the collective body also underscore dissolution—loosening the bonds of the old order in service of a new one—as a primary effect of pestilence.[25]

The altered mental state (*un délire*, 1964, 39) induced by the theater is similar to plague, in so far as its most powerful manifestation is a shared experience that makes the boundaries instilled by convention porous and ultimately fluid:

> For if the theater is like the plague, it is not only because it affects important collectivities and upsets them in an identical way. In the theater as in the plague there is something both victorious and vengeful: we are aware that the spontaneous conflagration which the plague lights whenever it passes is nothing else than an immense liquidation . . . The plague takes images that are dormant, a latent disorder, and suddenly extends them into the most extreme gestures; the theater also takes gestures and pushes them as far as they will go: like the plague it reforges the chain between what is and what is not, between the virtuality of the possible and what already exists in materialized nature. (1958, 27)

Artaud here draws a parallel between the plague's power, long written into narratives of its dissemination, to destabilize the familiar and upset the social order, powers specifically articulated through familiar tropes of reversing fortunes and collapsing hierarchies: the poor man becomes rich, the lecher becomes pure, the pious son kills his father—processes that, however devastating, often anticipate a clean slate, a cleansing of the old order (1958, 24). To emphasize this function Artaud frequently invokes the language of liquidation as here and later in the essay, where he likens the process of theater to that of draining a giant abscess (*pour vider collectivement des abcès*, 1964, 45). Thus the revolutionary potential ascribed by many readers to Artaud's theater as plague, a notion of theater at odds with many conventions of nineteenth- and early twentieth-century drama, but which would make a decisive impact on leftist theater groups (e.g., *The Living Theater*) that emerged in the 1960s.[26] Both theater and plague, by

[25] For Jannarone (2010, 34–5), there is a distinct ambiguity as to whether the plague/theater in summoning destructive forces re-harnesses them, or simply unleashes them, or, perhaps more sinister than both, allows a dictator/director figure to harness them; see further below.

[26] Jannarone (2010, 13–15). As Jennifer Cooke has observed, the beginning of the essay, in which Artaud cites "coups" as diverse as the revolution in Mekao, Japan in the 7th c.BCE and the Peloponnesian War, draws a suggestive link between historical outbreaks of plague and political upheaval (2009, 50).

compelling people to experience a break with old habits, release a powerful, formerly latent imagery in the minds of the people; the shared experience of such imagery can in turn forge a new sense of community. For many critics, Artaud's theater is not political in the narrow sense of agitating for a particular cause,[27] but rather in its relentless interrogation of conventional systems of belief, or, more precisely, of "epistemological formations and the structures of representation from which they spring" (Baker 2003, 2).

The absence of any restorative vision to follow in the wake of Artaud's theater as a giant abscess, to be drained collectively, has been questioned by recent critics, who detect echoes of fascist discourse in the actor/playwright's emphasis on the authority of the director as well as on the power of a collectivity, which dwarfs the will of the individual.[28] Whether or not we wish to detect twentieth-century fascist ideals in Artaud's thought, his overtures to the authority of a director, when used as a means of clarifying the expurgatory force of plague in Latin epic, productively align with social and political impulses in ancient Rome: from some vantage points, these impulses, and the waves of contagious internal conflict they propelled, would demand the remedy of an effective dictatorship in the figure of Augustus.

Two properties of Artaud's plague as metaphor emerge as paramount: loss of individuality and an emphasis on plague/theater as a kind of release, often articulated as a process of liquefaction. As I shall demonstrate in the following chapters, both properties constitute salient characteristics of Latin plague narratives. Lucretius emphasizes decomposition and its link with the dissolution of identity (explicit in Book 3,[29] but also implied in his use of *tabes*, "physical wasting away" (*OLD* 1), in his account of Athenian plague, 6.1201). Vergil introduces liquefaction into the symptomology of plague narratives, a symptom re-inscribed as a condition of the plague's *telos* in Ovid's *Metamorphoses*. Artaud's metaphor allows us to observe how such operations within the plague-stricken body function as a

[27] Hence his break with the Surrealists in their alignment with Communist party politics (Cooke 2009, 53).

[28] Jannarone (2010, 48). Cf. also speculation at the essay's conclusion on whether "... there can be found a nucleus of men capable of imposing this superior notion of theater, men who will restore to all of us the natural and magical equivalent of the dogmas in which we no longer believe" (1958, 32).

[29] Esp. *DRN* 3.580–5; see the discussion in Segal (1990, 144–70).

corollary of the dissolution of law and anticipate reversion to a pre-civilized state of existence (Artaud 1958, 30–1). The "true freedom" of plague is rooted in primordial eros, prior to the restrictions that bind sexuality to conventions; that freedom, moreover, reverts to cosmogony, to "all the magnificent Fables which recount to the multitudes the first sexual division and the first carnage of essences that appeared in creation," as the source of its own appeal:

> The theater, like the plague, is in the image of this carnage and this essential separation. It releases conflicts, disengages powers, liberates possibilities, and if these possibilities and these powers are dark, it is not the fault of the plague nor of the theater, but of life. (1958, 31)

In the passage Artaud imagines plague/theater as sparking a reversion in the human condition to a pre-Oedipal pause, humankind poised vulnerably in the process of separation from the maternal body and just prior to imposition of the Law. Or, from a less psychoanalytic perspective, we might say that Artaud's idealized plague/theater leaves human life stranded within an atmosphere of epochal evolution—pivoting between a Golden-Age absence of boundaries and their impending Iron-Age imposition—and faced with the liberty of choosing just how that evolution will unfold.[30]

For Artaud, theater as plague works ideally to dissolve those fetters of convention that bind human desire, facilitating the expression of an "orgiastic dream" (Foucault 2003, 47). Artaud's admirer Foucault, who develops his own theory of plague's significance in a 1975 lecture published in the volume *Abnormal*, concedes that literary discourses of pestilence frequently locate the moment when the law is forgotten and the "decomposition of individuality" prevails (2003, 47). At the same time, Foucault identifies, within a diachronic scheme charting the development of medico-legal authority, a point at which the practices of government and medicine used to manage plague-stricken populations also brought with them a kind of increased surveillance over identities (2003, 42): in contrast to former social practices of exclusion that defined the

[30] For the Latin Golden Age as emblematic of Lacan's Imaginary dyad, in which the subject is allowed full fusion with the object of desire, see Miller (2004, 126–8). While Artaud resists explicitly invoking Freudian paradigms, the nature of the liberties he discusses in other parts of the essay (e.g., patricide 1958, 24; incest 28) reflects the influence of Freudian psychoanalysis.

community of healthful individuals (e.g., the constitution of leper colonies), practices of population control and spatial partitioning (*quadrillage*), used initially in response to bubonic plague, emerge in the eighteenth century.[31] *Quadrillage* and related processes of distributing healthy vs. sick individuals within the larger community emblematize the invention of what Foucault describes as positive technologies of power (*technologies positives du pouvoir*),[32] exercised from within the community rather than being imposed strictly from above (as in, e.g., monarchical government)—technologies that function to establish qualifications and criteria of normalization (2003, 48–9; Wald 2012, 114; Cooke 2009, 2).

While Foucault is interested primarily in how these normalizing practices lead to the creation of abnormal sexuality, for our purposes his use of eighteenth-century responses to bubonic plague as a model of "discipline normalization" demonstrates one way in which contagious disease affects the exercise of power and its relationship to the articulation of the individual. On the one hand, as a response to plague we observe a relentless process of distinction, of "giving [individuals] their own place, of assigning places and of defining presences and subdivided presences" (2003, 46). On the other hand, such finely graded distinctions underscore how plague in its uncontrolled form (as an imaginative experiment) repeats constantly the transgression of status barriers and aims at homogeneity: "[P]lague appears as the moment of panic and confusion in which individuals, threatened by visitations of death, abandon their identities, throw off their masks, forget their status, and abandon themselves to the great debauchery of those who know they are going to die" (2003, 47). Foucault goes on to contrast plague as a catalyst for the abandonment of conventions and laws that determine the individual's place in society with plague as an instrument by which political authority is consolidated and "exercised to the full."

Epidemic disease, as such, prompts governmental oversight and partitioning of the population as a means (initially) to control the spread of disease, but gradually as a means of engineering and exploiting individuals as so many cogs in the machine. Despite the

[31] The practice is especially evident in Defoe's meticulous chronicle of increased surveillance in London, *Journal of the Plague Year*, set in 1665 but published in 1722; see below, Chapter 7, pp. 256–8.

[32] From the Gallimard edition of *Les anormaux* (1999, 44).

individualizing pressures of membership within a finely calibrated social order (one whose taxis Foucault likens to "the dream of a military society"; 2004, 47), the impetus behind such pressures is, as Foucault's larger argument in *Abnormal* demonstrates, a rigorous process of normalization. As I argue more expansively in Chapter 5, it is a similar rebirth into orthodoxy and identity defined entirely by the state that Ovid describes through the origin of the Myrmidons in his *Metamorphoses*. That rebirth, however, relies initially on the fantasy of collapse in order to issue a clean sweep and make a space for its newly calibrated citizenry, an ant-born population whose members lack former markers of identity (e.g., familial lineage) and are defined predominantly by state function (e.g., military service). Ovid thus offers us both dreams of plague and illustrates their interdependence in the process. Once we have peered beneath the poet's metaphoric veil of disease and dissemination to observe the path of civil war and its aftermath, we may better understand the very nature of the political catastrophe that Augustus' new order relied upon for its instantiation. Ovid's plague constitutes a twofold motion, the first of which performs the explosion of identity in the manner of Artaud's "orgiastic dream," and the second of which organizes the remaining matter into a normalized (proto-Fascist) citizen body.

While Foucault only glances at plague's literary formulations as a contrast to its function within the technologies of power governing the early modern state, Susan Sontag focuses intensely on the representational capacity of disease.[33] And yet she too recognizes how those representations—initially of cancer and tuberculosis, later of Acquired Immune Deficiency Syndrome (AIDS)—are constructed in ways that heighten individuality or, conversely, de-individualize the sick through their association with a larger community of the afflicted (1988, 133–4; Gomel 2000, 415). Medical metaphors, according to Sontag, far too often confuse tenor and vehicle and in turn cause us to conflate figurative language with lived and suffered experience, ultimately redoubling the exclusionary force of disease on the individual.

Cancer and tuberculosis are diseases thought to emerge from personal passions: Sontag cites numerous literary portraits that draw on the perception of tuberculosis as a disease of the breath (and by

[33] Sontag's *Illness as Metaphor* first appeared in 1978 in the *New York Review of Books*; she published *AIDS and Its Metaphors* in 1988. I rely on the combined version of the essays available from Picador (1988).

extension, the soul), especially evident in the Romantic poets; the same portraits inform our understanding of it as a disease of love that conferred on its victims "appealing vulnerability" and "superior sensitivity" (1988, 17–20). Cancer's origins in the passions she traces primarily to Wilhelm Reich who, in theorizing Freud's cancer, identified it as the "bio-energetic shrinking" that follows resignation and loss of hope (1988, 23). The two diseases have thus frequently conferred distinctive characteristics upon their victims. Sontag even goes so far as to suggest that it is through aestheticized literary portraits of the suffering tuberculosis victim (for instance, the heroine of Alexandre Dumas' *La Dame aux Camélias*) that "the idea of individual illness was articulated . . . and in the images that collected around the disease one can see emerging a modern idea of individuality" (1988, 37). While cancer victims have been distinguished by a less ethereal and frequently less attractive set of traits, the disease gradually assumed the privileged place held by tuberculosis as the condition that, in the twentieth century, isolated and further defined the individual, often by signaling those psychological characteristics (e.g., melancholy, sexual repression) that were thought to be the cause of the cancer. Such conflations of representational language about disease and the material realities of any pathogen, however, can also have the opposite effect, and erode individual identity by discursively creating sick communities.[34] Sontag observes that certain contagious diseases, such as cholera, bubonic plague, and more recently AIDS, "simplif[y] a complex self, reduce it to sick environment" (1988, 37).

Western cultures, especially American culture, have capitalized on the community-forging and stigmatizing rhetoric that attends the path of contagion, which makes visible otherwise invisible social interactions, telling a "hidden story" of who has been where and when (Wald 2008, 37): a moral judgment frequently haunts those afflicted with AIDS, since its primary means of transmission is sexual, through bodily fluids. Even those who deny the moral significance of AIDS often add ideological weight to the disease by assigning it a status, shared with lethal contagions throughout history, as grist for

[34] For a critique of Sontag, see Porter and Rousseau (1998), who argue that medical metaphors can positively heighten individual identity and expression of self. They concede, however, a more destructive force of illness metaphors in so far as they are applied to communities and collective groups.

the mill that produces doomsday scenarios. Such scenarios reflect a fascination with apocalypse as they repeatedly propose "radical endings and brand new beginnings," which Sontag defines as a peculiarly Western, and American, phenomenon:

> The taste for worst-case scenarios reflects the need to master fear of what is felt to be uncontrollable. It also expresses an imaginative complicity with disaster. The sense of cultural distress or failure gives rise to the desire for a clean sweep, a tabula rasa. No one wants a plague, of course. But, yes, it would be a chance to begin again. And beginning again—that is very modern, very American, too. (1988, 175)

Sontag's observation about the rhetorical utility of predicting the *telos* of one especially lethal virus at the end of the twentieth century sheds light on the function of another (proto) Western culture concerned with re-inventing itself, Augustan Rome. Though Augustus' concern with masking innovation by appeals to tradition and continuity has been well documented (cf. Zanker 1990; Galinsky 1996), the promotion of the Principate as a *novus ordo*, a revived Golden Age, operated under the premise that the age preceding it was one of Iron-Age atrophy and decline, of a slate that needed wiping clean.

As we shall observe in Chapter 4, Vergil tempers the horror of dystopian, plague-stricken Noricum with certain utopian features of the Golden Age, prompting readers to recognize how narratives that restore humans to a condition of harmony with the natural world often achieve that condition through prolonged suffering.[35] More recently, Elana Gomel has attempted to disentangle Sontag's clean sweep impulse, representative of some plague narratives, from those that resist closure by endlessly replicating the pains of transmission:

> The apocalyptic desire that finds satisfaction in elaborating fictions of the end is double-edged. On the one hand, its ultimate object is some version of the crystalline New Jerusalem, an image of purity so absolute that it denies the organic messiness of life. On the other hand, apocalyptic fictions typically linger on pain and suffering. The end result of apocalyptic purifications often seems of less importance than the narrative pleasure derived from the bizarre and opulent tribulations of bodies being burnt by fire and brimstone, tormented by scorpion stings. (Gomel 2000, 405)

[35] A cost of achievement that in turn prompts readers to question the value of the "Golden" Age, a question I explore in Chapter 4.

For Gomel, accounts of plague are frequently governed by a "logic of repetition": images of mortality repeat themselves to the extent that they imply constant deferral of closure and ultimately thwart the *telos* inscribed in so many visions of the apocalypse (2000, 409–10). The failed burials and squabbling over funeral pyres that constitute the final lines of Lucretius' *De Rerum Natura* conform to this pattern of plague as death constantly repeating itself. Thus the utopian transformation of the body politic ("the giddy hopefulness of endism") promised through the pestilential Fourth Horse of the apocalypse is challenged in the poem by the "backward-looking narrative of trauma" that defines plague in the post-apocalypse (2000, 408).[36]

When we view these competing impulses in tandem—as Vergil will allow us to do in the failed closure of the third *Georgic* and fourth's newly born apian community—we gain a heightened awareness of both the "aftermaths and remainders" of plague as lingering post-apocalypse and the dangerous allure of plague as a vehicle for a utopian final solution.[37] Vergil engages in an imaginative project that allows him to rethink Rome; an utter dismantling of civilization brings with it the promise of rebuilding, but also a need to reckon with remainders of an old order. In response, Ovid both fulfills and subtly denounces the promise of plague in the *Georgics* with his impossibly uniform population of ant-born Myrmidons.

Like Sontag, René Girard is concerned with the representational power of epidemic disease and how that power has a homogenizing, and potentially purifying, effect upon afflicted communities. Girard, however, focuses more intently on epidemics in the literary and mythic imagination and their role in staging social crises, eroding markers of distinction, and dramatizing the dissolution of the social bond (cf. Cooke 2009, 11). For Girard, moreover, the end point that interrupts the "process of undifferentiation, and destruction of specificities" (1974, 833) is not primarily a *tabula rasa*, but instead the

[36] I use the term "apocalypse" in accord with various senses discussed by Berger (1999, 5), but primarily as referring to the *eschaton* or "actual imagined end of the world," not only in Jewish and New Testament representations, but also in literary and cinematic visions of unparalleled worldwide disasters. Such disasters are "apocalyptic" in so far as they have a revelatory function, clarifying what forces brought about destruction. Lucretius, of course, was not writing under the shadow of Revelations, but he does direct readers to consider the ending of the status quo. As with other writers discussed in this project, he relies on the myth of the ages to frame possibilities of destruction and speculate on the potential for renewal.

[37] On aftermaths and remainders as defining features of post-apocalyptic narratives, see Berger (1999, xii), discussed further in Chapter 3.

identification of a sacrificial scapegoat, whose expulsion purifies the polluted social order, as with the figure of Oedipus in Sophocles' tragedy.[38] He observes how these narratives tend to transform the existing social order, conceived as a finely graded system of hierarchies, into an aggregate, a homogeneous mass. Where Foucault describes the subjective experience of disease as beginning among conceived aggregates or collectives that are gradually partitioned into specific identities through technologies of power, Girard's interest in the "literary dream" of plague concentrates on how these narratives orchestrate the collapse of distinctions in the first place.[39]

In reflecting on Artaud's physiologically misguided impressions of how the bubonic plague bacillus works to dissolve internal organs, Girard observes:

> This loss of differentiation is medically mythical but aesthetically powerful because it patterns the pathological symptoms on the breakdown of culture, producing an overwhelming impression of disintegration.
> (1974, 846)

However medically mythical liquefaction is with respect to bubonic plague, it is a symptom of contagious disease whose provenance we can trace to Vergil, who furthers the processes of dissolution already implicit in Lucretius' account of pestilence in Athens. Such collapse of distinctions (referred to as *gradus* or "steps"; Girard 1974, 838) within the social order is born from intense competitions for limited honors. Girard posits this competition for the same distinctions that results in a kind of mirroring between individuals (or "mimetic doubling") as one of three central features of the plague narrative: in addition to the disease pathogen achieving epidemic status (1), its narrative triggers rivalry among mimetic doubles, binaries that will collapse through transgression and a failure to differentiate (2); the process culminates in a sacrificial theme that may take the form of a scapegoat process

[38] For the logic of differentiation that structures myths of the scapegoat, see also Girard (1986, 24–44).

[39] Though, again, the two dreams are to some extent complementary: where Girard is interested in the process of systemic entropy initiated through plague, Foucault directs his attention to the opportunistic measures undertaken by the state to correct such entropy. At the same time, it is important to stress that Girard's model predicts a cure through expulsion, where Foucault observes the social order restored through management and recalibration of the population.

(3), in which the expulsion of an element deemed contaminated allows distinctions to reassert themselves (1974, 845).

All three elements offer insight into the workings of those accounts of pestilence generated during the civil wars of the late Roman Republic. Raskolnikov's dream of a plague in Dostoevsky's *Crime and Punishment* is highlighted by Girard as an illustration of the role of mimetic doubling in the larger scheme of the plague narrative. Raskolnikov describes how "new sorts of microbes" attacked the bodies of men:

> Each thought that he alone had the truth and was wretched looking at the others, beat himself on the breast, wept, and wrung his hands. They did not know how to judge and could not agree what to consider evil and what good; they did not know whom to blame, whom to justify. Men killed each other in a sort of senseless spite. They gathered together in armies against one another, but even on the march the armies would be attacking each other, the ranks would be broken and the soldiers would fall on each other, stabbing and cutting, biting, and devouring each other.
> (cited in Girard 1974, 835–6)

Dostoevsky sets up plague as a paradigm for civil war, a war among equals who gradually, while striving for complete autonomy, lose the ability to differentiate themselves. Girard translates this further into a scenario wherein plague emblematizes the mimetic nature of desire. When the desires of two individuals converge on the same object (we want what other people want, a tendency Girard sees as endemic in the social order), those individuals imitate each other, and a conflict inevitably arises between them (1974, 837); the expulsion of the one identified as the scapegoat resolves the crisis. For Girard, the homogenizing effect of various cultural crises and the need to differentiate in the wake of such homogeneity is the impulse behind mythmaking writ large as well as the force that drives the plague narrative.[40] A cultural crisis is frequently resolved through stereotypes of persecution that allow the collective to identify an individual (or subculture of individuals) who must bear responsibility for the crisis (Girard 1986, 24–44). While the restoration of the status quo is frequently the

[40] See esp. Girard (1986, 21), who no doubt overreaches here in his attempt to offer up a universalizing impulse behind myth, though he relies partly on the structural template for "lack of differentiation" theorized by Levi-Strauss. Hardie (1993) uses Girard's doubling and sacrificial scapegoat as a means of understanding (*inter alia*) the rivalry between Aeneas and Turnus, an argument I address further in Chapters 4 and 6.

consolation of Girard's master plague narrative, the purging of a community through a scapegoat can alternatively result in the birth of a new order (1986, 42).

This model offers a useful way of formulating the political strife of the late Republic, where powerful aristocrats, backed by increasingly powerful armies, vied with each other for command of Rome. We can detect Vergil's concern for the kind of intense competition for personal distinctions (*honores*) throughout the *Georgics*, especially in passages that address recent civil wars (1.489–514; cf. 2.495–512). When he revisits such conflict, veiled under the guise of disease in *Georgics* 3, sacrifice blatantly fails, and no scapegoat is identified to check the spread of contagion. The death of Aristaeus' rival Orpheus in the fourth *Georgic* and atonement for that death in the form of a violent ritual (the *bougonia*) play an important role in the restoration of Aristaeus' bees, beset by a similar epidemic. Girard's model allows us to better understand the relationship between contagion within the hive, the conflicting desires of Orpheus and Aristaeus that are its origin, and the nature of those remedies available. And yet, where Girard's model of plague and persecution would require the identification and expulsion of a single entity, allowing restoration or birth of a new order, Vergil's resolution is to reintegrate the individual perceived as culpable, Aristaeus (4.454–5), in such a way that forces us to question why it is Orpheus who suffers expulsion in the form of death and dismemberment. As such we observe mimetic doubles contending without a clear and morally infallible victor.

1.3. CAVEAT: ON THE DANGERS OF INVOKING PLAGUE DISCOURSE

From many of these perspectives, literature's intersections with plague have a salutary impact insofar as those intersections reflect on, and thus heighten awareness of, the threat that certain cultural practices pose to the larger community (e.g., the excessive competition for distinctions in the late Republic, reconceived as "pathological").[41]

[41] Cf. Healy (2001, 63), who observes how plague texts have been interpreted variously and often with conflicting agendas; while discourses generated during the

With varying degrees of didacticism the Roman poets under discussion operate with an underlying premise that a diseased society can somehow demonstrate (by foil or by imagined path to recovery) what a healthy one looks like. From other perspectives, the project of writing plague, or contagion more generally, and using it as a metaphor pose a more sinister threat. As Sontag's indictment of representational thinking about disease has made clear, not only will those experiencing the real, physical onset of illness suffer from the assumptions and images that surround a specific disease, but, as noted above, the metaphoric power of disease is frequently harnessed against a particular marginalized group, whom discourses of contagion can assist in further marginalizing.

In remarking on the status of contagion as a metaphor of choice and a repeatedly invoked heuristic tool over the past few decades, Magnusson and Zalloua question:

> What happens to the concept of contagion when it exceeds its original epidemiological context and starts contaminating other discourses . . . Is the contamination to be celebrated as a positive effect of cross-fertilization, that is, for the cross-disciplinarity that it affords? Or do we need to scrutinize more carefully the ideological underpinnings of its dissemination in contemporary debates (keeping in mind who defines contagion and what or who gets defined as contagious)? (2012, 4)

The editors situate their own inquiry in a post-9-11 climate characterized by terrorism commonly labeled as a contagion and are concerned with contemporary implications of that metaphor for the sovereignty of individuals as well as nations. With these caveats in mind and with the conviction that we cannot recognize pernicious use of any metaphor unless we have studied its transmission, I turn in closing to a contemporary trend in contagion discourse.

As I began formulating my own arguments about what plague meant to the ancient Romans and, in turn, how those meanings have impacted the Western tradition of plague narratives, the Zaire strain of the Ebola virus re-emerged in western Africa. Ebola, one of

Black Death, e.g., played a role in identifying Jews as scapegoats, other texts and interpretations have the potential for, "highlighting actual areas of, and reasons for, social fragility and keeping the excesses of the unscrupulous in check." See also Davis (2002, 831), who observes of the equation between contagion and cultural contact that contagion discourses have the potential to foster reflection on the "pleasures of contact" and other positive transformations enacted through cultural exchange.

the viruses that causes hemorrhagic fever, replicates within the blood cells with such intensity and determination that the internal organs of its host gradually liquefy. A victim of the disease will die from various causes (heart failure, brain damage, liver failure), but that death is often accompanied by bleeding from nearly every orifice of the body. From the initial outbreak reported in Guinea in March of 2014, the number of reported cases in Sierra Leone, Guinea, and Liberia peaked in transmission and fatality rates during December of 2014. By September of 2015 over 30,000 cases were documented with an average fatality rate of around 50 percent.[42] While transmission of the disease slowed significantly after 2015,[43] global media coverage, heightened screening and security protocols, well-publicized efforts to produce vaccines, as well as the World Health Organization's Phase 3 management of areas impacted by the disease, all attest to the reality of Ebola's brutal impact on the human population. At the same time, various imaginative strains of Ebola—that is, narratives of the disease's origins and spread—have been generated in order to make a non-human pathogen comprehensible in human terms, but also to address anxieties concerning our status as humans possessed of national and familial identities living in an increasingly global and porous world. Thus Ebola as a signifier has become implicated in a less tangible (but no less frightening) network of representations that foreground above all the dehumanizing effects of contagion.[44]

Consider a few passages from Richard Preston's *The Hot Zone*, a taut, non-fiction account of the threat of an earlier (1983) Ebola outbreak on U.S. soil. While Preston's investigative powers are as laudable as his documentation is thorough, his construction of a narrative that will generate fear and dread in his readership inevitably

[42] Statistics are drawn from the September 2015 situation report published by the World Health Organization (WHO): http://apps.who.int/ebola/current-situation/ebola-situation-report-30-september-2015.

[43] According to the WHO, June 2016 marked the end of the outbreaks in Liberia and Sierra Leone; see http://www.who.int/ebola/en/. In May of 2018 the Democratic Republic of Congo suffered an Ebola outbreak; thanks partly to coordinated efforts of local and international authorities, as well as to distribution of the vaccine developed during the 2014 outbreak, the WHO declared the DRC outbreak over in July of 2018.

[44] For instance, see an October 2014 piece in the *NY Times* on how family members from communities afflicted with Ebola are afraid to touch each other, a tendency encouraged by the larger set of protocols issued for effectively preventing the spread of the disease: http://www.nytimes.com/2014/10/05/world/africa/ebolas-cultural-casualty-hugs-in-hands-on liberia.html.

casts certain places as dangerously resistant to human intervention (central Africa, a primary "hot" zone); certain characters and institutions, moreover, are portrayed as occasionally irresponsible (the Centers for Disease Control; USAMRIID) or lethally indifferent (the virus itself). The book opens in Nairobi with the story of "Charles Monet," who in January of 1980 nearly instigated an outbreak of the Marburg virus, a filovirus, like Ebola, that causes hemorrhagic fever. The effects of Marburg upon its victims are described in terms reminiscent of contemporary cinematic discourses of the living dead:

> The host is possessed by a life form that is attempting to convert the host into itself. The transformation is not entirely successful, however, and the end result is a great deal of liquefying flesh mixed with virus, a kind of biological accident . . . [As blood clotting progresses, the victim] doesn't seem to be fully aware of pain any longer because the blood clots lodged in his brain are cutting off blood flow. His personality is being wiped away by brain damage. This is called depersonalization, in which the liveliness and details of character seem to vanish. He is becoming an automaton. Tiny spots in his brain are liquefying. The higher functions of consciousness are winking out first, leaving the deeper parts of the brain stem (the primitive rat brain, the lizard brain) still alive and functioning. It could be said that the who of Charles Monet has already died while the what of Charles Monet continues to live.
>
> (Preston 1995, 18–19)

With less literary flourish but a similar emphasis on the virus's power to reduce the human host to an indistinguishable mass of rapidly dissolving tissues, Preston notes that:

> It could multiply in many different kinds of meat. It was an invasive life form, devastating and promiscuous. It showed a kind of obscenity you see only in nature, an obscenity so extreme that it dissolves imperceptibly into beauty . . . It did not know boundaries. It did not know what humans are; or perhaps you could say that it knew only too well what humans are: it knew that humans are meat.
>
> (Preston 1995, 139)[45]

Evident in both passages is the virus's lethal lack of discrimination, a failure to recognize boundaries, which facilitates transmission and in

[45] Making a similar claim about the Ebola virus's voracious appetite and lack of discrimination, Preston notes that: "Ebola can't tell the difference between a human being and a monkey. The virus jumps easily back and forth between them" (1995, 67).

turn makes its victims indistinguishable as human beings: organic matter is simply and efficiently converted into meat. The threat of this particular villain in Preston's story lies in its power to rob us of our status as individuals—a powerful, best-selling rhetoric, but one we must parse carefully before allowing it to color our responses to actual victims of the disease and the "hot" areas most affected by it.

As noted, ancient Romans knew relatively little about the processes of contagion, and also lacked the twenty-first-century global transport systems that make the scenarios postulated in *The Hot Zone* (and with a bit more sobriety on CNN) imaginable, if not likely. As Pricilla Wald's work on contagion discourse has demonstrated (2008, esp. 3–28), rapid transport systems and policies of inclusion and exclusion from communities work in tandem to create much of the dread and desire that surrounds the potency of the contemporary outbreak narrative: identification of infected subjects and attempts to isolate them operate with a ruthlessness equaled by the power of diseases to undermine those efforts once they have harnessed the machinery of global mobility. And yet even without the very contemporary fear invoked by "Patient Zero," harbored in the constantly recycled atmosphere of a teeming 747 airliner, pestilence has proven itself a potent signifier of what it means to be human, with imagined autonomy, and how humans work collectively within the social order: it does this in Roman discourses, as in many contemporary ones, by testing the strength of our relationships as often as it exploits our hostilities; plague inverts the social order before suggesting tentative means for recovery, for re-inscribing what is left behind after pestilence enacts its worst-case scenario, the clean slate.[46] At the same time, the fact that the slate is never entirely clean—as Vergil, Ovid, and Lucretius constantly demonstrate—productively problematizes the wish fulfillment embedded in any dream of plague's potential.

[46] Cf. Preston (1995, 93), who characterizes Ebola as a complete "slate wiper."

2

Livy, *Pestilentia*, and the Pathologies of Class Strife

As noted in the preceding chapter, concepts of pestilence were shaped at least in part by medical writing, anecdotal comments on the vulnerability of certain places or populations, and metaphoric uses of disease in political rhetoric. Within documented attempts to identify causes of epidemics, such discourses mingled with, and were in some sense ancillary to, attitudes about supernatural forces and the role of the gods in both inflicting disease upon populations and curing it. When we turn to historians of ancient Rome, who were more attuned to the cultural impact of plague than its effects on the human body, we find significant evidence for perceptions of plague as divinely inflicted. Caroline Wazer's (2016) recent study of public health measures in the city demonstrates that an overwhelming number of epidemics recorded in the histories of the Republic were treated by the senate as divinely sent prodigies. Divine origins allow shades of moral judgment to color historical accounts, suggesting a correlation between the behavior of a population and its susceptibility to epidemic disease.

In contrast to the growing interest in contagious disease and its documentation in the later Roman empire, attention to the historiography of plague in early Republican Rome, prior to the period when the extent of the empire had mobilized and imported foreign pathogens on a regular basis,[1] has been somewhat limited: Crawfurd

[1] As was the case with the Antonine plague (Jackson 1988, esp. 40, 173–4); see also Harper (2017, 72–98) for a recent discussion of how imperial expansion and urbanization facilitated circulation of disease-causing microbes among immunologically vulnerable populations.

devotes two chapters of his 1914 survey of plague in Western literature and art to Rome's experience of plague as recounted in various historical sources, including Livy, Dionysius of Halicarnassus, and Plutarch. Crawfurd, who was a practicing physician, is attuned to symptomatology, and finds most Roman historiographic treatments frustratingly vague or unduly influenced by Thucydides' treatment of fifth-century Athenian plague (1914, 51, 58). His approach is not exacting philologically, and yet it is immensely valuable in its assembly of recorded incidents of plague in the early city and in the conclusions he draws from them: Rome is distinguished from Greece by the sheer frequency with which pestilence beset the population, a condition that indelibly impacted Roman religion and art (1914, 42). As I will demonstrate, historical sources, Livy's notices of recurring plague in particular, also imply that political ideals are fractured, broken, and re-constructed under the weight of contagious disease. As an Augustan historian who treats documented outbreaks thoroughly embedded in accounts of political upheaval (*seditiones*) and cultural innovation, Livy demonstrates the power of plague to reconstitute a fragmented population and prompt reflection on the health of the body politic.

Crawfurd makes the observation that Rome's early plagues would have necessarily been endemic, bred in surrounding swamplands, since the fledgling state did not have extensive intercourse with foreign nations until the Punic Wars.[2] The endemic condition of disease is important to this project not so much for helping identify the pathogens that caused different outbreaks as it is for clarifying the reactions of the Roman populace toward those outbreaks, since diseases ostensibly arising from within the community provoke different responses than those appearing to beset the community from without.[3] Rebecca Flemming's recent treatment of Imperial notices of the paths of certain illnesses demonstrates a "conceptual patterning" (2009, 21) by which disease-causing microbes originate on the fringes of Roman geographic hegemony and move inward (from "periphery to center," 30), toward Rome as a locus of power and corruption.

[2] A comment made almost in passing (1914, 42). For endemic vs. epidemic diseases, see also Hays (1998, 5–6).

[3] See Scheidel (2003, 169 and passim) for treatment of endemic malaria and on the conversion of certain pathogens from epidemic to endemic status during the Imperial period.

Charting this movement implicitly or explicitly allowed Imperial writers, especially Pliny the Elder, to make a correlation between disease and the increasing dependence of the Roman elite on foreign medical expertise; by such logic, Romans gradually relinquished mastery of their own environs and bodies and ceded them to external authorities. Such a correlation also allows Pliny to indict the ruling classes for their moral failings and imply their punishment through particularly shameful forms of disease (2009, 37). The path traced by Pliny and made evident in Flemming's analysis conforms to Sontag's observations that plague is often identified as an invasion and associated with the alien other (1988, 135–8). So too Thucydides tells us the Athenian epidemic was imported from Ethiopia (2.47),[4] and Livy follows suit in remarking (albeit with less precision) that one particular pestilence, "invaded the population" (*invasit populum*, 4.21.2); the outbreak occurs after the Romans have returned from territories of the Veientes and Falisci, bringing war captives and animals as booty with them.[5] At the same time, there is frequently a distinct ambiguity concerning the origins of a pestilence in the historical record of early Republican Rome. Livy and presumably his annalist sources frequently view contagious disease as simply arising and designate its presence with compounds of *orior* (4.52, 7.1, 7.27). On the one hand, such plagues would be attributed to the gods, who were punishing the people for a religious failure or transgression, a break in the *pax deorum* (cf. Wazer 2016, 137-9). On the other hand, disease arising from within the population would serve even more readily as a metaphor for strife in the Roman body politic.

While Plutarch records an account of pestilence as far back as the reign of Rome's second king, Numa Pompilius,[6] Livy's first narrative of an outbreak coincides with the death of the bellicose king Tullus

[4] Thucydides mostly evades the question of the plague's aetion and does not seem especially interested in corrupt air as an agent of disease. At the same time, as noted in Chapter 1 p. 25, he implicitly recognizes the role of contact in transmission of the plague by noting that doctors died frequently since they were the ones attending to the sick (47.4; see Rusten 1989). Crawfurd (1914, 37) perhaps unduly credits Thucydides with an understanding (rather than mere recognition) of contagion, as stressed by Longrigg (1995, 34).

[5] Livy does not make the correlation explicit, though his immediate transition from the war booty to the pestilence in Rome hints at a causal relationship between military conquest and the importation of disease; see further below, p. 56.

[6] See Plutarch's *Life of Numa*, where the plague is cited as an aetion for one of Numa's religious innovations, the noisy procession of the Salic Priests (Crawfurd

Hostilius. Flush from the success of defeating the Albans and Sabines, the king faces a *pestilentia* that cripples his fighting force at home, though he insists on campaigning as a way of alleviating the malady (*unde pigritia militandi oreretur, nulla tamen ab armis quies dabatur a bellicoso rege*, 1.31). When Tullus himself is afflicted, however, he consults Numa's *commentarii* to find a remedy, and seeks solace in secrets rites and offerings to Jupiter Elicius, a god of rain introduced to Rome by Numa. Failure to perform the rites correctly provokes the wrath rather than the beneficence of Jupiter, and Tullus perishes in a manner markedly contrasting with the deified Romulus and peacefully deceased Numa (Ogilvie 1970, 124).

Though Livy provides few details of the actual *pestilentia*, he does correlate its occurrence with the transfer of political power, and implicitly with the warmongering policies associated with that transfer; he also links pestilence to religious innovation, in this case fatefully misguided, as Tullus is described as a man who, while scorning *sacra* previously, "suddenly conducted his life devoted to all kinds of superstitions large and small, and even influenced the people by his religious practices" (*repente omnibus magnis parvisque superstitionibus obnoxius degeret religionibusque etiam populum impleret*, 1.31.6). Here we encounter the first glimmerings of Livy's addition to Thucydides' canon of human responses to plague: where the Greek historian notes the Athenians' unsuccessful exhaustion of all human and divine resources in effort to combat disease (2.47.2), Livy adds as a third response, recourse to *superstitio*, recognized as "irrational religious awe or credulity" (*OLD* 1), but etymologically signaling that which "remains" or is "left standing" after other resources have been depleted.[7]

Following Tullus' death and the succession of Ancus Marcius, Livy documents over twenty epidemics in the surviving books of *AUC*, evidence of how regularly plague had been sown into the historical imagination by the Augustan period. Plague, in Livy commonly

1914, 43; cf. Ogilvie 1970, 98). Livy records the institution of the *Salii* without mentioning the plague.

[7] For Livy's revision of Thucydides' account of Athenian responses to plague, see Stoclet (2007, 135), discussed further below, pp. 67–8. The coupling of political transition and pestilence is strengthened in the account of Dionysius of Halicarnassus (4.69), who records that a plague occurring during the reign of Tarquinius prompts the king to send his sons, along with Brutus, to Apollo—thus precipitating the end of the monarchy and ushering in the consular system of government.

referred to as *pestilentia*, signals an unspecified disease afflicting a large percentage of the Roman populace.[8] While the historian often includes only passing reference to a particular outbreak, when he chooses to expand on the circumstances of the plague and its effects on the population, he ties pestilence to a shift of power within the political *ordines* and to religious and cultural innovations. Notably absent from his treatment are details of individual moral transgressions—thieving, debauched behavior, doing in public what had formerly been kept private—fueled by perception of the rapid changes of fortune that accompany pestilence. Such absence is all the more glaring in light of a Thucydidean model detailing lawlessness in behaviors that secured immediate pleasures and illustrated disrespect for human and divine constraints (Th. 2.53.2). By shifting his focus away from pestilence as an instigator of moral degeneracy among individuals, however, Livy assigns plague a novel and occasionally salutary role, parallel to that of war and strife between political classes, in furthering the *res publica*'s early development.

In the following discussion, I focus on three outbreaks that are given particular attention by Livy: the plague of 463 BCE, during war with the Aequi; the plague of 399 BCE, when the *lectisternium* is introduced; and the plague that gives rise to the *ludi scaenici* in 364 BCE. In each of these incidents, the literally transformative effects of *pestilentia* on the human body emerge in conjunction with political and ideological transformation in the expanding *res publica*. I argue that plague variously heightens or levels status distinctions in a context where the powers granted to different *ordines* were hotly contested. Livy's narrative design implies that the Roman people respond to these shifts in relative status through innovations in the social order: not only does pestilence have a lasting impact on how power is distributed among the classes of free-born citizens, it instigates cultural practices that transform their collective *mores* as well. The three episodes under discussion represent the range of roles played by plague, by no means mutually exclusive, in recognizing fractures among the Roman citizenry and prompting coalescence. In the outbreak of 463, plague functions as a direct cause of

[8] He also frequently refers to epidemic disease as *morbus*. For a catalogue of plagues occurring during the period between 490 and 390 BCE, see Ogilvie (1970, 394–5), who remarks on terms for the epidemics as well as on the difficulty of identifying disease pathogens. For a more exhaustive list, see Grimm (1965, 61).

civic reorganization as mortality rates create a power vacuum in a vulnerable population; the same episode, in turn, offers a heuristic model for reading the many less detailed accounts of pestilence in the fifth century. The plague of 399 results in cultural innovation rather than political reorganization, but is contextualized within plebeian resistance, described as ideological *contagium*, to required military service, a context that informs the "promiscuity" and Saturnalian atmosphere of the *lectisternium*. The plague of 364 emerges in a notable absence of both *seditio* within and wars abroad, but the *ludi scaenici* ("stage plays") imported as a remedy bind contagious disease closely to a cultural phenomenon recognized as a *nova res* in its own right.

Such a reading of plagues in *AUC* recognizes an integration of disease metaphors within an overarching program of figurative language that, beginning with Livy's famous *Praefatio*, uses the human corpus to indicate the health of the body politic. Within the terms of that program, the project of history offers a "salubrious and productive" (*salubre et frugiferum*) approach to dysfunction within the civic body, dysfunction that the writer diagnoses at a time when Rome can no longer endure its "vices" or its "remedies" (*nec vitia nostra nec remedia*, *Praef.* 9–10).[9] The analogy between the human corpus and the Roman civic body is perhaps most clearly articulated in the speech of Menenius Agrippa, who attempts to persuade the *plebs* to return to Rome after their secession of 494 BCE by comparing the well-being of Rome to the health of a human body and illustrating how "*seditio* against the internal organs of the body was similar to the anger of the *plebs* against the *patres*" (*quam intestina corporis seditio similis esset irae plebis in patres*, 2.32.12).[10] As Dutoit observes (1948, 117–18), the speech employs the same *tabes* that Livy uses to describe the physical impact of plague in his notices of epidemics: Menenius' speech designates *tabes* as the emaciated condition of the collectively defined body resulting from attempts by lesser limbs to starve its commanding faculty, the belly, into submission (*ipsa una membra totumque corpus ad extremam tabem venisse*, 2.32.10).[11] As we will

[9] Frequently interpreted as moral failings, though the *OLD* primarily defines *vitium* as any "quality which impedes success, perfection, etc." (*OLD* 1).

[10] On the Greek origins of parables likening the human body to a larger community, see Ogilvie (1970, 312).

[11] Livy has prepared his readers to conceptualize dysfunction in the state as a diseased body not only in his Preface, but also in an event that sparks the secession, a

see, later uses of the word and its cognates connote the putrid decay ubiquitous in Rome beset by plague (3.6, 4.30; cf. 25.26), a connotation that retrospectively infuses Menenius' paradigm of the corpus as civic body with all the structural entropy and renovation that pestilence would come to mean in the evolving project of Livy's history.

Feldherr (1997, 142), in his contribution to Habinek's and Schiesaro's volume on *The Roman Cultural Revolution*, understands Menenius' speech as paradigmatic of Livy's larger interest in articulating a new relationship between the individual and the body politic: on Feldherr's reading, the speech defines the transition from Republic to Principate not simply as a shift from liberty to tyranny, but as marking a "fundamentally different interaction between the individual and the social entities that enclose him, and therefore a novel conception of individual identity." Livian plague, as it encroaches upon all levels of the social order, discursively binds Romans to a collective and cohesive civic body (the *totum corpus* of Menenius' parable). While the historian's narratives of epidemics often urge adherence to *concordia*, to a properly *hierarchical* arrangement of individuals within the civic body,[12] the drastic shifts in status and gradual homogeneity that often characterize a plague-stricken populace are frequently precursors to achieving that harmony; both conditions thus prove ultimately productive for the growth of the *res publica*.

2.1. PLAGUE AND *SEDITIO* OF THE FIFTH CENTURY

While other sources mention plagues of the monarchical period aside from the one that struck during the reign of Tullus (see n. 6), Livy

plebeian veteran's outcry over the debt-slavery in which the ruin of his livelihood has culminated: metaphoric and literal bodies collide in the veteran's complaint that debt (*id cumulatum usuris*) has taken over patrimony and property to the point where it at last has spread to his body as a form of *tabes* ("rot" or "disease"; 2.23.6, *postremo velut tabem pervenisse ad corpus*). Here Greenough suggests for *tabes*, "a cancer" (1988, 190). I am grateful to Dominic Machado for the observation.

[12] On Menenius Agrippa's parable as a reflection of Livy's political and social "dualism," as well as his commitment to the senate's priority within the Roman body politic, see Mineo (2015a).

does not revisit pestilence again until book three, where he offers an account of a plague of 463 BCE, and its impact on the environment, allies, and enemy forces as well as the citizens crowded inside the city walls:

> Grave tempus et forte annus pestilens erat urbi agrisque, nec hominibus magis quam pecori, et auxere vim morbi terrore populationis pecoribus agrestibusque in urbem acceptis. Ea conluvio mixtorum omnis generis animantium et odore insolito urbanos et agrestem confertum in arta tecta aestu ac vigiliis angebat, ministeriaque in vicem ac contagio ipsa volgabant morbos. (3.6.2, text is Ogilvie 1974, *AUC Libri I–V*)

> The season was difficult and the year was characterized by plague for the city and the countryside, to both men and flocks; the power of the disease increased because, out of fear of plundering, country dwellers and their herds had been brought into the city. That confluence of animals of all kinds mingled together distressed the city-dwellers because of the unaccustomed odor and the rustics because of the wakefulness and heat, since [the latter] had been packed into tight quarters; ministering to the sick and contact[13] with them tended to spread diseases.

Ogilvie notes the Thucydidean reminiscence, especially in Livy's observation that the crowding of rustics within the city walls aggravated the disease (Th. 2.52.1; Ogilvie 1970, 405; cf. Grimm 1965, 62). And, as with Thucydides, the crowding occurs within the context of a foreign army plundering or threatening to plunder the surrounding countryside (cf. Th. 2.47). Livy may also be influenced here by the belief, as we observed reflected in medical texts, that odors were a source of disease. While these conditions aggravate the pre-existing *pestilentia*, we are not informed that the disease was brought to Rome through a foreign agent.

Moreover, unlike Thucydides, who expands on the crowded conditions, then turns to the disruption of burial rites and other breaches of human *nomoi* (*anomias*, 2.53.1), Livy sets a scene in which the mixing together of humans and animals, rustics and city dwellers—generally indiscriminate intercourse as well as ministering to the sick and contact with those infected—offers an immediate backdrop for political disruption. Illness interrupts the usual political functions of

[13] See Dutoit (1948, 117) on reading *contagio* here, rather than *contagia* (plural of *contagium*), though both terms can refer to the transmission of disease (however imperfectly understood) as well as merely implying contact.

the city (*infrequens senatus*) and offers a visible sign of weakness to hostile tribes, the Volsci and Aequi, who proceed to plunder nearby territories, including those of Rome's ally, the Hernici. Where some, like Grimm (1965, 62), fault Livy's failure to draw a detailed portrait of the mental and physical anguish of the citizens, as Thucydides had done for Athens, to do so would also be to deny the Roman writer's power to telescope, within the monumental expanse of his city's history, the immediate impact of pestilence in destabilizing or empowering the political machinery of the fledgling city-state. Livy, perhaps more so than his predecessor, observes the status-leveling function of plague, as the disease kills Rome's consuls, leading citizens, and youth eligible for military service (*adfecti plerique principium, patrum maior pars, militaris fere aetas omnis*, 3.6.9); we later learn that the lower classes are equally afflicted as the disease moves "through unknown persons" (3.7.8, *per ignota capita*; i.e., those who were not property owners).

Rome can do nothing to assist her allies and answers a plea for help with a response that attributes the *pestilentia* to the wrath of the gods (*urbem Romanam subita deum ira morbo populari*, 3.6.5). Where Thucydides' excursus of the Athenian plague unfolds as a kind of suffering in isolation,[14] Livy's historiography ties disease within to a larger network of Italian allies and embeds the city within its physical environment. As hostile tribes approach Rome they encounter disruption among those georgic surroundings whose cultivation would become, in the Roman imagination, a contributor to the development of the city's character and its success (*perque omnia non praesidiis modo deserta sed etiam cultu agresti transirent*, 3.6.7).[15] Livy's account thus registers the current devastation by drawing on the celebrated correlation between a productive Italian landscape and the strength of the Roman people. The Volsci and Aequi who encounter the deserted countryside view such circumstances, where the land is deprived of both military protection (*praesidia*) and agricultural

[14] Thucydides mentions that the *nosos* afflicted populated areas near Athens, but does not indicate any intercourse between Athens and her neighbors (2.54.5).

[15] Livy's own history provides a strong testimony to the important role played by agriculture in shaping Roman ideals (cf. the legends of Cincinnatus and Horatius Cocles, the latter of whom was rewarded for his service to the state with as much land as he could plow in a single day, 2.10); Vergil's *Georgics*, as well as a variety of prose treatises on farm management, provides equal testimony to the perception that agricultural pursuits played a crucial role in shaping Roman *mores*.

stewardship (*cultus agrestis*), as another signal of Rome's debilitation, and perhaps one tinged with moral judgment, in light of the divine wrath thought to be the source of the pestilence.[16]

All the same, Rome's imposing appearance, combined with the eerily deserted, formerly teeming and productive landscape prompts the enemy tribes to abandon their plan of besieging the city and turn their attention to more prosperous locales. Commentators are divided over whether it is the plague or the site of Rome's imposing hills that causes the invaders' change of heart:[17]

> deserta omnia, sine capite, sine viribus, di praesides ac fortuna urbis tutata est, quae Volscis Aequisque praedonum potius mentem quam hostium dedit. Adeo enim nullam spem non potiundi modo sed ne adeundi quidem Romana moenia animus eorum cepit tectaque procul visa atque imminentes tumuli avertere mentes eorum, ut totis passim castris fremitu orto quid in vasto ac deserto agro inter tabem pecorum hominumque desides sine praeda tempus tererent, cum integra loca, Tusculanum agrum opimum copiis, petere possent, signa repente convellerent transversisque itineribus per Labicanos agros in Tusculanos colles transirent. Eo vis omnis tempestasque belli conversa est.
>
> (3.7.2–3)

> Everything was abandoned and without a head, without strength, but the gods as protectors and the fortune of the city watched over it, which gave to the Volsci and the Aequi the attitude of plunderers rather than enemies. For to such an extent did they not only give up the idea of gaining possession of Rome, but also of approaching Roman walls; and the roofs seen from a distance and threatening *tumuli* turned their minds away (from the prospect). Here and there in all their camps a murmuring arose as to why in a vast and deserted field, among the rot of humans and animals, they were indolently wasting their time without any plunder, when they might be attacking wholesome places and the best Tusculan fields. So they uprooted their standards quickly, and turned their journey through Labican fields and crossed over into Tusculan hills. For that reason the whole force and fury of war was turned.

[16] The Greek tradition had coupled famine and pestilence, using them as signals of moral corruption, since Hesiod in the *Works and Days* banished both from his just city and replaced them with bounteous fields, healthy flocks, and prosperous farmers (*WD* 225–37; cf. Sophocles *OT* 25–6).

[17] See Novàk (citied in Ogilvie 1970, 407) on the possibility that *imminentes tumuli* might refer to burial mounds, as an indication of the plague's death toll, heaped outside the city walls.

Just prior to Livy's focalization of Rome from the enemy's perspective, he has noted reshuffling among the political orders to create some semblance of security and governance: to compensate for a shortage of patricians, consular powers are assigned to plebeian aediles (3.6.10),[18] though the city is still left *sine capite*—that is, without the head that elsewhere in Livy signals leadership in the body politic.[19] Livy tempers the threat posed by Rome's imposing hills with language that points to its current underlying weaknesses, and not merely among magistracies: *tabes*, echoing its use in Menenius' image of a dysfunctional and atrophied body politic, signals the rot and decay of hardly distinguishable human and animal corpses.[20] The corrosive nuances are juxtaposed with productive fields and healthy places (*integra loca*) that are now preferable to Rome. By unfolding his narrative through the perspective of an advancing enemy, Livy shows us a sick city rather than sick individuals; and it is a general atmosphere of decay along with the disruption of civic functions, rather than individual suffering, that Livy foregrounds. As such the salvation of the city may also be credited to adjustments within the political structure—remedies at the level of the body politic rather than individual body.

Livy's explanation of the plague's eventual abeyance, which credits both the gods and a change in the atmosphere (3.8.1), reflects what was a commonly shared ancient belief about multiple causes and multiple remedies that should be considered when healing the sick body (Hays 1998, 12–13). In summing up the devastation experienced by both Rome and her allies, he invokes an equation—posited

[18] *Circumitio ac cura aedilium plebis erat; ad eos summa rerum ac maiestas consularis imperii venerat* (3.6.10, "inspection and care [of the posted guards] fell to the plebeian aediles; to them had come the highest power over affairs and the sovereignty of consular command").

[19] E.g., Camillus as *caput* (5.46), who prefigures more positive (non-monarchical) uses of the "head" and the need for a "head of state" to govern the Republic; on this point I am influenced by Julia Mebane's recent University of Chicago dissertation ("The Body Politic and Roman Political Languages," 2016).

[20] While Dutoit (1948, 117–18) emphasizes a contrast between the use of *tabes* here with its use in the medical metaphor of Menenius Agrippa's speech (2.32.10), where *tabes* indicates emaciation rather than decomposition, it is likely that both senses of the word resonate in each episode; moreover, use of the word in 3.7 prompts readers to search for common ground in Livy's application of the term to describe collective views of the Roman people. The medical writer Celsus equates *tabes* with the Greek terms *ἀτροφία*, *καχεξία*, and *φθίσις* (3.22), which variously stress the emaciation ("wasting away") and rot associated with the Latin term.

as early as Homeric *νόσος* in the *Iliad*—between war and plague: *haud minor Romae fit morbo strages quam ferro sociorum facta erat* (3.7.1, "the disaster from disease that occurred at Rome was in no way less than that which came to the allies from war"). At the same time, Livy innovates in stressing the relationship of the city to Italian neighbors, hostile tribes, and the surrounding physical environment, as well as in foregrounding *pestilentia*'s impact on Rome's political institutions: the plebeian aediles' assumption of consular powers, noted above, results in permanent modifications of their duties. As Ogilvie observes, Livy has anachronistically assigned to the aediles responsibilities that these officials could not have assumed until after the infamous Decemvirate (1970, 406). The historian's interest in designating this *pestilentia* as a cause for transformation of Rome's civic institutions has compromised the chronological precision of his account.

Rome would continue to experience plague regularly throughout the mid-fifth century BCE, incidents afforded fewer details in Livy's history than the outbreak of 463. In scattered notices throughout books three and four, he draws similar attention to the intersection between the emergence of plague and its effect on class privileges. In 453 BCE, plague erupts amidst a struggle between the tribunes and the patricians over the right to make laws, a conflict resulting initially in the decision to send an embassy to Athens to consult Greek law, and eventually in the founding of the Decemvirate.[21] We have already noted the outbreak of 436 BCE, characterized as an invasive force (*pestilentia populum invasit*, 4.21.2), perhaps an indication of the newly imported war captives and livestock gained in recent conflicts with the Veientes and Falisci. The disease disrupts the populace to the extent that they lack the resources to continue campaigning; meanwhile, a tribune of the *plebs* begins to stir unrest among the lower classes by making accusations against two prominent senators (*et seditiones domi quaesitae sunt*, 4.21.2). Internal weakness from plague and civil strife are nearly elided in the text, as the historian turns his

[21] *Perpetuo silentio tribunorum, quod primo legatorum qui Athenas ierant legumque peregrinarum exspectatio praebuit, dein duo simul mala ingentia exorta, fames pestilentiaque, foeda homini, foeda pecori*, 3.32.1–2. Dionysius of Halicarnassus treats the same pestilence with much more detail (10.53) and describes it as the most severe to date. Like Livy, Dionysius is interested in innovations prompted by the crisis, in this case, religious measures, though he readily pronounces them ineffectual.

attention to the hostile Veientes, who join forces with the Fidenates to launch an ultimately unsuccessful attack against Rome.

In the same decade, plague prompts the Romans to vow a temple to the foreign god Apollo, after they have consulted the Sibylline books (4.25; 434/33 BCE).[22] The outbreak occurs again during an episode of strife (*contentiones*, 4.25.1) between the patricians and the tribunes of the *plebs*, who block the consular elections in order to ensure the election of military tribunes with consular power. Pestilence is described as occurring during a momentary respite (*otium*) from the hostilities, and results in indiscriminate death of humans and livestock: *magna tamen clades in urbe agrisque promiscua hominum pecorumque pernicie accepta* ("still, there was great disaster in the city and the fields, with indiscriminate loss among humans and animals," 4.25.5). The leveling effects of pestilence in this case function in subtle opposition to the class divisions sharpened through political wrangling.

Five years later, and soon after the temple is dedicated (4.30, 427 BCE), again within the context of the plebeian tribunes' attempt to have military tribunes with consular powers elected, contagion (*contactus*) erupts, spreading from animals to humans in the countryside and eventually within the city walls (*scabie alia absumpta, volgatique contactu in homines morbi*, 4.30.8). The disease's origins are located in Rome's rural environs, as drought aggravates conditions for scabies among the livestock. While the city is filled with disease (*impletur*), it is also besieged by religious innovation viewed as a foreign threat:

> Et primo in agrestes ingruerant servitiaque; urbs deinde impletur. Nec corpora modo adfecta tabo, sed animos quoque multiplex religio et pleraque externa invasit, novos ritus sacrificandi vaticinando inferentibus in domos quibus quaestui sunt capti superstitione animi.
>
> (4.30.8–9)

> At first disease fell upon the rustics and slaves; from there it fills the city. Not only were their bodies afflicted with rot (*tabum*), but frequently manifold and foreign religious practices penetrated their minds, with people importing new rites for sacrificing by means of augury in the homes of those whose minds were seized at a profit by *superstitio*.

[22] Ogilvie (1970, 574) recognizes this as one of a series that occurred throughout Latium in the late 430s.

Foreign religious practices launch a sinister and potentially corrosive invasion among the Romans, one quickly checked after it has penetrated the upper echelons of the social order. At the behest of the political leadership (*primores civitatis*), aediles are charged with restricting worship to only Roman gods, and only in a traditional manner (*neu quo alio more quam patrio colerentur*, 4.30.11).

Livy's syntax implies a structural parallel between *tabum* and *multiplex religio*, and the historian writes of *superstitio* in a disparaging tone, since only *pudor* among the leading citizens, *primores civitatis*, can check it.[23] Where Thucydides had indicated a range of pleasure-seeking behaviors that contributed to Athenian *anomia*, Livy singles out deviations in religious practices as the only form of lawlessness in the city. It is important to keep in mind, however, the comparatively salubrious religious import, worship of the god Apollo, whose temple has in the narrative just been dedicated. For Livy, contagious disease (here the historian makes a specific correlation between illness, proximity, and transmission, *vulgatique in homines morbi*, 4.30.11) is presented as a social crisis that in turn provokes experimentation, tampering with the traditional order of things. As such it operates on a stage parallel to the dramas enacted among political orders, where *seditio* and, as we shall observe, *novae res* are both detrimental and necessary safety valves for managing the pressures of an expanding population.

2.2. PESTILENCE AND THE *LECTISTERNIUM* OF 399 BCE

The correlation between *seditio* and contagious disease is made even more evident in Livy's narration of a plague that erupts in the early fourth century. In the historian's treatment of fifth-century plagues, we have observed political and cultural innovation as a direct response to disease (powers granted to plebeian aediles, worship of the god

[23] On *superstitio* in Livy and its regulation by the state, see Scheid (2015, 84–5). Scheid counters the notion that suppression of *superstitio* in *AUC* appears motivated in order to safeguard aristocratic privilege. While that may be the case in general, Livy's account here does suggest antagonism between the practitioners of the new rites and the *primores* charged with restricting them.

Apollo, introduction of foreign *superstitiones* and their suppression by *primores civitatis*). We have also noted a tendency to contextualize these notices within the larger struggle between the patrician and plebeian orders, particularly in the plague (453) that erupts just prior to the foundation of the Decemvirate, and during those of 433 and 427, concurring with efforts of the *tribuni plebis* to have military tribunes elected from their own order. Guided by a similar impulse, Livy explains the aetiology of the Roman *lectisternium*, a ceremony in which certain gods are invited to participate in a sacrificial feast,[24] as a direct response to the pestilence of 399 BCE. The origin of the custom is embedded in a broader narrative of internal strife focalized partly through the perspective of the patrician Appius Claudius Crassus, who predicts fractures in the hard won *concordia ordinum* as the result of ideological contagion.

Appius' speech (5.3–6) represents the view of the patrician military tribunes recommending the continued siege of Veii during the winter, and comes as a response to the *tribuni plebis*, who oppose year-round campaigning forced upon a largely plebeian army. His rhetoric likens the possibility of unrest in the camps to a *contagio*, one that Rome's enemies would surely welcome: *an est quicquam quod Veientibus optatum aeque contingere possit quam ut seditionibus primum urbs Romana, deinde velut ex contagione castra impleantur* (5.6.11; "is there anything that could happen so pleasing to the Veientes than that first the city of Rome, and then the camps, should be filled with political factions, as if by contagion?"). In describing the movement of *seditio* as a "contagion" Appius summons the earlier use of *contagio* to describe the pestilence afflicting Rome while the city was threatened by the Volsci and Aequi (3.6.3, *ministeria . . . ac contagio ipsa volgabant morbos*). The ideological dissent rebuked by Appius also parallels the outbreak of 427 BCE, as dissent threatens to "fill up" the camps (*impleantur*) in the same way that Rome was "filled up" by disease—spread through "contagion" (*contactus*) from livestock to humans—in the earlier episode (*impletur*, 4.30.8).

The link between ideological and nosological contagion is further emphasized through Appius' description of the *tribuni plebis* as bad doctors who have a need for a sick patient, that is, the *res publica: sic hercule, tamquam artifices improbi, opus quaerunt qui [et] semper*

[24] See Ogilvie (1970, 655) for details and possible Greek origins of the custom.

aegri aliquid esse in re publica volunt, ut sit ad cuius curationem a vobis adhibeantur (5.3.6, "Thus, by god, like bad doctors they seek out work, since they always want there to be some illness in the Republic, so that there might be something you might summon them to cure").[25] By relying on the same body-politic metaphor drawn by Menenius Agrippa, Appius recalls the model of a healthy citizen body as one whose functions are properly distributed: the body sick from ideological contagion has implicitly lost its properly hierarchical operations, due to the demagoguery of the plebeian tribunes.

Subsequent disaster experienced by the Romans at Veii turns popular opinion in favor of Appius and his advocacy of extended military service: equestrians, followed by infantry men, vow to serve the *res publica*, events that forge within the narrative a direct link between external threats and renewed *concordia ordinum* (5.7), the "harmony among the political orders" recognized as one of Livy's premier civic virtues (Walsh 1961, 66–9).[26] Ideological contagion within the city walls, by contrast, emerges as a pernicious force, and the direct opponent of *concordia*. It is worth noting, however, that in this case accident rather than Appius' leadership achieves *concordia*, and it is broken nearly as easily as it is forged. Within the next two years, circumstances at Veii remain undecided and the plebeian tribunes successfully prosecute the military commanders Sergius and Verginius for mismanaging the campaign, while also preventing the collection of tribute needed to pay the army in the field. The result is renewed *seditio*, again likened to a contagion, which threatens once more to extend well beyond the city walls and into the military *castra* (5.12.7, *haud procul erat quin castra quoque urbanae seditionis contagione turbarentur*).

It is in this immediate context, well woven with metaphorical links between contagion and civic unrest, that pestilence again besets the Roman people in 399 BCE. After describing the success of the plebeians at electing military tribunes from their own order, Livy notes a harsh winter followed by a summer "oppressive and disease-bearing for all living beings" (*gravis pestilensque omnibus animalibus aestas,*

[25] Appius again likens the tribunes to bad doctors for the body politic near the end of his speech, at 5.5.12: *haec sunt, tribuni, consilia vestra, non hercule dissimilia ac si quis aegro qui curari se fortiter passus extemplo convalescere possit, cibi gratia praesentis aut potionis longinquum et forsitan insanabilem morbum efficiat.*

[26] For the pronounced thematic resonance of *concordia* in Appius' speech and throughout book five, see Oakley (2015, 232).

5.13.4). The Roman people, unable to determine the origins of the "incurable danger" (*insanabilis pernicies*), look to divine causation: consultation of the Sibylline books yields a recommendation that the Romans hold the first *lectisternium* and honor Apollo, Diana, Latona, Mercury, Hermes, and Hercules by arranging images of the gods on couches before a feast. The event is accompanied by a generally convivial atmosphere, one in which traditional class distinctions are ignored.[27]

> Tota urbe patentibus ianuis promiscuoque usu rerum omnium in propatulo posito, notos ignotosque passim advenas in hospitium ductos ferunt, et cum inimicis quoque benigne ac comiter sermones habitos; iurgiis and litibus temperatum; vinctis quoque dempta in eos dies vincula; religioni deinde fuisse quibus eam opem di tulissent vinciri.
>
> (5.13.7–8)

> Throughout the whole city doorways were opened and there was indiscriminate enjoyment of all things arranged out in the open; they say that here and there known and unknown strangers shared hospitality, and that greetings were exchanged in a civil and kindly manner even among personal enemies. There were restrictions against quarrels and lawsuits; prisoners were released from their bonds in those days; and it was a matter of religious objection for those whom the gods have given such help to be bound again.

Livy concurs with Dionysius of Halicarnassus (12.9) here in stressing the intermingling of all citizens, conceived of in *AUC* as a collective entity (*tota urbs*), an identity reinforced through language stressing the removal of physical barriers (*patentibus ianuis, in propatulo posito*). While both authors are relying on Piso, as Ogilvie notes (1970, 657), the Saturnalian atmosphere is likely false, and did not accompany subsequent *lectisternia*. And yet the historian's use of *promiscuus* to describe the shared enjoyment of the feast is pointed: as we have seen in a similar plague context, the word indicates the devastation that afflicts humans and livestock "without distinction" (433 BCE, 4.25), though it also frequently refers to a lack of discrimination between orders in more explicitly charged political contexts, when privileges are contested (4.56.12; cf. 29.17, 34.44 on privileges of watching *ludi*). As in other accounts of plague, Livy passes over the

[27] All gods are perhaps invoked for their healing powers; but see Ogilvie (1970, 656) on the peculiar assortment of deities.

symptomatology of the disease and the suffering of individuals in order to demonstrate cultural innovation, in this case a remedy that relieves tensions in the social order, as the festival, homeopathically mimicking the status-leveling effects of pestilence, temporarily neutralizes hostilities between citizens.

In the following year, the patricians will interpret the plague (*pestis*) as a sign of the gods' displeasure over the fact that under their auspices, "offices were shared and the distinctions among families were confused" (*honores volgari discriminaque gentium confundi*, 5.14.4). The historian has already assigned to the patricians less than honorable motives in making such claims (i.e., they wish to keep the offices of military tribune among their order), so it would be wrong to infer Livy's patrician sympathies in this instance.[28] What we can say with more certainty is that the historian uses plague and the promiscuity that results from it as a means of reflecting on more deeply ingrained class tensions. The tendency of an epidemic to force those tensions to erupt on the surface of the body politic grants plague an expurgatory role that is both detrimental and salubrious to the well-being of the state. If, as I hope to have demonstrated, pestilence is metaphorically resonant of the struggle of the orders, we need not conclude that strife between *patres* and *plebs* is necessarily harmful to the Roman people. Rather, Livy's narrative design encourages us to view it as critical to Rome's development: the (controlled) promiscuity of the plague-inspired *lectisternium* is one answer to the ideological contagion spread by self-serving doctor-tribunes advocating for (uncontrolled) promiscuity among the orders.[29]

It is worth noting that Livy is not alone in his perspective on the salutary effects of class strife and *seditiones*: Cicero echoes it in the words of *De Oratore*'s Antonius, who, outlining his defense of Norbanus, argues that episodes of civil discord (*seditiones*), while bothersome, are sometimes just, necessary, and a *salus huic*

[28] For Livy's ambivalent depiction of the *patres* in the first pentad, see Miles (1995, 115–16).

[29] The regular correlation between plague and class strife speaks to Livy's frequently overlooked talents as a keen, and fairly systematic observer of Rome's development. Luce (1977, esp. xvii–xxv) offers an overview and rebuttal of negative assessments of Livy's powers as an historian, especially in the area of structural design. See also Vasaly (2015) on the structural integrity of the first pentad. We might consider *pestis* among Vasaly's character types or *personae* whose repetition gives shape, predictability, and unexpected twists to the narrative (221).

civitati (2.199). Even more pertinent to Livy's correlation of epidemics with sedition are comments in Cicero's *De Legibus*. In the dialogue, Quintus invokes disease metaphors in his inquiry concerning the origins and impact of the *tribuni plebis*, whose power (*potestas*) he describes as a twice-born deformed child, "plague-bearing... born in civil strife and tending to civil strife" (*pestifera... in seditione et ad seditionem nata sit, Leg.* 3.19). Cicero concedes the potential for abuse within the office, but argues in response that the tribunate on the whole functioned as a restraint to rebellion among the *plebs*, fostering the perception of a civic body in which power is more equitably distributed, and deserved to be recognized as a *salus civitatis* (3.24). Livy's view of *seditio* and the tribunes tied to its eruption is thus conditioned to some extent by late-Republican political theorizing on the matter.[30] His talents as an historian, however, situate the salutary impact of political disruption within contexts of epidemics in such a way that guides readers to a clearer understanding of how a "plague-bearing" political innovation often invigorated the body politic.

2.3. PLAGUE AND ROME'S *LUDI SCAENICI*

Livy's account of the origins of *ludi scaenici* ("stage plays") posits a historically integral relationship between an outbreak of pestilence in the year 364 BCE and the foundation of theater as a Roman institution (7.1–3; cf. Val. Max. 2.4.4). By linking disease to the importation of Etruscan music and dance, the episode may be understood as part of a larger program we have been charting, one of sustained correlation between contagion and cultural innovation. In describing plague's impact on the development of the theater, Livy makes a less direct link between disease and the political structure, though (as I discuss further below) the theater itself, in marking some as eligible or ineligible for citizenship, does widen the division between Romans and foreigners. As Gruen has argued, the theater will become increasingly important as an arena for giving voice to and reflecting on political upheaval (1992, 184), particularly by the late-Republican era. In marking the initial importation of *ludi* as a *nova res*, inconsistent

[30] I am grateful to Dominic Machado for the references; for further analysis of the parallels between Ciceronian and Livian political philosophies, see Mineo (2015, 133–5).

with formerly bellicose habits, Livy locates within the very origins of theater (and implicitly the plague that begets it) a fundamental role in shaping the collective *mores* of the Roman civic body—in a way that Artaud (who channels Livy through Augustine) will eventually recognize as the premier illustration of the transformative effect of theater as plague.

The historian's account of the introduction of theater among the Roman populace in 364 BCE has been cited by scholars of Roman literature as evidence for the nature and conditions of early dramatic performances (cf. Feldherr 1998, 180; Duckworth 1952, 4–7; Oakley 1998, 40–72). Aside from recognizing that, as an attempt to restore the *pax deorum*, Roman theater, like that of the Greeks, emerges from a religious context (Fantham 2013, 16–18; Gruen, 1992, 185), scholars have left the function of these initial performances as a remedy for an especially severe *pestilentia* largely unexplored. Livy does not speculate on why such performances occurred to the Romans as a means of propitiation, though it is possible that music here assumes its traditional function as an agent of healing, as has been argued for innovations in the language of fifth-century Athenian tragedy after the plague of 430 BCE (Mitchell-Boyask 2008, 8–17).

Feldherr has understood the cultural impact of the *ludi* in negative terms, an extension of Livy's tendency to polarize the pernicious effects of dramatic spectacles with the more salubrious images effected through historical *exempla*. As such the excursus on drama functions programmatically, like Livy's *Praefatio*, and allows the historian to contrast history and drama as "two systems of representation" in terms of their "effect on their audiences" (1998, 179); plague, within that excursus, emerges for Feldherr as ironically and prophetically announcing the misguided remedy intended to cure it.[31] I would like to turn attention away from the ramifications of this remedy as they extend into Rome of the first century BCE, which Livy unequivocally condemns, to the immediate causal relationship binding plague and *ludi scaenici*: in doing so, we observe how plague, in book seven as elsewhere, maintains its role as a challenge to the Roman people, but

[31] See esp. Feldherr (1998, 182): "Since the drama was imported originally to cure a pestilence, the description of drama as an *insania* itself points out the extent to which the practice has failed to fulfill the social and religious function for which it was designed."

one that unifies them and prompts comparative evaluations of the civic institutions wrought to remedy it.

Livy's account of *pestilentia* and Roman drama should thus be read as one of a series of endemic plagues allowing the historian to illustrate the ingenuity of the Romans, ingenuity paralleled in earlier accounts by the addition of a god to the pantheon or by new ritual practices or by redistributing privileges within the political order. In this particular episode the plague-inspired *ludi* assume the function of political upheaval—their explicit designation as a *nova res* echoes usage of the term to describe constitutional changes and revolutionary movements effected within the tumultuous years of the late Republic.[32] Like other endemic outbreaks, the plague that necessitates Rome's *ludi scaenici* simply "arose" (*pestilentia ingens orta*, 7.1.7),[33] but does so during a remarkable period of absence of class strife (*seditio*) or war with a foreign enemy (*bellum*). In opening book seven and setting the political scene, Livy describes the concession made to the *plebs* that curile aediles be chosen from that order, a concession eventually altered further so that candidates were allowed to stand for the office from either patricians or *plebs* "without distinction" (*postea promiscuum fuit*, 7.1.6). These concessions no doubt contribute in 365/4 to the lack of *seditio*, which we have observed frequently concurring with *pestilentia*. Similarly, Rome at the time was conducting no wars abroad:

> Inde L. Genucio et Q. Servilio consulibus et ab seditione et a bello quietis rebus, ne quando a metu ac periculis vacarent, pestilentia ingens orta. Censorem, aedilem curulem, tres tribunos plebis mortuos ferunt, pro portione et ex multitudine alia multa funera fuisse; maximeque eam pestilentiam insignem mors quam matura, tam acerba M. Furi fecit. (7.1.7)
>
> After that, during the consulship of Lucius Genucius and Quintus Servilius, when affairs were at rest from both war and class strife, lest the situation ever be free from fear and danger, a huge pestilence arose.

[32] See *res OLD* 10; cf. Cic. *Agr.* 2.91; Caes. *Gal.* 1.9.3; Hor. *Epod.* 16.6; Sal. *Cat.* 37.1. Cf. especially Livy's use of the phrase at 23.14 to describe the feelings of the *plebs* at Capua, who were eager for the "change in government" (*novae res*) that would attend breaking the city's alliance with Rome in favor of Hannibal.

[33] In 411 BCE (4.52) pestilence "arose" (*coorta*) just as Lucilius Icilius incites *seditiones* among the *plebs* by promoting agrarian laws. In 347 (7.27) a *pestilentia* arises (*adorta*), resulting in another *lectisternium* and the consultation of the Sibylline books.

> Sources say that a censor, a curile aedile, and three tribunes of the *plebs* died, and that there were a proportionally large number of deaths among the rest of the populace; and in particular the death of Marcus Furius, harsh even though tardy,[34] made that plague noteworthy.

Livy renews a familiar triangulation of terms (war abroad, civil strife, and plague), but alters the dynamics between them: where the occurrence of plague has in earlier references operated as a metaphor for concurrent illness in the body politic, here we have it functioning as an alternative to *seditiones* and *bellum* against foreign enemies (*metus hostilis*), both of which are more commonly identified as agents of Rome's development.[35] By implicitly stationing these three forces on equal footing, and then shifting plague to the fore, the historian assigns pestilence a potentially progressive function, explicitly described, like *bellum* and *seditio*, as a condition that constantly tests the mettle of the Roman people.

In remarking on the impact of the plague Livy continues his practice of minimizing or overlooking altogether symptomatology and psychology. His few remarks on the suffering of the populace *in toto* are largely restricted to the mention of a few unnamed officials, whose function within the state supersedes their individual identities. Such practice, on the one hand, is consistent with the generally dehumanizing effects of pestilence, a tendency observed most compellingly in the work of Sontag (1988) and Girard (1974).[36] On the other hand, Livy does not treat all *funera* equally, deeming the deaths of those men who play important roles within the state as more worthy of commemoration than the rest of the population.

Rather than overlooking individual suffering altogether, he confines his comments on the mortality rate to the impact of the disease on Rome's governance, by offering one of only a handful of death notices in *AUC* (Oakley 1998, 35), that of Marcus Furius Camillus: the loss of the former dictator Camillus is distinguished (*insignis*) because of how it affects the stability of the city's leadership, in the case of a man so crucial to Rome's well-being that he is described as a second "founder" (*conditor*). Indeed, the historian's emphasis on

[34] For variations in the manuscripts and suggested translations, see Oakley (1998, 35).

[35] See Walsh (1961, 52–3) on Livy's use of final clauses (here, *ne ... vacarent*) to convey the idea that trials constantly beset the Romans early in their history, "so that they may become physically and morally capable of world-leadership" (52; cf. Oakley 1998, 34).

[36] See Chapter 1, pp. 34–40.

Camillus' death as a casualty of the plague lends even more weight to the role played by contagious disease in advancing *novae res.* If Camillus' well-being and role as head of the body politic (*caput*, 5.46.5) secured Rome's second founding after its sack by the Gauls, then his death marks, if not a new political regime, at least a growing pain in the maturation of the civic body.[37]

Livy's history has been characterized as one "preeminently concerned with individuals" (Walsh 1961, 82), and indeed his interest in the deaths of leaders like Camillus, as opposed to the physical and psychological trials of the Roman people, would confirm such an assessment. Plague's tendency to fracture and forge collectivities, however, also allows the historian to reflect on what motivates or restrains certain political groups.[38] In contrast to the class fissures exposed in earlier treatments of pestilence, the plague that prompts the importation of the *ludi* forges a uniform coalescence among the entirety of the *populus Romanus*, in so far as it impacts their collective *mores*. After the death of Camillus, pestilence continues into the following year, again (though in this case less explicitly) in the context of an absence of internal or external conflict (*eo nihil dignum memoria actum*, 7.1.2). After noting that another *lectisternium* fails to appease the gods, Livy recalls Thucydides' formulation of resources summoned in times of plague, *humana concilia* and *divina ops* (cf. Th. 2.47.4); and as in his account of responses to the plague of 427 (4.30; cf. 1.31.6), he adds a third term, *superstitio*, among which he includes the newly imported *ludi*:[39]

> Et cum vis morbi nec humanis consiliis nec ope divina levaretur, victis superstitione animis ludi quoque scenici, nova res bellicoso populo—nam circi modo spectaculum fuerat—inter alia caelestis irae placamina

[37] For Camillus as *caput*, see Mebane, cited above, n. 19. Camillus' structural significance within book five and in the first pentad have been stressed in recent studies by Oakley (2015) and Vasaly (2015), respectively; in the same collection of essays, see also Mineo, who explores Camillus' role as a *conditor* and embodiment of Livy's political ideals (2015b, 146–7, with significant bibliography on the topic).

[38] Miles (1995, 115 n. 20) remarks on the influence of Walsh's view of Livy's interest in exceptional individuals, but suggests that such influence "may obscure [Livy's] significant, even if secondary, interest in political groups and classes, and their distinctive character and roles."

[39] See Stoclet (2007, 135–6); Livy's addition of *superstitio* to *consilia humana* and *ops divina* in his account of reactions to the plague of 364 BCE introduces a particularly Roman tendency to initially rely on human planning and traditional reverence for the gods, but, when pressed, to turn "to supernatural powers outside the recognized or dominant canon, and invoke them in various ways" (136).

> instituì dicuntur; ceterum parva quoque, ut ferme principia omnia, et ea ipsa peregrina res fuit. (7.2.3)
>
> And when the virulence of the disease was alleviated neither by human planning nor divine aid, after minds had been overcome by superstition, stage plays (*ludi scenici*) also—a new custom for a warlike people (for up to that point there had only been the circus spectacles)—are said to have been instituted among other means of placating the anger of heaven; but even these were small at first, as is the case of nearly all beginnings, and the custom itself was foreign.

From here Livy offers his famous excursus on the early development of Roman theater, which began as rudimentary dances accompanied by the *tibia* (*ad tibicinis modos*) imported from Etruria. Such performances, described as musical "medleys" (*saturae*), were eventually assigned to professional actors and evolved into comedies with plots.[40]

Particular controversies surrounding the veracity of Livy's account and his reliance on an earlier source, perhaps Varro,[41] are not as important to our discussion as his observation of changes in the social order effected by this *nova res*. The arrival of the *ludi* are not accompanied by redistribution of class distinctions, but instead by a sharpening of the division between citizen and non-citizen individuals, one that unifies the collective Roman civic body in opposition to the foreign, Etruscan other. Livy notes that in the second phase of the evolution of *ludi*, young Romans (*iuventus*, 7.2.5) began to imitate the Etruscan dancers and add to the performance rude jests in "undisciplined verses" (*inconditis versibus*), which the historian likens to Fescennine verses (*Fescinnino versu*, 7.2.5–6).[42] Later, however, professional actors (*histriones*) resumed control over the art, dropped the rude jesting, and performed *saturae*. As the discrepancy emerged between staged performances of *ludi* by professional actors and the earlier jesting of the Roman youth, the

[40] Famously crafted first by Livius Andronicus; the passage is often compared with the account given in Hor. *Ep.* 2.1.139–63; see Duckworth (1952, 4–7).

[41] See Oakley (1998, 42–4) for bibliography on Livy's sources; the account of Valerius Maximus is similar, though perhaps because Livy is his primary source; see also Waszink 1948 (cf. Feldherr 1998, 180) on problems with reconstructing Livy's sources for the excursus.

[42] In Varro's account, rude jesting predated the importation of the Etruscan performances (cf. Waszink 1948, 234–5).

young men abandoned the performance of *ludi* altogether and turned exclusively to rude jokes in what was eventually known as Atellan farce, a comic form unique in its capacity to allow its performers to maintain their citizen privileges:[43]

> quod genus ludorum ab Oscis acceptum tenuit iuventus nec ab histrionibus pollui passa est; eo institutum manet ut actores Atellanarum nec tribu moveantur et stipendia, tamquam expers artis ludicrae, faciant (7.2.12).
>
> The youth took charge of this kind of *ludi*, having received it from the Oscans, nor did they allow it to be polluted by the involvement of professional actors. Once established the custom has persisted that those acting in Atellan farces are not removed from their tribe and they maintain their eligibility for military services, as if they are untainted by the actor's *ars*.

While the custom of *ludi* and its evolution does not directly address tensions between citizen *ordines*, it does point to a causal and sequential link between plague, cultural innovation, and eventual reconstitution of the qualities that determine citizenship through army enlistment and membership in a tribe.[44]

More important for developing Livy's pattern of correlating pestilence with transformation in the body politic is the historian's speculation concerning the impact of disease-inspired *ludi* upon the collective Roman *mores*. The unusual length of this digression in *AUC* suggests to Oakley (1998, 41) a "moral and didactic purpose," signaled in the historian's summary comment on the current state of *ludi* in the Augustan era:

> inter aliarum parva principia rerum ludorum quoque prima origo ponenda visa est, ut appareret quam ab sano initio res in hanc vix opulentis regnis tolerabilem insaniam venerit. (7.2.13)

[43] Cf. Horace's account of Fescennine verses among Roman youth and their gradual regulation in *Ep.* 2.1.139–55. While Livy recognizes the Oscan origins of the closely related Atellan farce, Horace implicitly links this type of performance with Roman identity, in contrast to non-native poetic forms (e.g., those imported from Greece).

[44] For Feldherr this exemption allowing the performers of Atellan farce to retain their citizen status further highlights the status of the *histriones* and their *ars* as foreign purveyors of a "distracted and disconnected" social phenomenon (1998, 181). Thus plague functions to redistribute membership within the citizen body, but also redefine elements external and threatening to the citizen body.

> It seems that among the modest beginnings of other things, so too we must place the first origin of the *ludi*, so that it is clear how from a healthy beginning the practice has become this sickness hardly able to be supported by wealthy kingdoms.

Livy's statement contrasting early theater with the current excess that characterizes the *ludi* (*inter aliarum parva principia*, 7.2.13) returns readers to the notion of small beginnings (*ceterum parva quoque*, 7.2.4) and, with those beginnings, to the original situation of pestilence (*vis morbi*) that prompted the importation of theatrical performances in the first place. We are thus implicitly asked to evaluate the "force of the disease" and its concomitant importation of *ludi* in light of the "madness" (*insaniam*) that now accompanies the Roman theater: Livy uses a term that refers to mental illness, but whose root, *sanus*, frequently indicates physical well-being, as we are reminded in the historian's assertion of an initially salutary impulse behind the performance of the *ludi* (*ab sano initio*). Feldherr is right to register the author's disdain for the current practice of *ludi scaenici*, especially as a foil to the *monumentum* of an historical record (1998, 184–5). Still, the *sanum initium* must give us pause, signaling a healthy start in an etymologically pointed contrast to its currently morbid conditions.

In fact the excursus in its entirety, with its references to conditions of health and well-being (*sanus, insania*), as well as its language of origins and development (*origo, principia, initium*) and its embedding within a plague context, are better understood if we view them as extensions of those priorities outlined in the preface. Livy's programmatic defense of history implies that the historian's craft is one of the few *remedia* Rome's current conditions will tolerate; as noted above, he describes his work, especially his goal of representing exemplary conduct, as "health-giving and profitable" (*salubre ac frugiferum*, Pr. 10), a means of addressing maladies in the body politic (Woodman 1988, 133–4 and 2009, 52). In constructing a cultural history that charts a transformation of one *ars* from a condition of relative health into sickness, Livy poses the question of whether the theater (as the *ludicra ars*) should be reckoned among those *artes* that augmented Roman *imperium*, which the historian promises to chronicle at the start of his account (*per quos viros quibusque artibus domi militiaeque et partum et auctum imperium sit*, Pr. 9). Even if the answer in this case is resoundingly negative, the episode confirms the role of *pestilentia*—as crisis within the body politic *par excellence*—in motivating the Roman people to reevaluate their social structure, their *mores*, and the cultural practices that subtend them.

Ludi scaenici as a remedy for plague fail initially and are only the second of a tripartite attempt to appease the gods, beginning with the *lectisternium* (7.2.2), like the one celebrated in 399, and ending with a ceremonial "driving of the nail" (7.3.3–9). The latter practice, revived from an earlier outbreak of pestilence (perhaps in 435 BCE), will be repeated during a subsequent quasi-pestilence, in which a number of Roman *matronae* are charged with poisoning after various leading citizens fall ill (8.18.11–12). Livy does not comment explicitly on the efficacy of the ritual,[45] but as with earlier remedies proffered to combat epidemic disease, his narrative artistry forges a link between plague, experimental measures, and the effect of such measures on the overall *concordia* of political orders.

The driving of the nail, probably originating as a means of keeping time, but also assuming early on an apotropaic function, involved appointing a dictator to fix a nail in the right side of the temple of Jupiter Optimus Maximus. The dictator chosen in this instance, aptly named Lucius Manlius Imperiosus, promptly abuses his power and attempts to levy troops for war against the Hernici. His efforts are successfully countered by the united *tribuni plebis*. Thus, we must evaluate the remedial function of appointing a magistrate "for the sake of driving the nail" (*causa clavi figendi*) with caution; its efficacy in resolving the crisis of the plague remains implicit, overshadowed by one dictator's abuse of his authority. Origins of the ritual continue to be debated, and Livy's history adds to the confusion by referring to the institution elsewhere as a practice that originated not with plague (as its first notice in book seven indicates) but with an incident of internal political strife.[46] Such confusion in the text, however, only adds to the cumulative impression that plague and political sedition are closely linked in Livy's historical imagination.[47]

[45] Cf. Feldherr (1998, 184), who sees it as efficacious, though Livy never mentions whether the innovation worked.

[46] See Oakley (1998, 73–46) and Liv. 8.18.1–13, where, in his second account of the practice, Livy remarks that it had been recalled not from the *pestilentia* of 364, but from an earlier instance of plebeian secession.

[47] Scholars have had difficulty reconciling the apotropaic function of the rite (whether in warding off *seditio* or *pestilentia*) with its chronological function; see Bodel (1995, 290–1). Livy's annalist sources may have explained the (apparently

Livy's expansion on the origin of the practice (7.3.5–9) performs a function similar to his account of the theater, in so far as it has the effect of relativizing the foundations of the city's cultural institutions in terms of contemporary Augustan Rome. The practice had fallen out of use in the late Republic; Augustus revived the practice of "driving the nail" (cf. Dio 55.10.4), but did so in the recently dedicated Temple of Mars Ultor (*c.*2 BCE) and commissioned "those who completed the census" to accomplish it—that is to say, the Princeps. As Bodel remarks (1995, 291; cf. Feeney 2007, 176), Livy's account confirms a popular association during the Augustan Principate of driving the nail, the dedication of a temple to a chief state deity, and the beginning of a new form of government. By appropriating and transforming the practice, Augustus assumed a crucial role in the apotropaic function of the ritual, not least of which was historically linked, as we have just seen, to the aim of warding off *pestilentia*. Moreover, the Augustan resonance of the episode would prompt readers to interpret the crisis of 364 BCE within a late first-century context fraught with its own articulations of internal strife. The *pestilentia* that opens book seven, claims Camillus as its victim, and begets a series of "new" practices offers the historian opportunities to narrate the missteps, successes, and innovations that have led to current excess: as such, and when interpreted in light of the larger programmatic metaphor positing the *res publica* of the late first century as body politic in need of the right *remedia*, the episode functions as a *mise-en-abyme* of Rome's development, encouraging reflection on the (re)founding of Rome under a novel form of leadership.

* * *

In *De Civitate Dei* ("City of God"), Augustine identifies an irony in the fact that the Romans had introduced *ludi scaenici* in order to appease gods during a time of plague, since such measures had corrupted the very character of a community in order to remedy a merely physical malady. On this point, Augustine draws heavily from Livy's account of various responses to the plague of 364 BCE, but intensifies the historian's cynicism concerning the excesses of contemporary spectacles. As we have observed, Livy's digression places

extraordinary) measure of appointing a dictator by linking it to a time of crisis (Oakley 1998, 76).

the evolution of stage plays, and all *spectacula* implicitly, within a larger arc of Rome's imperial progress, asking readers to evaluate the role of this particular cultural innovation in the fortification or deterioration of Roman *mores*. His *Praefatio* makes clear that the empire can no longer tolerate certain *vitia*, and we are to imagine that such spectacles might be among them.

Augustine, having witnessed the recent sack of the city by Alaric in 410 CE, is equally concerned with how the Roman cultural heritage has affected its current social and political instability. Where defenders of the old ways, the Roman aristocracy, attacked Christianity and its role in turning citizens away from worship of the pantheon, Augustine in *De Civitate Dei* locates within reverence to the "pagan" gods themselves the source of Rome's misfortunes, for they are the entities who authorize a spiritual plague in order to remedy a physical one. As part of his immediate polemic, Augustine draws on Livy's aetiology of Roman *ludi* in order to detract from the reverence given to Rome's deities, while conceding that even some Romans, such as the prudent Scipio Nasica, recognized the corruption of *mores* that the theater promoted:[48]

> Si aliqua luce mentis animum corpori praeponitis, eligite quem colatis! Neque enim et illa corporum pestilentia ideo conquievit quia populo bellicoso et solis antea ludis circensibus adsueto ludorum scaenicorum delicata subintravit insania; sed astutia spirituum nefandorum praevidens illam pestilentiam iam fine debito cessaturam aliam longe graviorem, qua plurimum gaudet, ex hac occasione non corporibus, sed moribus curavit immittere. (*De Civ.* 1.32)
>
> If by any clear rationale you prefer the mind to the body, choose whom you would worship! And not even (by such a measure) did that disease of the body abate, because a dainty madness (*insania*) for stage plays took possession of a warlike people and one accustomed only to the games of the circus before; but the cunning of malicious spirits, foreseeing that the physical plague would cease soon by an established end,

[48] Augustine's interpretation of Scipio's motives for condemning the *ludi* may occlude other dynamics driving Scipio's campaign to block the building of a permanent theater in Rome (cf. Liv. *Per.* 48). Gruen argues that the senatorial class, led by Scipio, wished to preserve its authority over regular production of *ludi*, an authority diminished in the case of a permanent theater (1992, 209). The possibility of such a motive shines a rather different light on the power of the theater to promote cohesion within the Roman body politic.

took care, during this opportunity, to introduce another plague more serious by far not into their bodies, but into their customs.

The theologian's appropriation of Livy's narrative of *pestilentia* in 364 BCE makes explicit the metaphorical relationship binding a shared physical crisis to a communally experienced ideological one. As I have demonstrated, however, Livy had already primed pestilence for use as a metaphor for ideological contagion. Plague, weighted with implications of shared suffering, transformation, and innovation, aptly reflects the shared experience of theatrical performance because both theater and plague spread indiscriminately to reorient a community's values. Artaud will make much of Augustine's appropriation of Livy in his celebration of theater's explosively expurgating and transformative power, which not only "affects important collectivities and upsets them in an identical way," but also "disturbs the senses' repose, frees the repressed unconscious, incites a kind of virtual revolt . . . and imposes on the assembled collectivity an attitude that is both difficult and heroic" (1958, 27–8). For Livy, the heroism of the Roman people lies partly in their ability to constantly suffer revolts from within, but emerge from the trial in a more concordant formation.

Livy colors his accounts of pestilence with different shades than his epic counterparts—as noted, he is generally not interested in symptomatology or the drama of individual suffering. Nor does the historian elaborate on the traditional forms of lawlessness and criminal neglect as observed by Thucydides. By painting his canvas with broader strokes, he offers a cumulative impression not only of how plague gradually enacts the collapse of the social order, but of how its various challenges to the fledgling *res publica* strengthened the city's development. He does so by relying on a discourse of health and infirmity in the civic body that his epic contemporaries exploit to full advantage. The historian's use of pestilence as an agent of political and cultural transformation is consistent with his dynamic understanding of the past in relation to the present: rather than constructing Rome as a static entity best preserved through an idealized view of the past, Livy gives his reader, "variety, complexity, and change in Roman history and leaves a wide range for political innovations" (Miles 1995, 119).

Epidemic disease in Livy culls the ranks of humans to isolate those whose function is pertinent to the state (as with Camillus and the unnamed officials). At the same time, Livy's *pestilentia* develops for all Romans a new understanding of national identity, in so far as it rehearses the ideologies that have alternatingly sharpened divisions and forced novel coalescence among citizens bound by an awareness of what it means to be Roman and the stumbling innovations that have shaped the *res publica*. The new arts, customs, and offices introduced as a response to plague are made meaningful in the larger scope of Livy's history, as institutions that would collectively transform the character of the Roman people—often for the better, occasionally for worse. If indeed, as Feldherr suggests (1997, 142), Livy's history played a key role in shaping citizen identity, at a time when that ontology was especially unstable, the historian's plague narratives function to define Rome as a community and orient the individual's sense of responsibility to that community. As we have seen, plagues repeatedly devastate the body politic, but also force it to acknowledge a kind of elasticity that will admit *novae res*.

Part II

Experiments in Apocalyptic Thinking

3

Human and Civic *Corpora* in Lucretius' Athenian Plague

Lucretius' *De Rerum Natura* concludes with the discomfiting image of citizens brawling over the burial of kin who have died in the Athenian plague of 430 BCE, risking death rather than abandoning their *corpora* (6.1280–6). Critics have responded antithetically to this passage, as a conclusion to both Book 6 and the poem *in toto*. Some have found the lines, admittedly abrupt and absent any gnomic reflections on the travesties described, to be an indication of the poem's incomplete or unrevised condition.[1] Others have defended the ending of Book 6—the brawling as well as the account of plague that precedes it—as a test for the enlightened Epicurean, a challenge to the reader's *requies* and validation of the poet's method: has Lucretius' *callida musa* enabled the reader, "to contemplate with a mind that has found its peace the scene of the dissolution of the highest form of human society" (Clay 1983, 256)?[2] If we view the plague as a final challenge, the poet's interest in material disintegration

[1] Esp. Bignone (1945, 318–22), who argues that a segment on theology would have followed the plague; cf. Kenney (1977, 22–33) and Sedley (1998, esp. 157–65). Clay (1983, 257 and 341 n. 199) considers other scholarly attempts to propose a more appropriate conclusion to the poem.

[2] Similar views are endorsed by Segal (1990, 169 n. 17), P. Fowler (1997, 138), and Morrison (2013, 223). Cf. Nichols (1976, 178) on plague as a "test for the piety of the reader." Müller (2007, 252–4) also offers a defense of the poem's conclusion based largely on the way that the ending of Book 6, like the endings of the other five, contrasts the delusions of unenlightened humans with the truths of *natura* illuminated through Epicurean doctrine. Stoddard (1996, 107) allows that the plague constitutes a test for the reader, but does not agree that Lucretius made final intended revisions to the poem.

throughout *DRN* prepares his reader for the social, cultural, and indeed narrative disintegration that defines the end of the poem.

Another approach to explaining the undeniably dismal tone with which the poem concludes is to understand the plague and its impact on Athens as representative of the human condition, whether as an "emblem of mental or psychological states" (Commager 1957, 109) or as a commentary on "la vie des non-épicuriens" (Schrijvers 1970, 315).[3] Commager in particular stops short of calling the plague a deliberate or systematic metaphor (1957, 114 and esp. 117 n. 23), but his interpretation recognizes that Lucretius' account of disease among the Athenians conveys an idea different from, or in addition to, the lesson it purports to convey—that is, it does more than simply illustrate how hostile atmospheres spread the seeds (*semina*) of disease (6.1090–7).[4] Agreement that the ending is designed to elicit interpretation requires tacit recognition of the Athenian plague's representational capacities, and, given the determinative relationship between a narrative's closure and what that narrative means, the stakes for understanding the plague's function at the end of the poem are reasonably high.[5]

Peta Fowler's (1997) defense of the ending's propriety aligns scholarly interest in content (why the plague?) with concerns over structure (why the plague here, at the end of Book 6?): *De Rerum Natura*'s closure in veritable decomposition invokes and subverts comparable

[3] Schrijvers in fact begins with and furthers the arguments of Commager for the plague's function as a symbol of psychological and spiritual malady (1970, 314). He is much more explicit, however, concerning the plague's applicability to moral and social dysfunction within Rome of the late Republic (esp. 319–21). Interpreting the ending of the poem as a test and arguing for the symbolic value of the plague are, of course, by no means exclusive. Cf. also Gale (1994, 209), who stresses the polyvalency of both Venus at the poem's opening and the plague at its conclusion.

[4] Cf. S.T. Kelly (1980, 96), another advocate for the propriety of the final lines of Book 6, on the poet's tendency to "see sermons in stones."

[5] See especially Ricoeur (1984), who observes that conclusions furnish "the point of view from which the story can be perceived as forming a whole" (67). Lucretius' poetry is, of course, not unproblematically narrative, though his plague episode is developed with some linearity and includes temporal markers that suggest its kinship with more traditional methods of emplotment. Cf. Hutchinson (2001, 160): "The poem, though decidedly refusing to be a narrative poem, gestures in various ways toward elements of narrative." Volk (2010), drawing partly from D. Fowler (2000), also observes the narrative features characteristic of Lucretius' poem, and of the proem in particular. As D. Fowler (1997, 3–4) has demonstrated, the very term "closure" is equally problematic. Here I rely primarily on a rather limited sense of the word: "the concluding section of a literary work," Fowler's first sense of the term.

closural devices in ancient literature, especially those of Homer's *Iliad*.[6] In manipulating such devices and literary conventions, Lucretius enhances the meaning of plague for his newly converted Epicurean audience. The plague's use in *DRN* as a metaphor for moral or psychological failings (variously defined), however, also imbues the transmission of the plague (*contagia*, 1236)—its rapid spread through social proximity—with a gradual, but totalizing power that would prove adaptable for writers who wished to address the ideological corruption of the late Republic. Commenting on the closural affinities between the poem's ending and Sallust's concluding images of corpse-strewn battlefields in *Bellum Catilinae*, Fowler observes early evidence for the impact of Lucretius' metaphoric swerve: "It is not insignificant that Sallust takes up in the *Catiline* the metaphor of plague for moral corruption. It does not figure in literature before Lucretius as prominently as the simple disease metaphor, and it carries connotations not available to the commoner image, of a collective crisis and of contagion" (1997, 135).

Fowler has made explicit the metaphoric innovation implicitly credited to Lucretius by Commager, Schrijvers, and others.[7] This metaphor, with its particular ability to articulate a collectively experienced crisis in Roman *mores*, in addition to conveying ideas of spiritual malaise or life without Epicurean philosophy, offers the poet a means of indicting civic strife and the competitive strivings that fueled it. By drawing from Thucydides' Peloponnesian War, cast as a war fought by Greeks against one another and serving as a model

[6] Although Fowler's argument for the *Iliad*'s resonance here depends partly on the transposition of lines 1247–51 to the very end of the poem (first suggested by Bockemueller 1873), after the struggle over the corpses described at 1282–6. While her arguments, based on literary convention and Lucretius' own language of closure throughout the poem, are largely convincing, she does not review scribal errors that would account for the repositioning of the lines. Bright also defends Bockemueller's transposition, arguing that the move would better reflect the sequence of events presented in Thucydides. See also Müller (2007, 251) whose argument in defense of the ending was one of the earliest to note the antithesis it creates with the opening book (cf. Schrijvers 1970, 323–4).

[7] Lucretius' role in such development is perhaps somewhat inconsistent with his espoused aversion to poeticizing treatments of health and well being, 3.124–35, cited by Sontag as an early indictment of metaphorical thinking about disease (1988, 95–6); see above, Introduction, p. 8 n. 9. For the history of scholarship on Lucretius' inconsistencies and the attempts to emend or resolve them, see O'Hara (2007, 55–76).

for Roman depictions of their own civil wars (Pelling 2010, 107–9),[8] Lucretius prompts his reader to listen for hints of internecine strife murmured beneath the more clamorous disaster of disease.[9] The poet of *DRN*, however, conveys these hints in an idiom all his own and one that engages directly with a Roman language of bodily and societal collapse.[10] Where Thucydides glances toward the status-leveling effect of a disease that "no particular constitution . . . proved sufficient in itself to resist, but carried off all indiscriminately" (51.3), Lucretius transfers that effect from a democratic context to one more reflective of the pathologies afflicting a fiercely competitive aristocracy. In the first section of this chapter, I demonstrate that Lucretius stages the transformation of the collective citizenry under the impact of plague as a two part process: initially, boundary disintegration erodes distinctions within the body and between citizens, resulting in relatively homogeneous *corpora*; bodies are then amassed in chaotic heaps, unstructured elevations littered throughout the city and described in repetitive language that strengthens the poem's resistance to narrative closure.

Lucretius' interest in bodily dissolution and repetition anticipates the constant stripping away of identity in death that will characterize numerous subsequent plague narratives. And yet it is not just the ubiquity of death that the poet lends to his successors—ubiquity also observed, if to a lesser degree, in Thucydides. The *DRN* poet also injects accounts of pestilence with an Epicurean, materialist agenda that confronts readers with their own corporeal selves:

> Death by pestilence, thus, is particularly efficacious—or brutal—in confronting the individual with the irreducible fact of corporeality.

[8] See above, Introduction, p. 9. Stoddard (1996, 127) addresses the matter of Lucretius' choice of Thucydides more specifically, arguing that the contrast between the idealized Athens of the funeral oration and the polis in the grip of plague in the *History* bolsters the connection in *DRN* 6 between Athens depicted as the height of civilization at the book's beginning and its utter devastation at the book's conclusion.

[9] As studies of the plague metaphor in recent history have revealed, associative links between disease and war are just as important for exposing where similarities fail as for demonstrating where they prevail (cf. Cooke 2009, 41–3): for Lucretius in particular, disease is an altogether natural, inevitable process; war, and civil war in particular, is not.

[10] See McConnell (2012) on the poet's adaptation of the Greek concept of *stasis* to language reflective of Roman politics, though he denies that Lucretius' comments on civil strife (necessarily) address specific contemporary events (e.g., 116), an argument I address further below, p. 98.

> But pestilence shatters the symbolic defenses of the individual self and dissolves the boundaries of the individual body. Contagion, moving from one person to another, often crossing boundaries of species, creates an impersonal intimacy in which the ecological community is felt as an irrecusable fact: not, however, the fact of living together, as in ecofantasies, but the fact of dying together. (Gomel 2000, 416)

As we shall observe, boundary dissolution during the plague is an extension and recapitulation of concerns about our material and perishable selves addressed throughout the poem, but such dissolution during the plague narrative bears important implications for the Roman body politic as well as the human corpus.

In section two of this chapter, I observe how the poet balances the failed "symbolic defenses of the individual self" and graphic accumulation of anonymous citizen *corpora* against the familial relationships that are confirmed under the pressures of contagious disease, a counter to the plague's totalizing force that will emerge often poignantly in later Latin poets. In a clear and somewhat inconsistent departure from Thucydides, Lucretius depicts kin struggling to bury each other (Stoddard 1996, 125); and selfish avoidance of "one's own" is matched by an intimate portrait of families succumbing together to illness and death. The impetus that propels this tradition of narrating plague as a family tragedy is generated largely from Lucretius' interest in foregrounding the conflict between individual sovereignty and communal safety. As disease spreads, citizens struggle to define themselves and make claims for autonomy, but do so according to a familial identity whose interests are not always consonant with the well being, the *communis salus* (2.43), of the body politic.

As noted in Chapter 1,[11] while both Romans and Greeks indicated awareness of the role played by physical interactions in spreading disease, Lucretius' use of *contagium* signals the peculiarly Latin nuances of "touch" and physical proximity in spreading the *pestilitas*: his rendering of plague in Athens shines new light on how plague works in contradictory ways to disrupt kinship networks (through fear of contagion and death) while also affirming the strength of those relationships in the face of contagion and trauma. I suggest that Lucretius' evocative treatment of the family in the plague, delicately recalling the specificities and identities lost in the face of an epidemic,

[11] See Chapter 1, pp. 25–7.

is born from a peculiarly Roman sense of familial devotion (or *pietas*) and intensifies the metaphoric bond between the plague and Roman civic strife of the late Republic. Such strife conceptually originates within Rome's legendary first family, Romulus and Remus, and is revisited throughout Latin literature in accounts of rivalry between brothers, family members considered to be a kind of second self (*frater inquit est dictus quasi fere alter*, Aulus Gellius, *NA* 13.1046).[12] The shoring up of "one's own" that attends efforts to preserve the family lineage betrays in Lucretius more aggressive bids for autonomy, often at the expense of *both* family and community.

In charting a process by which competitive claims for autonomy gradually yield to unstructured and indistinguishable masses of human remains, Lucretius' plague narrative draws from the same thematic cluster that Girard identifies in other examples of the Western plague topos, a "process of undifferentiation, a destruction of specificities" (1974, 833), which transforms the hierarchically structured society into an aggregate, lacking the differences of degree that ensure the social order's proper functioning. Raskolnikov's dream in *Crime and Punishment*, in which a mysterious disease inspires individuals to believe that they are possessed of an infallible and unique truth, worth defending to the point of death, serves as his premier example.[13] The plague narrative symbolizes social pathologies emerging from the rapid transmission of imitative violence—violence, as a kind of contagion, almost always begets further violence—born from conditions that encourage individuals to desire the highest honors and privileges for themselves: "this desire implies a contradiction; it aims at complete autonomy, at a near divine self-sufficiency, and yet it is imitative" (1974, 836). Such conditions aptly describe the competitive ambitions of Rome's leading aristocrats in the late Republic:[14]

> To imitate the desires of someone else is to turn this someone else into a rival as well as a model. From the convergence of two or more desires

[12] For discussion of the quote and its implications for fraternal *pietas*, see Bannon (1997, 64). Bannon also stresses the brothers' status as twins, suggesting an identification between them that further supports Girard's fusion of the rival with the mimetic double in his analysis of plague narratives (172 n. 109).

[13] See Chapter 1, p. 39, for further discussion of Raskolnikov's dream.

[14] Cf. McConnell on *invidia* within the Roman aristocracy (2012, 111–12), where the author also notes major scholarly assessments of competitive (and destructive) politics of the elite during the period.

> on the same object, conflict must necessarily arise ... Mimetic desire cannot keep its illusions alive without falling in love with its own disastrous consequences and focusing more and more on the violence of its rivals. The mimetic attraction of violence is a major topic of Dostoevskian art. Thus, violence becomes reciprocal. In the dream of the plague, the expressions "each other, one another" recur constantly. (1974, 836–7)

From a Girardian perspective, unchecked *ambitio* gradually corrodes the different functions assigned to individuals within a community, as each individual seeks the same limited honors for himself: "as these ambitions are mimetically multiplied, reciprocal violence grows and the differences dissolve" (1974, 839). The proliferation of sameness, of doubling through *mimesis*, is quashed only through sacrifice, the elimination of one party to mimetic violence that will allow the double to emerge as a singularity and restore the degrees of difference integral to the social order. Lucretius leaves us with no such resolution in his narrative, which instead closes by intensifying its focus on Athenians, each attempting to bury his own (*quisque suum ... humabat*, 6.1281) and brawling with fellow citizens in the process. In this way, the poet's adamant interest in the dissolution, rather than restoration, of the civic body in the final lines of Book 6 replays the dissolution of individual bodies dramatized earlier in the narrative. This internal physical process will be conjured 2000 years later by Artaud and described by Girard as an esthetically powerful means of dramatizing cultural entropy (1974, 846). Lucretius' resistance to closure and lingering vision of a deteriorating civic body suggest that the social order itself, rather than needing restoration through sacrifice, is somehow beyond recovery.

3.1. TRANSGRESSING THE THRESHOLD OF DEATH

Lucretius' account of the Athenian plague relies heavily on the language of dissolution, decay, and liquefaction, particularly in passages where he diverges from his source material in Thucydides. As noted, for the Greek historian, the plague's homogenizing effect is restricted largely to its indiscriminate nature: it levels status distinctions within the body politic, in so far as it affects all citizens equally (51.3); it also results in drastic, if temporary, changes of status and behaviors, as citizens observed "all dying without distinction" (53). The disease's corrosive operations within the human form, however, remain largely unobserved, despite the historian's careful attention to symptomatology. Thucydides avoids the kind of affective language—verbs of rotting and putrescence[15]—that signals the body's decomposition. As Bright notes (1971, 609), in contrast to Lucretius' account of steady deterioration, Thucydides confirms that the victims' bodies tended to resist the process of wasting away (49.6). Bodily decomposition in the Lucretian account is consistent with a larger goal in the poem: as Charles Segal (1990) has shown, the philosopher-poet's descriptions of decay serve as armament in his desire to tackle basic human fears concerning the dissolution of identity—threats to "the integrity of the self" (144)—fears that ultimately spring from a fear of death. Anxieties surrounding the dissolution of the physical form are directly addressed in Book 3's arguments on the mortality of body and soul, but the language of bodily transformations reemerges in the plague episode to indicate that the poet is addressing and allaying similar fears there. The plague's assault on the individual bodies of Athenians as well as on the Athenian polis constitute parallel processes illustrating the kinds of decay and deterioration that fuel our fear of "primary boundary violation" (148).

Lucretius' persistent concern with the topic reflects Epicurean tenets on the permeability of the human body, and its susceptibility to external forces: "Against other threats it is possible to provide security, but on account of death all of us humans inhabit a city without walls."[16] Epicurus' statement ingeniously reverses the usual terms of the body politic metaphor, so that the city functions as a vehicle to express the material conditions of the human body, the tenor. For Lucretius' plague victims the body as wall is experienced as an increasingly tenuous "threshold of death" (*limen leti*). The vulnerability of the body is not only demonstrated through rot and decay, but also through the increasing confusion between life and death. The poet puts a border (*limen*) between them only to show repeatedly how it is crossed.

[15] For the language of rot in both Greek and Latin discussions of disease, see Chapter 1, pp. 26–7.

[16] From the sayings of Epicurus recorded in the *Sententiae Vaticanae*, cited in Clay (1983, 186 and 265).

DRN's account (*ratio*) of disease initially draws on the familiar language of seeds (*semina*), both noxious and nourishing, air- and earth-borne. Echoing the Hippocratic idea of diseased atmospheres, the poet locates the origins of plague in an alien sky (*caelum*), which is stirred up to become hostile (*inimicus aer*, 1120)[17] and eventually falls upon the food and water supply, or lingers in the air to be inhaled by humans. Readers confront as an example of the process, "a death-bearing current within the borders of Athens" (*mortifer aestus/finibus in Cecropis*, 1138–9). In narrating the plague, Lucretius follows a tripartite structure used by Thucydides and observed with some variation by subsequent Latin poets: origins (aetiology), symptomatology, and epidemiology, though the latter two parts, effects on the body and effects on the populace, are occasionally intertwined. He introduces both the disease and its victims as dwelling in defined territories (*finibus* 1139; cf. *finibus* 1141), only to demonstrate how vulnerable borders are in the context of the plague. More importantly for our purposes is language in the aetiological passage that urgently anticipates the epidemiological outcome of virtually dissolved bodies amassed in confused piles:

> haec ratio quondam morborum et mortifer aestus
> finibus in Cecropis funestos reddidit agros
> vastavitque vias, exhausit civibus urbem
> nam penitus veniens Aegypti finibus ortus,
> aëra permensus multum camposque natantis,
> incubuit tandem populo Pandionis omni.
> inde catervatim morbo mortique dabantur.
> (6.1138–44)

Once within the lands of Cecrops this cause of disease and death-bearing current rendered fields deadly, devastated the roads, and drained the city of its citizens. For after arising deeply within the borders of Egypt and coming forth, it travelled through much of the upper air and the swimming plains, (and) it lay down at last upon the entire people of Pandion. Then they were given over in heaps to death and disease.

[17] For diseased atmospheres as a cause of plague, see above, Chapter 1, pp. 23–4. See Bailey (1947, 1138) on other sources, especially Hippocratean, that may have informed Lucretius' account. Vallillee (1960, 177) notes that Lucretius is responsible for importing the language of "hostile" (*inimicus*) *aer* (6.1120) into the lexicon of Latin plague narratives. Certainly the language of personal enmity is absent from Thucydides' account of the pestilent atmosphere.

This noxious current enacts a figurative liquidation of the city. While *exhaurio* is by no means limited to connotations of draining fluids, its primary definitions describe processes of drawing off and draining liquid substances (*OLD* 1–1b).[18] *Catervatim*, moreover, not only signals a confused process of piling up bodies, it does this frequently in military contexts (cf. Sal. *Jug*. 97.4, Liv. 23.27.5), importing a martial resonance to use of the word here, and later when Vergil will use it in his own account of plague in Noricum.[19] *Vasto* further personifies the disease as a military force (Godwin 1991, 173), and, as Schrijvers observes, may summon civic strife of the late Republic by evoking Cicero's familiar collocation of *pestis/pestilitas* with forms of *vastare/vastitas* (1970, 320–1). Lucretius' introduction to the Athenian plague thus fuses aetiology with teleology, signaling that dissolution, accumulation, and military resonance will shape his subsequent treatment of the disease.

In turning to symptomatology, Lucretius elaborates *signa* of the disease in excruciating detail, signs that cumulatively point to an inevitable *telos* in death. Breath is proleptically described as corpse-like: *rancida quo perolent proiecta cadavera ritu*, 1155. Here the poet inflects his predecessor's "foul-smelling" (δυσώδες, 49.2) breath with the macabre rot associated with decaying bodies. Again we are reminded of the perpetually liminal state in which victims exist, *corpus leti iam limine in ipso*, 1157. Thucydides had succinctly demonstrated the Athenian plague's power to intermingle living and dead bodies, a process dramatized in the crowded enclaves and huts of the city where, "dead and dying were piled on top of each other, and half-dead creatures staggered around every fountain" (52.2). Lucretius expands and innovates by staging (and initially confining) the transgressive confusion of life and death within the body of the individual plague victim. He will return insistently to this confusion after moving on to epidemiology, where victims scattered throughout the streets roll about with bodies "half-dead" (*semanimo*, 1268) while "buried" (*sepulta*) in "foul ulcers and dirt" (*ulceribus taetris . . . sorde*, 1271).

[18] Bailey (1947, 1726) observes the striking quality of the verb, noting a parallel in Livy's *exhausta funeribus* of the plague in *AUC* 3.6.

[19] Cf. *iamque catervatim dat stragem atque aggerat ipsis/in stabulis* (V.*G*. 3.556), and Rouse/Smith's translation of *DRN*, "in troops" (1992, 578).

Within the realm of symptomatology, however, Lucretius further modifies his source to stress the tendency of Athenian *corpora* to waste away in a process of uninterrupted decline. As noted (cf. Bright 1971, 609), Thucydides observes how the bodies of plague victims remained surprisingly resilient throughout the course of the disease and were not "extinguished" or "weakened" (*οὐκ ἐμαραίνετο*, 49.6) when death came, usually after six to eight days; weakness only attended those who survived beyond this point to experience severe diarrhea and subsequent death. Lucretius, by contrast, omits reference to the body's persistent strength and expands on the effluences experienced by the victim, followed by the disease's migration into the limbs and genitalia:

> quorum siquis, ut est, vitarat funera leti,
> ulceribus taetris et nigra proluvie alvi
> posterius tamen hunc tabes letumque manebat,
> aut etiam multus capitis cum saepe dolore
> corruptus sanguis expletis naribus ibat:
> huc hominis totae vires corpusque fluebat.
> profluvium porro qui taetri sanguinis acre
> exierat, tamen in nervos huic morbus et artus
> ibat et in partis genitalis corporis ipsas.
> (6.1199–1207)

And if any one of them had avoided an end in death, as happens, still later on rot and death, with foul ulcers and a black discharge from the bowels, awaited him, or else a good deal of corrupted blood went forth from his stuffed nostrils, often along with a headache. In this, the whole strength and person/substance went forth. Moreover, for anyone who had survived the severe outpouring of foul blood, the disease still went forth into his limbs and sinews and the very genitals of his body.

While Bright explains the revised trajectory of the disease as a way to "shut out any hope of survival and intensify the horror of the disease's advance" (1971, 612), it is important to note that the poet not only alters the course of the disease, but the symptoms as well. In the passage just preceding, Lucretius recounts the frigid hardness of the skin and taut forehead that defined bodies of victims, *frigida pellis/ duraque* (6.1194–5), language of rigidity not found in Thucydides:[20]

[20] Though, as Bailey notes, comparable, if not identical symptoms are found in Hippocr. *Progn.* 2.114, where the skin is described as rough/tight (*σκληρόν*) and dry (1947, 1732).

this sets up a stark contrast with the softening, erosion, and decay that the victims experience here, on the verge of death, a juxtaposition of opposites that indicates a body at war with itself and, as we shall observe, an influence on Vergil's account of Noric plague. There is, moreover, no equivalent of *tabes* in Thucydides' account,[21] though it is an important indicator of bodily decay throughout *De Rerum Natura*, and its implications of putrifying and dissolving human flesh are amplified through the language of liquefaction (*fluebat*) and bodily fluids (*proluvie, profluvium*) that conclude the lines.[22] The poet's reference to decay prior to death (*tabes letumque*) may be a hysteron-proteron, since decay usually follows death (Godwin 1991, 178), but in this case the reversal also redoubles the forces of deterioration already at work in the body, an aggressive intrusion of death into the realm of life.

The final flux of death here is the culmination of a language of dissolution and flow experienced internally during earlier phases of the disease, as its force "had flooded" (*confluxerat*, 1152) a mournful "mind" (*cor*), and its constant retching had wearied sufferers to the point of "breaking them down" (*dissoluebat*, 1162).[23] There is no analogous comment in Thucydides that compounds the language of flux and dissolution with an explicit observation of how the boundaries that structure the internal operations of the corpus (the "bolts of life") were collapsing: *omnia tum vero vitae claustra lababant* (6.1153).[24] This may be in part an effect of transferring the episode

[21] For Bailey (1947, 1734), these lines (1202–4) constitute the "chief part of Lucretius' misrepresentation of the original." While I would stop short of referring to the passage as a misrepresentation, his comment underscores the fact that it is in the language of fluidity and decay that Lucretius makes his clearest departures from his source. Godwin (1991, 178) also cautions that Lucretius may be working from other sources in addition to Thucydides.

[22] Thucydides offers a source for the poet's liquefaction in his stress on the diarrhea suffered by victims, though Lucretius' location of "all the strength and the body of the man" suggests a total evacuation of the self, not paralleled in the historian's account.

[23] The verb is used elsewhere to describe "dissolution of a compound," and that is what Lucretius has in mind here (Bailey 1947, 1729).

[24] As Craik has argued (2001), Thucydides indicates his awareness of "flux" as it refers to the balance and imbalance of bodily humors, as well as the movement of the disease through bodily channels. I use the term, in accord with Clay (see below), primarily in reference to the processes of rot and liquefaction experienced by the diseased body, but also in accord with the flow of atoms observed throughout the poem.

from a Greek discursive context to a Latin one (Bailey 1947, 1723). For Clay, the innovative flux of matter that determines the symptoms of Lucretius' plague allows the poet to defend his larger philosophical claims of a world whose atoms are in constant flux (1983, 265; *iure igitur pereunt, cum rarefacta fluendo/sunt*, 2.1139–40). At the same time, when such fluidity of matter is articulated within the immediate context of contagious disease, it does more than simply add to the armament of a staunch materialist: it observes the collapse of boundaries (both bodily and social) and diagnoses collective, contagious behaviors as the origins of such collapse. The plague's corrosive power is initially enacted in Lucretius at the level of the human body, but the Epicurean premise that all humans "inhabit a city without walls" looks forward to the transference of those operations from the body to the body politic.

As noted, dissolution and liquefaction in the plague are qualities that import an earlier poetic context. In Book 3, *tabes*, its compounds, and the relationship of "rot" to liquefaction emerge as salient features of decomposition (cf. Segal, 1990, 148):

> et veluti manus atque oculus naresve seorsum
> secreta ab nobis nequeunt sentire neque esse,
> sed tamen in parvo liquuntur tempore tabe,
> sic animus per se non quit sine corpore et ipso
> esse homine, illius quasi quod vas esse videtur,
> sive aliud quid vis potius coniunctius ei
> fingere, quandoquidem conexu corpus adhaeret.
> (3.551–5)

And just as hands or eyes or nose, when separated apart from us, are not able to feel or exist, but instead are dissolved into putrefaction in a short time, thus the spirit in and of itself is not able to exist without a body or the person him/herself, which seems to be a container for it, or if you wish to imagine instead something more closely joined, since the body clings to it in close connection.

While this passage deals specifically with the rot associated with severed limbs, rather than the corpse *in toto*, the analogy posited (*sic*) suggests a similar liquefaction experienced by the body without the *animus*. In fact, lines following shortly thereafter address the condition of the body upon the soul's departure: *denique cum corpus nequeat perferre animai/discidium quin in taetro tabescat odore* (3.580–1). *Tabescat* illustrates the processes that lead to a substance inevitably (*quin*) overtaken by *tabes*, and accompanied by the same foul odor (*taetrum odorem*) that emanates from the still living plague victims in Book 6 (6.1154). As we shall see, the epics of Vergil and Ovid also invoke bodily decay (e.g., V. *G*.3.481, 556–8, Ov. *Met.* 541), frequently referred to by *tabes* or its cognates, as a way of anticipating the liquefaction that will soon characterize the bodies of the deceased.[25]

The intertexuality that binds plague symptoms in Book 6 to the body's post-mortem condition in Book 3 should confirm the equanimity with which we encounter the sufferings of the Athenians: the dissolution of bodily integrity, the decay of the self, and gradual incorporation of the individual among heaps of other *corpora* will supply a new cycle of atoms bound for regeneration. We should, moreover, accept this loss of identity (that of the Athenians and ourselves) with relative aplomb since, as Book 3 has also demonstrated, death is nothing to us (*nil igitur mors est ad nos*, 3.830). Indeed, the poet's insistence on severing our attachment to personal identity clamors for attention with or without a *telos* in death and decay. Drawing from Thucydides (49.8), he stresses how plague survivors forgot themselves or experienced permanent disfigurement through bodily mutilation (6.1208–14). On this point he has transformed the Greek's observation that,"many lived on, having lost genitals, fingers, and toes," into a more explicit reference to castration, one that foreshadows the self-mutilation of Vergil's plague-stricken horses in *Georgics* 3. Rather than leaving unstated (as in Thucydides) whether the disease itself or human intervention resulted in loss of genitals, castration here appears a willful act motivated by fear of death (Bright 1971, 612; Stoddard 1996, 119). Again, death is figured as the other side of a boundary that plague victims, unaware of the processes of dissolution already vigorously at work within their bodies, are afraid to cross (*metuentes limina leti*, 1208). Desperate acts, and their collocation in the text with comments on survivors who suffered amnesia, imply a fundamental instability at the core of human identity: what secures "the self" under assault from a disease that interrupts memory and psychological continuity, while also visibly corroding bodily integrity?

[25] So too does Livy use "rot" (*tabes*) to indicate deterioration in plague-stricken bodies and in the body politic of Menenius' parable; see Chapter 2, pp. 50–1.

3.2. REPETITION, ACCUMULATION, AND ITERATIVE MORTALITY

As a complement to his sustained depiction of bodily decomposition at the level of the individual, the poet directs his readers to observe the constant and repetitive accumulation of citizen bodies. This process is met with occasional resistance, as individuals reassert themselves or the poet recalls relics of former identities, a challenge I discuss further in section 3.3 of this chapter. The overall process, however, is one that gradually dehumanizes the Athenian population, leaving behind masses of virtually indistinguishable *corpora*. From his comments on those plague victims who survived without their bodies or their memories intact, Lucretius broadens his poetic scope to the realm of epidemiology, and describes the spread of disease among the population as well as the social pathologies that accompany it. The poet's intense preoccupation with the presence of the dead, the transformation of funeral rites, and the impact of both on the psychology of the afflicted contributes to the poem's overall interest in confronting the fear of death, as observed earlier with reference to bodily decay (Commager 1957, 112; Segal 1990; Morrison 2013, 224–32). Lucretius' fixation on the body count, however, also drives the plague's dramaturgy toward homogenization and accomplishes a macabre coalescence of the body politic.

The response of beasts and birds of prey to the epidemic allows the poet to introduce the image of the unburied dead, an image to which he will insistently return:

> multaque humi cum inhumata iacerent corpora supra
> corporibus, tamen alituum genus atque ferarum
> aut procul absiliebat, ut acrem exiret odorem,
> aut, ubi gustarat, languebat morte propinqua.
> (6.1215–18)

And although upon the earth a great number of bodies lay upon bodies unburied, nevertheless the races of birds and wild beasts either leapt far away, to keep at a distance from the foul odor, or after they had tasted of it, soon languished in death.

Here, Lucretius draws from Thucydides' comment that animals avoided human flesh "although many bodies lay unburied," issued as a succinct genitive absolute (πολλῶν ἀτάφων γιγνομένων, 50.1) leaving readers to fill in "bodies" from the substantive πολλῶν. Lucretius explicitly articulates his many *corpora*: the elision in the first foot of line 1215, in conjunction with the repetition of *hum-* from *humi* within *inhumata* and the enjambment of *corporibus* in 1216, works to concretize in hexameters the proliferation, confusion, and entanglement of human forms.[26]

The body count increases as the process of *contagium* relentlessly does its work:

> quippe etenim nullo cessabant tempore apisci
> ex aliis alios avidi contagia morbi,
> lanigeras tamquam pecudes et bucera saecla; 1245[27]
> idque vel in primis cumulabat funere funus.
> (6.1235–7)

For at no time did the contagion(s)[28] of the greedy disease cease from spreading (lit. cease from "attaching itself to," or "reaching out after"), from one person to another, just as woolly sheep and the horned herds; and that especially piled funeral upon funeral.

The poet transforms the historian's reference to citizens who attended the sick and spread the disease in the process (Th. 51.5–6) into a personified menace, "the contagion of the greedy disease" (*avidi contagia morbi*, 1236). The end result of rapid transmission is the dehumanization of the plague's victims, who are likened to sheep in both Thucydides (τά πρόβατα, 51.4) and Lucretius. In *DRN*, however, the sheep are modified by epic epithets whose elevated style creates a striking contrast with the degradation experienced by plague victims (Godwin 1991, 182). Such dehumanization is underscored by a verb of accumulation (*cumulabat*), of piling in a heap one funeral virtually indistinguishable from another; we might detect a hint of irony as well, since the funeral constitutes the ultimate ceremonial expression of an individual's life. Repetitive language mirrors the process of contagion, as the disease is spread from "some to others" (1236, *aliis alios*; cf. *inque aliis alium*, 1247), replicating itself while

[26] Cf. Godwin (1991, 180), who suggests that verbal repetition in the passage, "suggests the physical accumulation of the corpses."

[27] Following Bentley, Rouse/Smith transpose 1245 to follow directly after 1236 (1992, 586).

[28] Consistent with the majority of translators, I'm inclined to treat *contagia* as a poetic plural, though it is worth noting that the plural form conveys the very notion of replication and multiplicity that the process of contagion enacts.

emerging from within the household into the wider civic arena (*funere funus*).[29]

As Gomel argues in defining the relationship between plague, apocalypse, and post-apocalyptic scenarios, the contagious and thus repetitive nature of pestilence forges cohesion within the body politic ("tenuous and moribund" as that body may be; 2000, 406). In such a way, it offers a solution to division in the social order. At the same time, at least in the post-apocalyptic version of the plague narrative, that solution is never final, but threatens to repeat itself without end:

> Pandemic, in its interminable duration, generates the text of fragments rather than sequels: an accumulation of repetitive episodes, deferring any kind of meaningful closure . . . And indeed many—though not all—plague narratives are structured by the logic of iterative mortality that undermines the teleological progression of the apocalypse. (409–10)

While Lucretius' Epicureanism is not responding to the Judeo-Christian notion of a final unveiling, the poet is perhaps the first in the tradition of plague writing to use contagious disease to address eschatological concerns, that is, to direct readers to contemplate the endings of things. Somewhat paradoxically, however, Lucretian eschatology plays itself out with endless repetition and accumulation.[30]

Indeed, an imagery of accumulation, mimicked by the verbal repetition of *corpora* in the text, directs the poet's (and reader's, *videres*, 1268) vision as the plague moves beyond the household and into the streets of Athens. The rustic population flows from the countryside into the city (*confluxit*, 1260), and because of this seething influx (*quo . . . aestu*, 1262), "death was piling them up all the more in such a way packed together in heaps" (*confertos ita acervatim mors accumulabat*, 1263). Language used earlier to describe the liquefying operations of disease within the individual body (*fluebat*, 1204, *profluvium*, 1205) is here echoed in the compound *confluo*, used to describe movements within the polis and marking the poet's

[29] Wills (1996) cites the line, along with 3.71 (*caedem caede accumulantes*) as examples of Lucretius' use of "accumulation," a figure of repetition that employs polyptoton. He observes how the figure underpins aspects of the poet's philosophical argument: "Much of Lucretian polyptoton involves continuities and accumulations in nature" (192).

[30] These elements are also consistent with another feature of the post-apocalyptic narrative, the "aftermaths and remainders" identified by Berger (1999, xii) in late twentieth- and early twenty-first-century examples of the genre; see Chapter 1, p. 37.

shift of focus from body to body politic, but also underscoring the metaphorical relationship between them. The poet follows this observation with graphic, repetitive demonstration of *corpora* littered throughout the city:

> multaque siti prostrata viam per proque voluta
> corpora silanos ad aquarum strata iacebant
> interclusa anima nimia ab dulcedine aquarum,
> multaque per populi passim loca prompta viasque
> languida semanimo cum corpore membra videres
> horrida paedore et pannis cooperta perire
> corporis inluvie, pelli super ossibus una,
> ulceribus taetris prope iam sordeque sepulta.
> (6.1264–71)

Many bodies prostrate from thirst lay throughout and over the road, rolling about, strewn before fountains of water, their life's breath cut off from the excessive sweetness of the water. And you would see clearly throughout many public places and roads languishing limbs of a body, half-living, bristling with filth and covered in rags, dying in the impurity of the body, with skin alone covering their bones, nearly buried in foul ulcers and dirt.

Corpora crowd around fountains (1265); limbs of half-dead bodies (*semanimo . . . corpore*, 1268) and unwashed bodies (*corporis inluvie*, 1270) are crowded in streets and public places. The trifold repetition of *corpus* in various forms is matched by other forms of verbal repetition: *viam/vias*; *aquarum/aquarum*; *multaque/multaque*. Collectively such duplicated images underscore a fundamental similarity in death, despite ostensibly disparate conditions.

As the poet builds upon an imagery of corporeal accumulation, we observe temples stuffed full of abandoned bodies (*corporibus . . . exanimis*, 1273) and cadavers (*cadaveribus*, 1274). Shifting the scene within the *templa caelestum*, Lucretius expands on Thucydides' comment that, "the sanctuaries in which they had encamped were full of corpses—people dying there were not moved: all sacred and secular constraints came to be ignored under the overwhelming impact of the disaster, which left men no recourse" (52.3). The poet's rendering affords him a final wry comment on the efficacy of religious devotion:

> omnia denique sancta deum delubra replerat
> corporibus mors exanimis, onerataque passim
> cuncta cadaveribus caelestum templa manebant
> hospitibus loca quae complerant aedituentes.

> nec iam religio divom nec numina magni
> pendebantur enim: praesens dolor exsuperabat.
> nec mos ille sepulturae remanebat in urbe,
> quo prius hic populus semper consuerat humari.
> (6.1272–9)

Finally, death had filled all the sacred shrines with lifeless bodies, and here and there all the temples of the heavenly gods remained burdened with corpses, places which the temple keepers had filled with guests. Neither did worship of the gods nor their divine powers matter greatly. Urgent grief superseded everything. Nor did there remain in the city that custom of interment by which earlier this population was accustomed to be buried.

Beyond illustrating the failings of religion, the final infringement of corpses within the sacred space of the temple enacts the collision of sacred and profane in a way that suggests the utter collapse of the social order. Julia Kristeva has argued in her *Pouvoirs de l'horreur* that the corpse is the ultimate taboo—its abjection (or "casting away") is integral to constituting the self and the community (1982, 109), the very process abhorrently reversed as bodies intrude within sacred precincts. Here we have a topographical demonstration of the final collapse of boundaries (*omnia denique*) that have already occurred within the body of the plague victim (*omnia tum vero vitai claustra lababant,* 6.1153) and an apt prelude to the brawling over funeral pyres (6.1283)—a last ditch effort to reclaim a boundary that distinguishes self from other—that concludes the poem. Such language is a symptom of an adamantly materialistic view of the universe, and the plague a tool to demonstrate how readily *corpora* at both atomic and societal levels can be shuffled around. At the same time, plague as a force of reshuffling is not arbitrary: its workings through *contagia* and ability to show up the tensions inherent in Roman political life—grounded in intense individualism and the rivalry it provokes—prove fundamental to the poet's message.

3.3. CONTENDING FOR "ONE'S OWN": FAMILIAL DEVOTION AND CIVIC DISCORD

As I hope to have shown in the preceding discussion, the *DRN* poet has staged the Athenian plague as a drama of dissolution and chaotic accumulation: the status-leveling and homogenizing effects that are evident in Thucydides' history and that will become critical to the plague topos in the West are articulated in Lucretius through a language of decay, the utter failure of boundaries, and the heaping up of indistinguishable *corpora*. Yet that process is not without interruption. As Cabisius argues in her analysis of the reciprocally metaphoric relationship between social and atomic alliances throughout the poem, human behaviors during the plague are initially marked by intense discord and fragmentation as individuals recognize the solitary condition of their plight (1984, 118; cf. 6.1231–2, *quod ubi se quisque/videbat implicatum morbo*); so too, as individuals fight for rights to bury "their own" (*suum*) a language of individuality and isolation defines their efforts (*unus quisque*, 6.1280–1). The struggle to define one's self and one's kin against the totalizing force of the epidemic is manifested in both intimate and hostile interactions, but it is frequently the contentious efforts to assert identity that concern the poet—efforts that reflect upon and underscore the turbulent and ephemeral nature of alliances at the atomic level (cf. Fowler 1989, 145). Various scholars have aligned the strained political and social structures alluded to in *DRN* with the threat of civil war that cast its shadow over the decade in which it was published: Hutchinson (2001) in fact argues for a relatively late publication date, just after war erupted between Caesar and Pompey (49 BCE), based largely on language of the proem that frames the *fera moenera militiai* ("savage works of war," 1.29) Venus is invoked to quell within specific temporal circumstances (1.41–3).[31] While a number of arguments have pushed back against the notion of the poet's concern with specific individuals and events attending the civil war (Volk 2010; McConnell 2012), there is general agreement that the poet is concerned with internal strife and that such concern is expressed through cultural idioms of the late Roman Republic.[32]

Critics as early as Commager (1957, 112) and as recent as Pope (2016) have, moreover, tied the language of the plague in Book 6 to

[31] These lines address the poet's inability to complete his poem at a "troubling time for the fatherland," *patriai tempore iniquo*; such circumstances (*talibus in rebus*) also keep Memmius' attention directed to the safety of the commonwealth, rather than devoting himself to Epicurean principles. As Volk (2010) observes, however, some of the language of the proem is conventional and may suppose a hypothetical, rather than actual crisis. Lucretius does after all continue with his poem, and does so with Memmius as his addressee.

[32] See esp. Fowler (1989, 134–41 and passim).

the quest for honors and self-aggrandizement associated with civil war elsewhere in the poem. For Pope, Lucretius' reference to *sudare sanguine* as a symptom of the Athenian plague (6.1147–8) echoes the only other use of the phrase in *DRN*, in Book 5's indictment of ambition that drives men to acquire power over others at the expense of the common good:

> nequiquam, quoniam ad summum succedere honorem
> certantes iter infestum fecere viai,
> et tamen e summo, quasi fulmen, deicit ictos
> invidia interdum contemptim in Tartara taetra,
> invidia quoniam, ceu fulmine, summa vaporant (1131)
> plerumque et quae sunt aliis magis edita cumque; (1132)
> ut satius multo iam sit parere quietum (1127)
> quam regere imperio res velle et regna tenere.
> proinde sine incassum defessi ***sanguine sudent***,
> angustum per iter luctantes ambitionis . . .
> (5.1123–30, text Rouse/Smith 1992)

[Men grasp at power] in vain, since, by struggling to attain the highest honor, they made their way of life threatening, and still envy, with contempt, like a thunderbolt, casts them down now and then from the heights into foul Tartarus. Since by envy, just as by a thunderbolt, the highest places are scorched in smoke; so too is often the case with those things that are elevated more than others; so that it is much better to obey in peace than to want to possess kingdoms and govern with *imperium*. So let them sweat with blood, wearied to no purpose and struggling along the narrow path of ambition.

As Gale notes, the language of envy and the struggle to ascend the path of a political career, suggestive of the *cursus honorum*, would have a distinct resonance for Lucretius' audiences of the first century BCE, when rivalry among elites was coming to a head (2009, 193; cf. Fowler 1989, 143–4). In the same context from Book 5 we observe the social order dissolve under pressures aptly accounted for by Girard's notion of mimetic rivalry: *imperium sibi cum ac summatum quisque petebat* (5.1142, "when each one sought for himself power and the highest honor"). The echo of "sweating with blood" (sudabant *etiam fauces intrinsecus atrae*/sanguine) in Book 6 thus imports the phrase's original context of destructive rivalries in Book 5, and strengthens the plague's association with civil strife (6.1147–8). Use of the phrase outside the poem in teratological contexts, in addition, lends both uses of *sanguine sudare* in *DRN* a portentous effect, striking a literally ominous note as *signa* "symptoms" of disease semantically resound with signs (*signa* as omens) of an impending civic crisis (Pope 2016, 50).

Taken collectively, these observations at the least demonstrate the poet's awareness that the Athenian plague as civic crisis *par excellence* would offer some lessons applicable to other polities in crisis, including Rome, whose dysfunction (however vaguely or precisely defined) has by the poet's own confession nearly driven him to distraction. I would go further, however, and argue that it is Lucretius' particular emphasis on families under pressure from the plague that allows him to address the internecine strife of the late Roman Republic:[33] beginning with its assault on the individual, *avidi contagia morbi* works its way through the larger community, relying on networks linking individual and family, as well as those binding the family to the *res publica*, often demonstrating in its progression a discrepancy between the needs of the individual and those of the family, as well as a discrepancy between the interests of the family and those of the state.[34] As plague instigates the dissolution of the family, nucleus of Lucretius' social order described in Book 5 (cf. 5.1011–18), and as the bonds of *amicitia* that tied the family to the larger community are dismantled, readers are left with newfound skepticism of the language of the *res publica*, terms like *gloria*, *honor*, *pietas*, and *nobilitas*, signaling ideals that had formerly secured the stability of the state.[35]

[33] The extent to which *bellum civile* might be construed as a familial affair is reflected in roughly synonymous terms used to describe the phenomenon of internal discord: *bellum intestinum* and *bellum domesticum*. For the interchangeable use of (esp.) *bellum civile* and *bellum intestinum*, see Jal (1963, 33–4), who also cites a number of references to civil strife in the late Republic as *bellum domesticum* (e.g., Cic. *Catil.* 2.1.1; 4.7.15).

[34] This discrepancy in turn disrupts the long-cherished analogy between family and state—one concretized through the Roman *pater*'s easy transference into political patronage (as *patronus*) and governing authority (as among senatorial *patres*); see Minyard (1985, 11).

[35] Minyard has in fact read the entire plague episode as a satire of faith in and adherence to Roman civic institutions (1985, 60–1). While I would argue that the affective dimension of Lucretius' poetry in the episode transfers it outside the traditional parameters of Roman satire, Minyard's general thesis, that the poem is attempting to indict the failures of former categories ("collapse of categories in the polity," 14), those linked to Roman communal identity, is supported by political terminology within the poem as well as the language of political crisis used in contemporary literature. Fowler (1988) rightly observes significant flaws in Minyard's approach, while affirming some of the book's basic ideas concerning Lucretius' critique of contemporary Roman society. Nugent (1994, 188 n. 45) is equally critical: she notes that Minyard's attempt to have Lucretius redefine signifiers critical to Roman ideology

Failures of Roman civic values enabled (or left a vacuum for) new systems available to explain the world and one's position in it, systems such as Lucretius' Epicureanism.[36]

Despite the plague's power to demonstrate the advantages of Epicureanism, Lucretius' evocative and affective imagery of families in crisis also develops an uncomfortable paradox that he will not resolve within the terms of his narrative: the source of transmission of the *pestilitas* afflicting the Athenians is the very attendance to family members that within a healthy community fortifies the social order, as the poet has shown us already in his own excursus on the development of early society (5.1011–18), in which human bodies were gradually softened by protection from the elements just as their minds were softened by the coaxing words of children. Nugent, however, reads the "softening" that attends the genesis of the family as part of a larger system of deteriorative imagery conceptually aligned with the "feminine" in *DRN* (1994, 202–3). Such deterioration reaches its apogee in pestilence emanating from *mater terra* and impressing its corrosive, softening powers upon human bodies. Thus it may be that reliance on the family as the bedrock of the social order is already compromised and fraught with its own vulnerabilities.

At the same time, Lucretius gives readers no viable alternative to the family unit as the genesis of the social contract, and (more importantly for our estimation of kinship behavior in the plague) he paints family behaviors with a distinctively, if inconsistently sympathetic brush. Both Thucydides and Lucretius, in their accounts of families under pressure from plague, acknowledge the ironic outcome of either privileging claims for autonomy and self-preservation or

(*pietas*, *gloria*, etc.) overlooks the poet's *criticism* of such revisions of meaning in a lover's discourse. Lucretius' disparaging judgments of one practice (in the erotic realm), however, does not necessarily preclude (or render inconsistent) his own attempts at redefinition in the political realm. Comments on linguistic instability might equally articulate an understanding that signifiers are always vulnerable to re-appropriation, but that some conditions align these acts of appropriation more consistently with Epicurean values.

[36] For a reading of Lucretius' attitude toward politics that views the poet as far less reactionary to or engaged with the particular dysfunctions of Roman values, see Nichols (1976). Nichols generally sees Lucretius as disparaging of political life (144–8), since it is primarily fueled by fear of punishment according to the rule of law (5.1151). Voluntary *amicitia* by contrast is a worthier pursuit, though it is not always clear how to prevent communities bound by friendship alone from expanding into larger political bodies (5.1019–27).

nobly attending to one's own (*suos aegros*, 6.1238; cf. Th. 52.3, family members disposing of "their own" corpses, τὸν ἑαυτῶν νεκρὸν): either course concluded in death. But where Thucydides avoids using terms that recognize explicit biological kinship,[37] Lucretius refers to specific familial relationships among the dead and dying. As Commager observes (1957, 108), Lucretius' language of retribution for the selfish, plaintive laments from the weary, and death for the noble foregrounds the obligatory, as in "binding," force of kinship. Such language makes moral obligations among kin a more salient feature of the plague narrative.

The poet summons the affective dimension of those obligations, rephrased as voluntary familial devotion, in his description of bodies intertwined in death in the rustic community outside the city walls:

> . . . penitusque casa contrusa iacebant
> corpora paupertate et morbo dedita morti.
> exanimis pueris super exanimata parentum
> corpora nonnumquam posses retroque videre
> matribus et patribus natos super edere vitam.
> (6.1254–8)

And deeply within the house bodies lay about given over to death from disease and poverty. Sometimes you would see the lifeless bodies of parents lying over their lifeless sons, and children yielding up their life over their mothers and fathers.

Godwin observes how the misplaced *super* in 1258 reflects the chaos of the heap of bodies (1991, 184), identifying a visually evocative artistry that would lend itself to a multitude of artists painting images of plague from the sixteenth century onwards. Despite the chaos, the poet has stressed the relationships that structure the family unit, using an excess of terms denoting kinship: parents, mothers, fathers, children, sons—a partial recapitulation of terms that marked the origins of the family, and the emotive bonds that secured it, in Book 5 (cf. *puerique parentum . . . pueros . . . muliebreque saeclum*, 1017–21). As Morrison observes (2013, 225), the lines also recall the grief for departed family members depicted earlier in the poem, especially in

[37] The historian makes no specific references to parents or children and instead uses general terms that somewhat ambiguously indicate either close friendship or familial connections: ἐπιτήδειος (49.8, 53.4); οἰκεῖοι (51.5); φίλοι (51.5).

the well-known Iphianassa passage (1.84–101) and the imagined mourners of the dead father in Book 3 (3.894–911). The passage expands on Thucydides' clipped comment that "the dead and the dying were piled on top of each other" (52.2), contributing to the poet's portrait of hopelessness and "total and unrelieved horror" (Bright 1971, 615; cf. Clay 1983, 263).[38] Lucretius' reference to individuals within the family unit, loyal until death, however, also suggests an exemplary, if not exaggerated, form of *pietas*. On the one hand, it may be significant that the scene of familial devotion is placed beyond the city walls and, by implication, beyond the corruption that has tainted the polity within it. On the other hand, the boundary between city and country has already proven itself permeable and will continue to do so in the narrative of the disease's progress.

In passages where death has expanded its dominion throughout the city and the social fabric has begun to unravel, the absolute value of *pietas* is cast in an increasingly darker light. This recasting is initially evident through the hasty execution of funeral rites as well as the failure of friends and family to attend them: *incomitata rapi certabant funera vasta* (1225). As Bailey and others have noted (Bailey 1947, 1736), line 1225 is awkward where it stands and may need transposing to a point later in the text, perhaps to discussion of burials at 1247–51, a passage which some critics would move to the end of the poem (see n. 6 above). Whatever their original positions, both references to burial practices, at line 1225 and again twenty-two lines later, rob the process of its usual communal context (*incomitata*), and inject it with a rivalry within the community not evident in Thucydides' original observations on Athenian social dysfunction. Lucretius here has in mind the casual disposal of corpses in the history (Stoddard 1996, 124), but challenges the indifference of participants in his predecessor's account through evidence of effort despite the odds. Line 1225's observation of citizens "struggling" (*certo*) to perform unaccompanied funerals is echoed with a more precise account of the familial relationships that motivate the struggle in 1247: *populum sepelire suorum/certantes; lacrimis lassi luctuque redibant* ("[those] struggling to bury their kin, they kept returning

[38] Cf. Rho (1966, 144), who also remarks on the affective dimension of the portrait of death in the countryside.

wearied with tears and grief").[39] Taken in conjunction, the two references to burial counter Thucydidean apathy and instead indicate friction within the community generated from efforts to preserve familial identity (*populum . . . suorum*).

If the second passage (1247 ff.) belongs at the end of the text, it crowns another moment of contention among citizens to which we shall return. For now it is worth observing that the struggles of the Athenian citizens (alone and against each other) to bury *corpora* of their kin mirror the equally futile efforts of the politician despised ("looked down upon") in the well-known opening to Book 2, a correspondence that ties the pathologies of the plague to those of the Roman political order.[40] The Epicurean can take comfort in watching from a distance the struggles of others:

> . . . certare ingenio, contendere nobilitate,
> noctes atque dies niti praestante labore
> ad summas emergere opes rerumque potiri.
> (2.11–13)

[as they] contend in talent, contend in renown/lineage, and struggle night and day with exceptional toil to rise to the highest wealth and gain mastery of affairs.

As the poet extols the comforts of Epicurean *ataraxia*, he surveys the pathological behaviors that define the Roman *cursus* to emerge pre-eminent in wealth, talent, and *nobilitas*, that combination of offices and familial connections that secured prestige for the elite Roman male.[41] Viewed from the poet's ivory tower, there is little distinguishing the *certamina* (2.6) of destructive warfare from rivalries over innate talent (*certare ingenio*), since neither mind nor body has need for the objects of such struggles. Book 5's comment that those

[39] While the lines (1247 ff.) follow a lacuna in Rouse/Smith's text and are possibly misplaced, they undoubtedly expand on the notion of the struggle mentioned at 1225; cf. Rho (1966, 143–4).

[40] On the Epicurean antipathy toward politics as expressed in Lucretius' *DRN*, see Nichols (1976, discussed on p. 101 n. 36 above). His attitude is generally confirmed in Fowler (1989, 122–33), who discusses various qualifications to the poet's antipathy and rebuts various attempts to demonstrate the Epicurean's advocacy of a particular form of government (e.g., kingship, as argued by M. Gigante and T. Dorandi [1980]).

[41] While at some periods personal achievement may have been more important than ancestral lineage in securing *noblilitas*, familial identity (and the offices held by ancestors) was clearly a critical component of one's *nobilitas*, esp. in the late Republic; see Hellegouarc'h (1963, 224–7).

men "sweating with blood" while seeking to attain the highest honor "made the journey of life hateful as they struggled" (*certantes*, 5.1124) conveys an even more precise echo of the participial form of *certo* used in the plague passage, in an identical metrical position.

Despite the implications of positive contention for supremacy in *virtus* or artistic achievement that this verb occasionally conveys (e.g., Hor. *C.* 4.1.31; Luc. 6.255), Lucretius consistently uses it to describe destructive (2.119) or inane (3.779) pursuits.[42] As such, the apparently well-intended efforts of kin to respect the honors traditionally accorded are questioned within the sureties of Epicurean doctrine: the struggle is futile after all, since the plague has reduced all family members to virtually identical *corpora*. Beyond the futility of such efforts lie the threats of destruction they pose: the internally destructive struggles that mark efforts to bury dead relatives early in the poet's epidemiology erupt into hostile brawls at the end of it, in the poem's final lines:

> perturbatus enim totus trepidat, et unus
> quisque suum pro re et pro tempore maestus humabat.
> multaque res subita et paupertas horrida suasit;
> namque suos consanguineos aliena rogorum
> insuper extructa ingenti clamore locabant
> subdebantque faces, multo cum sanguine saepe
> rixantes potius quam corpora desererentur.
>
> (6.1280–6)

For the entire population was disturbed and on edge, and each one gloomily kept burying his own as his occasion and situation allowed. Unforeseen circumstances and poverty persuaded many horrid acts. For they were often placing their own blood relatives upon the built-up pyres of others with a loud clamor; and they put torches beneath, often brawling with much bloodshed rather than have their bodies deserted.

The language concluding the poem may contain a double entendre, according to Kelly (1980), whose interpretation of *corpora* in the final lines suggests that the "bodies" in the passage invoke the atomistic view of a *corpora*-filled universe detailed throughout the poem.

[42] The "struggles" of the *DNR* anticipate use of *certare* in the nearly contemporaneous *Bellum Catilinae*, where we find the verb used to indict the very socio-political pathologies diagnosed by the Epicurean poet. For Sallust, *certo* marks a turning point in recent political life, following the restoration of the tribunician power during the consulship of Pompey and Crassus (70 BCE), when men "pretending to act on behalf of the public good, were in truth working for their own advancement" (*bonum publicum simulantes pro sua quisque potentia certabant*, *Cat.* 38.3; cf. 54.6).

Reference to *corpora* also marks a final refrain of the indistinguishable *corpora* littered throughout the streets of Athens. Such a finalizing assertion of nearly interchangeable bodies, however, must contend with the blood relatives who, in a clear departure from Thucydides' depiction of citizens hurrying off after secretly disposing of bodies, fight to preserve something of their kin and of their own identities as expressed through kinship. Repetition of the reflexive third person adjective *suum . . . suos* gestures toward self-preservation as well as preservation of "one's own." In this case, such efforts appear justified through shared bloodlines (*consanguineos*), and yet here, familial ties, rather than inspiring the emotive and sympathetic bonding in death observed among the rustic community, motivate social dysfunction categorized by the poet among *multa horrida*.

The deteriorative violence in the poem's final lines answers the generative power of Venus in the opening proem, and correspondences between the two sections have been duly observed.[43] I would like to stress, however, the quality of this particular articulation of violence, which depicts a community turned against itself in defense of familial bonds, a community in which civic solidarity has been replaced by division and difference (*aliena*).[44] As we have seen, Thucydides records the presence of pyres and abandoned bodies, but Lucretius ignites them with discord. Camus recognized the distinction in his own rendering of plague's imaginative potential. As readers of *La Peste* apprehend the onset of plague in Oran, Dr. Rieux calls to mind, "the pyres that, Lucretius tells us, the Athenians built on the sea-shore when they were stricken with illness. The dead were brought there at night, but there was too little space and the living would fight with each other with burning torches to put their loved ones on the pyres, engaging in bloody struggles rather than abandon their dead bodies on the beach" (2001, 32–3).[45]

Lucretius has brought the family to the fore in a way that will have an irrevocable impact on subsequent plague narratives. Despite the

[43] By, e.g., Müller (2007, cited above); cf. Gale (1994, 224–6); Minadeo (1965) argues that the poem's architecture is consistently structured according to nature's cycles of destruction and creation.

[44] Cf. Pope (2016, 53), who observes that, "[t]he internal sweating with blood symptom with which Lucretius discusses the onset of the disease almost presages this external blood, or perhaps *civilis sanguis*, to use a phrase from earlier in the poem."

[45] See Stephanson (1987, 230–2) on how Camus' novel develops plague's "imaginative potential."

family's initial affective value, by the end of the poem kinship emerges as a means to defend "one's own" identity and a source of strife within the community. In fact, efforts to preserve the bonds among blood relations at the end of Lucretius' account of the plague are tinged with irony in light of the poem's earlier indictment of civil discord, whose most sinister orchestrations occur within the family. In Book 3, for instance, the relationship between brothers is defined as especially vulnerable to personal ambitions. After describing the desire for wealth and distinction, rooted in the fear of death and driving men to transgress the law, the poet addresses civil war:

> unde homines dum se falso terrore coacti
> effugisse volunt longe longeque remosse,
> sanguine civili rem conflant divitiasque
> conduplicant avidi, caedem caede accumulantes,
> crudeles gaudent in tristi funere fratris
> et consanguineum mensas odere timentque.
> (3.68–73)

From here (=*leti portas*) while men, driven by false fear, wish to flee and remove themselves far away, they build up property through civil bloodshed and greedily they double their wealth, heaping slaughter upon slaughter; they rejoice cruelly in the dismal death of a brother and they loathe and fear the tables of their kinsmen.

Forms of *consanguineus* are used on only three occasions in the poem, and only twice, here in Book 3 and at the end of the plague narrative, to refer to human blood ties.[46] In both passages the ambiguity of shared "blood"—designating the source of the bond as well as the violence resultant from the bond—is intensified through reference to *sanguis* shed over discord within the community (3.70, 6.1285). Such an echo, however faint, underscores the frailty of any bond within the social order: destructive desire to destroy the community to preserve the family is easily converted into bloodshed within the family for the aggrandizement of the individual.

The problematic nature of interfamilial relationships in the plague, in which citizens contend with each other (*certare*) to bury their own as often as they avoid tending to "their own" who are in the grip of the disease, reflects on a larger (and largely destructive) context of

[46] The other instance, also in Book 6, metaphorically describes the moisture in the sea as "akin" to the moisture in the clouds, 6.475.

late-Republican alliances of family and *amicitia*, forcing readers to question which relationships are worth privileging at the inevitable expense of the others. As suggested earlier, the family, as a source of security as well as a microcosm of internecine strife, is a paradox that can only be resolved by adopting Epicurean principles, that is, by disavowing the greed that compels brother against brother and accepting that death may well come with attendance to those we love. For the fully converted Epicurean, moreover, no relationship is worth a struggle in the face of inevitable and impersonal death. Readers who are not fully convinced, however (Vergil and Ovid among them), will exploit questions latent in the *DRN* and use them to problematize such relationships in the face of the newly emerging model of familial and political life in the early Principate.

Lucretius' language of familial bonds demonstrates a force of resistance against the totalizing and leveling effects of the plague, but also reflects on the kind of mimetic violence, as each one contends for "his own," that is the source of the plague in its metaphoric implications of civil war. Subsequent chapters in this project will demonstrate how this very language is adapted by poets of the early Principate who wish to address the reciprocally destructive relationships that fueled civil strife at the end of the Republic: in balancing the homogenizing effects of plague with familial claims to identity, these poets invoke the poignancy and security of the kinship bond as often as they reference its liabilities. Using divergent narrative strategies, they consider the possibilities of mending communal fractures by allowing a single individual and a single family—that of Augustus—to emerge as both object of devotions and panacea, a *communis salus* for a newly recovered *res publica*.

3.4. TERMINATING THE INTERMINABLE: SAECULAR AND LITERARY EVOLUTIONS

This chapter has identified Lucretius' sensitivity to the vulnerability of the human body, along with the chaotic accumulation of citizen *corpora*—in spite of dramatized resistance at individual and familial levels—as integral components of his rendering of pestilence in Athens and his chief bequests to the Latin tradition of narrating plague. The body's vulnerability, however macabre and grotesque, is also of fundamental importance when the property extends to the metaphor of the civic body, allowing for that body's disintegration and reconstitution in imaginative and productive ways. For later Latin poets, bodily decomposition and collapse into homogeneity, as integral to a plague's symptomatology and epidemiology, will issue a blow to those competitive drives that fuel the pursuit of an autonomous and fiercely individual self. The melting of discrete citizen bodies into a homogenized mass of rotting *corpora* and *cadavera* functions as a comment on the collapse of the social order in times of civil discord and a necessary prelude to restructuring a revised and, by some accounts, more cohesive, concordant citizen body. Vergil and Ovid will offer remedies for plague, ways of restructuring the aggregate to build a more or less satisfactory relationship between the individual and the greater community. All the same, successors in the plague tradition will find it hard to shake Lucretius' cynical attitude toward rehabilitating the Roman Republic, an attitude most clearly expressed through the claims for identity—a futile clinging to remnants of the self and "one's own"—that persist, despite the ubiquity of death.

When poets of the Principate recreate plague as civil war and impose variously satisfactory (and variously postponed) conclusions to its devastation, they are in effect attempting to answer the question left open-ended by Lucretius, whose post-apocalyptic scenario threatens to repeat itself ad infinitum. As observed in Chapter 1, "plague" was widely recognized as incurable. Since it arises from the commonly breathed air and affects all constitutions, it was considered beyond the scope of Hippocratic regimes; its status as such may have contributed to Lucretius' decision to end his poem with the Athenian plague. The concluding image of a polis, formerly the pinnacle of human civilization, in irrevocable decline has led one scholar to postulate that the episode functions as a depiction of the end of the world, which the poet had earlier promised his reader (Nichols 1976, 179). Monica Gale, who assigns to the plague the function of "warning and protreptic" (1994, 228) as much as that of a test, has stressed the timeless, mythic dimension of the episode.[47]

By such assessments, the plague fits comfortably into well-established Greek and Roman mythic traditions that seek to explain the gradual, but constant change in humankind's relationship with the gods, with

[47] Bright also stresses the plague's universalizing and mythic implications (1970, esp. 615, 622).

nature, and with itself, that is, the myth of the ages. The collusion of poetic closure with the representation of interminable and incurable disease, I suggest, serves as fodder for a new variety of epochal thinking that will color treatments of plague in the Augustan period—that is, the tendency to associate plague with the degeneration and regeneration that propel the cycle of the ages. The formerly sturdy farmer who languishes from disease just outside the walls of Athens (*robustus curvi moderator aratri*, 6.1253) summons the ghost of that figure not yet present in the primitivism theorized in Book 5, when a "heartier human race" (*genus humanum durius*, 5.925–6) lived off the land, content with what the earth provided of its own accord, *sua sponte*: "not yet did any sturdy guide of the curved plough exist" (*nec robustus erat curvi moderator aratri/quisquam*, 5.933). Vergil will codify the sturdy ploughman's role as an index of epochal evolution in his fourth *Eclogue*, as a *robustus arator* loosens his oxen from the yoke amidst a spontaneously productive earth (4.41). In the context of *DRN*, this figure's re-emergence in Book 6, as an epidemic besets one pinnacle of human civilization, marks the progress and inevitable decline of the ages.

The same farmer poised outside the walls of Athens also evokes, in a less obvious manner, the figure of closure haunting Book 2 of Lucretius' poem, the *grandis arator* (2.1164) who surveys deterioration from a better age, this time nature's evanescence rather than that of the human species and the social order thought to transcend her.[48] This aged farmer, along with a disheartened cultivator of the vine (*tristis sator*), bears witness to a decline in the ages: it is primarily the waning natural resources that bring scorn upon an entire *saeculum* (2.1169), though shades of moral decay also color his current vision and his longing for a former age, one "filled with *pietas*":[49]

[48] Commager draws attention to the similarity of the two figures (1957, 108). For Book 2 as a rival to Book 6 in tone and thematics, see Müller (2007).

[49] As Gale suggests (2013, 31), reference to *pietas* may be a jab at traditional notions of respect for the Roman pantheon ("nostalgic claptrap"). I would argue, however, that use of the word is somewhat ambivalent. *Pietas* throughout the poem (as I have indicated) refers equally to interfamilial relationships, and specifically fraternal ones. The poet unequivocally condemns infractions against this kind of *pietas*. And given the fraternal relationship that dominates Lucretius' Hesiodic model, it seems that waning *pietas* might be cause for the poet's and our consternation.

iamque caput quassans grandis suspirat arator
crebrius, in cassum magnos cecidisse labores,
et cum tempora temporibus praesentia confert
praeteritis, laudat fortunas saepe parentis.
tristis item vetulae vitis sator atque vietae
temporis incusat momen saeclumque fatigat,
et crepat, antiquum genus ut pietate repletum
perfacile angustis tolerarit finibus aevom,
cum minor esset agri multo modus ante viritim;
nec tenet omnia paulatim tabescere et ire
ad scopulum, spatio aetatis defessa vetusto.
(2.1164–74)

Now the old ploughman shaking his head sighs time and again, that his great efforts have been in vain, and when he compares the present times to times gone by, he often praises the fortunes of his father. So too the sad cultivator of the old and shriveled vine accuses the passage of time and criticizes the age, and he rattles on about how an ancient race, filled with reverence, supported an easier way of life within a narrow plot of land, although the measure of a field for each man was much smaller; nor does he grasp that all things decay little by little and "go to the reef of destruction,"[50] worn out by the ancient passage of time.

The calamity of plague is, of course, a much more abrupt shift in the order of things than nature's faltering productivity. But as the farmer is reassigned from his role as observer of nature's indifference in Book 2 to its casualty in Book 6, we are encouraged to assimilate the destruction of the plague with saecular evolution. The assimilation of these two figures holds out promise for further deterioration, but also for eventual renewal, whether in the form of nature's persistent regeneration of *corpora*[51] or as a political mechanism to revitalize a morbid body politic.

[50] For the translation, see Rouse/Smith (1992, 187).

[51] Cf. 1.215–16: *huc accedit uti quidque in sua corpora rursum/dissolvat natura neque ad nilum interemat res.* Minadeo (1965, 445) stresses the importance of the lines in his argument concerning Lucretius' goal of demonstrating the balance between nature's destructive and generative movements.

4

Plague, Civil War, and Epochal Evolution in Vergil's *Georgics*

However one chooses to defend the ending of Lucretius' *De Rerum Natura*, the sheer quantity of scholarship amassed to explain why a champion of *ataraxia* would conclude his treatise with such stirring images bears witness to the consistently sympathetic response of readers who confront his portrait of human suffering in the plague. Perhaps the most striking feature of Vergil's Noric plague in *Georgics* 3 is the similar response it has evoked, despite the fact that its devastation is confined largely to livestock, in a region fairly remote from Rome.[1] While the value of his treatment and its potential as a metaphor for the human condition have been frequently observed, most critics agree that Vergil's account is a fiction and, unlike Lucretius' re-presentation of Athenian plague, has no historical counterpart in antiquity.[2] This chapter offers an understanding of why the *Georgics* poet engaged in this particular imaginative

[1] Various critics, especially those following Harrison (1979), have understood Vergil's depiction of plague as something foreign and applicable to Rome's enemies; cf. Foster (1988, 33), who stresses the "topical urgency" of the passage and its representation of Alpine tribes recently subdued by Octavian. At the same time, the threat of *contagium* is introduced before the plague and presented as a realistic threat to the life of the Italian farmer (*videris*, "should you see . . . " 3.465). Thomas (1988, 129–30) suggests that Vergil's geographic sketch locating the plague North-East of Italy brings the disaster close to home.

[2] On the plague's implications for the human condition, see, e.g., Liebeschuetz (1965, 73–7); Putnam (1979, 215–35); Thomas (1988, 131); cf. Mynors (1990, 251). Servius (at *Georgics* 3.487) thought that Vergil's account described an outbreak of the same fifth-century plague that afflicted the Athenians. Harrison (1979) summarizes the prevailing opinions on the historicity of Vergil's plague and offers convincing evidence against those few critics who view the poet as describing what was an actual event in Noricum. See also Thomas (1988, 129).

experiment, and does so by examining the Noric plague in light of other references to contagious disease, primarily in Vergil's oeuvre. In the first *Eclogue*, the threat of *contagium* distinguishes the uncertain fortune of Meliboeus from the recovery boasted by Tityrus, reflecting on the circumstances of civil war and its aftermath that have marred the Italian landscape. In the *Aeneid*, the pestilence that incites the Trojans to uproot their settlement in Crete provides a coda to the Noric plague, remedying its open-ended connotations of civil discord in the *Georgics* with the narrative possibility of a fresh start, though one that glances back at the remainders lingering in the wake of a new order.

It is however within the larger context of the *Georgics* themselves that we find Vergil most clearly addressing the unresolved calamity that strikes the inhabitants of Noricum. The cattle plague ends with hints of the disease's impact on the human community, but the problems of contagion in Book 3 are extended and resolved, in some readings, by the *bougonia* of Book 4, in which bees, also beset by disease, are miraculously restored (Otis 1995, 188; West 1979, 26).[3] These readings diverge from interpretations, especially those of Thomas and Ross, that stress the impractical and fantastical nature of the *bougonia*, a custom that "has no place in the real world of the Italian farmer" and thus "cannot stand as the solution to the problems of man and beast in the world of *labor*" (Thomas 1988, 196; cf. 1982, 84–5; Ross 1987, 215–17).[4] As Perkell has noted, the process of killing a calf in order to produce bees is not a resurrection (the former hive is irretrievably lost), but is, rather, "an exchange of death for life" (1978, 219). Vergil leaves his readers to question whether the exchange will prove useful (the new hive likened to summer showers, 4.312–13) or destructive (the hive likened to Parthian arrows, 4.313–14).

In the following, I offer a close reading of Vergil's Noric plague that demonstrates the poet's dependence on a metaphoric relationship

[3] Cf. Gale (2000, 111), who suggests that "the *bougonia* acts as a kind of answer to the problem of pain and suffering raised at the end of book 3 and, less explicitly, throughout the poem." Morgan (1999) views the answer of the *bougonia* as a hopeful one, while not denying the violence that the practice relies upon; cf. Miles (1980, esp. 254).

[4] Thibodeau (2011, 192) resists commenting on the tone that surrounds the closure of Book 4, conceding that, "there is no indication that the ritual was a regular part of Mediterranean life"; for T., the *bougonia* is a kind of marvel that charms readers and functions usefully within Vergil's larger didactic program.

between plague and civil war. My discussion foregrounds the language of liquefaction, dissolution of identity, and Golden-Age eradication of the farmer's *labores* as conditions of pestilence in *Georgics* 3. In his concern with liquefaction and dissolution, Vergil is especially indebted to Lucretius, whose own account of plague, as observed in Chapter 3, emphasized processes of decay and the collapse of boundaries within *corpora* (e.g., *DRN* 6.1153). Such language, used in a broader discursive context that equates human and animal *corpora* with larger civic bodies,[5] addresses those transgressions of structural boundaries (within families, communities, and civic life) that characterize a population at war with itself.

Vergil's post-Actium treatment of pestilence, however, in contrast to his predecessor's account of Athenian plague, is shaped by the specific concerns of a citizen body embarking on a process of recovery under what would be known as the Augustan Principate. As an expression of those concerns, his account relies on imagery of Golden-Age plenitude that intersects provocatively with roughly contemporary poetic discourses, especially Horace's *Epodes*, where *contagium* and civil war are explicitly linked to the Iron-Age world that the poet hopes to relinquish. While Vergil's imagery is inverted to dystopian rather than utopian effect, it should be read within the larger set of signifiers that spoke of a revived Golden Age under a new *ordo*.[6] While the moment in the Principate ripe for using the Golden Age to give "permanent expression to th[e] mood of optimism" (Zanker 1990, 167) had not yet arrived when the *Georgics* was published (*c.*29 BCE), use of such imagery drew on an established tradition upholding the Golden Age as an alternative to the failures of an old system. Epochal thinking had been in the air throughout the 40's BCE, when a new *saeculum* was expected after Julius Caesar's victory had resolved the civil strife between his own partisans and the forces of Pompey Magnus, and more specifically following the

[5] For the human body as an indication of the body politic, and one vulnerable to disease, especially in late-Republican discourse, see above, Chapter 1, pp. 17–21, and Chapter 2, pp. 50–1.

[6] For observation of the plague's Golden-Age characteristics in Vergil, see Harrison (1979, 20–1), who views the Golden Age in the third *Georgic* as a response to Horace's *Epode* 16; discussed further below. See also Ross (1987, 182–3); Perkell (1989, 119–23); Nappa (2005,152–8); cf. Putnam (1979, 227). The Golden Age as a symbol revived and manipulated by the Augustan Principate has been extensively treated; see esp. Zanker (1990, 167–92) and Galinsky (1996, 93–140).

appearance of a comet, the *sidus Iulium*, after Caesar's assassination (Coleman 1977, 130).[7] Reluctance to invest too heavily in the potential of a new age, however, is evident in the shifting tones that surround its anticipation in the *Eclogues* (most famously, the fourth *Eclogue*) and Horace's *Epodes*.

In the third *Georgic*, Vergil adopts the abundance and lack of human *labores* associated with the Golden Age, as well as its absence of an organizing social hierarchy,[8] in order to indicate the collapse of the old order. While the plenitude of dystopic Noricum might be harnessed and redirected in the service of a new order, the promise of that plenitude is left jarringly unfulfilled within the context of Book 3. Vergil defers containment and resolution until we are forced to apprehend a similar disaster among the apian community in Book 4, where he presents a strikingly uniform hive born from the liquefied remains of a calf: the resulting *monstrum* (cf. *G*.4.554) suggests that something novel will issue from the homogenized rot of disease. But the utility of that *monstrum* depends upon sharply curtailing differences among members of the community, a process that Vergil's sympathetic portraits of individual suffering in the plague may leave readers reluctant to condone.

4.1. PLAGUE AND THE (POST-)APOCALYPSE: INVERTING THE AGES IN VERGIL'S NORICUM

As noted in the previous chapter, Lucretius' *De Rerum Natura* draws on the metaphoric relationship between plague and war in the Greek tradition, especially Thucydides.[9] For the historian, the war that contextualizes the plague, though fought between competing *poleis*, is an internal one, among Greeks, in contrast to wars waged against an invasive other (1.18, 23). The historical, martial context of the plague of 430 BCE encourages readers of Lucretius' poem to detect

[7] See also Jal (1963, 245–51), who observes that episodes of civil strife extending as far back as the wars between Marius and Sulla were interpreted as indications of a new age.

[8] As Perkell notes (2002, 20), the Golden Age's characteristic lack of social hierarchy is a distinct innovation of the Roman poets.

[9] Cf. Parry's (1969, 115) insightful reading of Thucydides' poeticizing treatment of plague: "The Plague is a pathos, and it is equated with the War."

hints of Rome's internal conflict in the account that closes Book 6. In addition, Lucretius' rendering of the Athenian plague constructs a causal relationship between contagious disease and internal strife, as citizens fight amongst each other for funeral pyres (*multo cum sanguine . . . rixantes*, 6.1285–6) in the tableau that abruptly concludes the poem. In Livy's account of Rome's origins we have observed how contagious ideas spark conflict within the city: the *novae res* that destabilize harmony between *ordines* are regularly (if tentatively) contained in a way that mirrors the containment of physical pestilence arising in Rome. In some cases, a causal link attributes outbreaks of pestilence to offices improperly distributed among the *ordines* (e.g., 5.13–14); at times, and conversely, a redistribution of offices results from the need to reassign leadership during a time of pestilence (e.g., 3.6); both narrative trends in *Ab Urbe Condita* demonstrate a tight conceptual link between *discordia* and disease, foundational to the historian's explanation of Rome's expansion and gradual dominance over the Italian peninsula.

Thus Lucretius and Livy, from different historical vantage points, imbue disease with the colors of civic strife. It is within this discursive context that Vergil prompts readers of the *Georgics* to search for common ground between the many natural disasters experienced by the farmer and Roman civic disasters (Miles 1980, 254). The civic disaster that looms largest in the poem is Rome's internal discord: the poet's initial digression on Roman civil war (1.466–514) is echoed on two occasions in scenes of conflict between heavily anthropomorphized oxen and bees (cf. 3.215–36; 4.67–87). While Miles has identified the conflict among *tauri* in Book 3 and the apian conflicts of Book 4 as direct reflections of Roman civic strife, he also observes nuances of civil strife in the plague, in particular, verbal echoes between the onset of pestilence and the portents that usher in civil war at the end of the first *Georgic* (1980, 220). Relying on the familiar contamination of plague discourse with the discourse of war, Vergil asks his readers to reimagine the natural disaster that besets the people of Noricum, an especially virulent *pestis* (3.472), in terms of the civil wars that Rome experienced in the years prior to the publication of the poem.

Vergil prefaces his account of pestilence in northern Italy with a general treatment of disease, one that introduces the notion of contagion and its increased threat through the very proximity that defines the herd. While his discussion promises the revelation of symptoms (or "signs") and causes (*te causas et signa docebo*, 3.440), it evolves rapidly from conditions manageable at the individual level (e.g., *scabies*, 3.441–54) to the kind of *pestis* that threatens the whole flock and is only remedied through slaughter. Discussion of topical diseases shifts to less easily marked behavioral changes, listlessness and lack of appetite, signs of communicable disease in livestock who must be slaughtered before contagion spreads:

> quam procul aut molli succedere saepius umbrae
> videris, aut summas carpentem ignavius herbas
> extremamque sequi, aut medio procumbere campo
> pascentem, et serae solam decedere nocti,
> continuo culpam ferro compesce, prius quam
> dira per incautum serpant contagia vulgus.
> (*G.* 3.464–9)

Should you see a sheep far off either withdraw too often in the gentle shade, listlessly picking at the highest blades of grass and following at a distance, or recline while grazing in the middle of the field, or withdraw alone late in the evening, immediately suppress (or "confine") the offense (*culpam*) with a knife, before dreaded contagion creeps through the unprotected flock.

Vulgus, in this context, easily registers livestock, though we have seen the term's coupling with contagion, in reference to the Roman people in Livy (3.6; cf. 5.12), where contagion itself flexibly connoted the transmission of ideological as well as physical pathogens within the urban populace and military *castra*. Nelson observes that the passage illustrates a general pattern in Book 3 according to which, "Vergil has created a double vision, which sees simultaneously the demands of the whole and the claim of the individual" (1998, 144). Thus details about the sheep's listlessness, for which he is hardly to blame,[10] obstruct our perspective on the good of the whole that the farmer must keep in view.[11] And it is with this double vision that we attempt to focus the calamity of the Noric plague, in which the

[10] A depiction that echoes Vergil's treatment of the stallion, worn out by old age, at 3.95–100. Servius comments on the sheep's lack of culpability (ad 3.468); cf. Mynors (1990, 249) and Nelson (1998, 144).

[11] The ambivalence which with Vergil portrays the sick sheep here is clarified by Grattius' comparable Augustan treatment of disease among dogs in the fragmentary *Cynegetica*. Grattius offers no details of behavior or perspective in recommending the single dog who must be killed to prevent *scabies* from spreading: *sed una/pernicies redimenda anima, quae prima sequaci/sparsa mala est, ne dira trahant contagia vulgus* (410–12). From there Grattius turns (as Vergil had before him) to the problem of a

impersonal and uniformly destructive force of the plague competes with the livestock who assert themselves as individuals—mindful of fading honors, tragically self-destructive, and mourning for kin.

Julia Hawkins, in her forthcoming treatment of the *Georgics* poet as healer, has usefully raised the question of prevention, arguing that the precepts offered here (excision of topical ulcers, slaughter of ill livestock) constitute a means by which the disaster in Noricum might have been prevented. While the question itself is critical, the circumstances of disease in Noricum, as we shall see, reflect a process of transmission more consistent with miasma theory, and establish implicit *limits* on the power of medical precepts to combat the plague: the very environment in Noricum is tainted, from its air to its fodder to its water supply. The poet turns away from the possibility of identifying individually stricken animals (those whom disease seizes "one by one") to *morbi* that infect entire herds. Some illnesses may originate with a Patient Zero—an individual culprit (*sola*), however blameless, who has the power to usher in pestilence—but the Noric disaster revises the serpentine crawl of contagion on an apocalyptic scale:

> non tam creber agens hiemem ruit aequore turbo,
> quam multae pecudum pestes. nec singula morbi
> corpora corripiunt, sed tota aestiva repente,
> spemque gregemque simul cunctamque ab origine gentem.
> (*G*.3.470–3)

Not with such intensity does the whirlwind driving on winter storms rush from the sea as do the many diseases of cattle. Nor do diseases seize upon bodies one by one, but suddenly [seize] the summer's whole brood, and the hope and herd together with the race from its origins.

Transmission through proximity will remain a key element in the poet's plague dramaturgy, one essential to intimations of civil strife that color the account. And yet here the force of disease moves irresistibly, and with such speed as defies the careful recognition granted to the shepherd and his listless sheep: its victims are seized

more widespread plague: he observes with some confidence the power of *experientia* (427) and, failing that, faith in and sacrifice to Mars Ultor, whose power to help those not tainted by the sins of civil war (451–4) the poet celebrates. Grattius' treatment throughout thus stands in sharp contrast to that of Vergil, whose Noric plague is irremediable and whose representation of sacrifice offers no clear answers concerning the cause of or remedy for the disease.

en masse, eradicating the herd collectively (*nec singula, tota, cunctam*) and leaving no trace of its past, present, or future.

Vergil's interest in the promise or "hope" of the flock extends back to the first *Eclogue*, where Meliboeus, displaced after land confiscations following civil discord (*civis discordia*, 1.71), presumably that at Philippi (DeVeau 1935, 2–5), laments the loss of two newborn goats (*spem gregis*, 1.15). In reckoning Tityrus' relative good fortune at having found lands and *libertas*, he marvels over his interlocutor's freedom from both foreign pastures and contagion from neighboring flocks:

> non insueta gravis temptabunt pabula fetas,
> nec mala vicini pecoris contagia laedent,
> fortunate senex, hic inter flumina nota
> et fontis sacros frigus captabis opacum.
> (1.49–52)

No unaccustomed fodder will assail your ailing,[12] pregnant ewes, nor will the baneful contagion(s) of a neighbor's flock harm them, fortunate old man! You will take cooling shade amid well-known streams and sacred fountains.

From Meliboeus' perspective, Tityrus enjoys a kind of Golden Age, where cooling shade and streams are readily available. While the need to provide fodder to flocks marks an Iron-Age world, such animals will not suffer from foreign pasturage.[13] Coleman (1977, 82) has noted the possible allusion here to Horace's *Epode* 16, where a similar absence of *contagium* defined the poet's imagined haven from civil war:

> nulla nocent pecori contagia, nullius astri
> gregem aestuosa torret impotentia.
> Iuppiter illa piae secrevit litora genti,
> ut inquinavit aere tempus aureum.
> aere, dehinc ferro duravit saecula, quorum
> piis secunda vate me datur fuga.
> (16.61–6)

No contagions harm the flock, the seething fury of no star scorches the herd. Jupiter has set apart those shores for a reverent race, after he sullied an age of

[12] As Coleman notes, *gravis* (as synonymous with *gravidas*) is somewhat redundant with *fetas*, and the adjective is often used to describe poor health (1977, 82).

[13] This will be the same source of disease among horses that Lucan will draw on in his *Bellum Civile*, and eventually the cause of plague among Pompey's men (Luc. 6.80–83); see Chapter 6, p. 190.

gold with bronze. With bronze, and from there he hardened the ages with iron, from which a fortunate escape is allowed to the reverent, with me as seer.

As an alternative to an age of constant attrition through civil strife (16.1, *altera iam teritur bellis civilibus aetas*), Horace constructs an escapist fantasy colored explicitly with shades of Golden-Age satiety, and imagined as a means of preserving a *pia gens*. The atmospheric conditions of "seething fury" that the poet banishes from these pristine *litora*, reflecting medical thought concerning links between climate and disease, also gesture toward the cool shade that defines Tityrus' new quasi-golden life. While priority between the *Eclogues* and the *Epodes* is difficult to establish, the cumulative impact of the verses is one that not only correlates contagious disease with an Iron-Age existence, but also sets them against a backdrop of civil war that threatens the continuity of the Roman *gens*. Thus, when the conditions of physical contagion assert themselves in the *Georgics*, we are tempted to find them fringed with reminders of internal conflict and upheaval, located in a distinctly fallen world.

When the *Georgics* poet turns from the general topic of the effects of disease on the *gens*, to illustrate the power of contagion through an account of the Noric plague, he invokes the same torrid atmosphere that Horace linked to his Iron-Age world, marred by civil strife:

hic quondam morbo caeli miseranda coorta est
tempestas totoque autumni incanduit aestu
et genus omne neci pecudum dedit, omne ferarum,
corrupitque lacus, infecit pabula tabo.
nec via mortis erat simplex; sed ubi ignea venis
omnibus acta sitis miseros adduxerat artus,
rursus abundabat fluvidus liquor omniaque in se
ossa minutatim morbo conlapsa trahebat.

(*G*.3.478–85)

Here once arose a season pitiable for the diseased atmosphere, and throughout all the seething of autumn it glowed white hot and gave over every kind of beast to death, and every [race of] wild animals, and it got hold of the lakes and stained the food supply with decay. Nor was there a uniform path to death; but when a fiery thirst driven throughout all the veins shriveled the wretched limbs, again a dissolving liquid flowed in excess and absorbed all the bones little by little toppled with disease.

Here we find the same fiery heat (*autumni aestu*), usually associated (as in Horace's *Epode*) with the rising of the Dog Star and the onset of autumn (*aestuosa impotentia nullius astri*, *Ep*.16.61–2), the usual season of pestilence in Rome.[14] While scholars rightly note that the *Georgics* poet has distanced his plague from Rome geographically, readers of Livy (and the historian's sources) may recall the various endemic plagues that the *Urbs* experienced in her infancy, which the historian marks as "arising" (*orta est*; cf. 4.52, 7.1, 7.27), in contrast to pathogens that invade the populace (*invasit*, 4.21); such plagues were frequently interpreted as originating within the population and the result of divine displeasure. This is not to suggest that the poet has in mind a particular outbreak or transgression among the people of Noricum. In fact, Vergil prompts us to look for a culprit only to deny us the pleasure of finding one: unlike the recognizable sheep as *culpa* who threatens the flock in the precepts prior to the cattle plague, no individual in Noricum is allowed to bear the responsibility of such widespread devastation. At the same time, Vergil's language of origins (*coorta est*, 3.478) tempts us to probe within the civic body and examine its composition for the aetiology of pestilence, suggestive of *discordia* within rather than an external threat.

The episode's evolving account of symptoms offers more of a sustained, evocative series of contrasts than an eyewitness account of physical processes. Vergil remarks on the lack of uniformity that defined the initial symptoms of the epidemic (*nec . . . simplex*), and, to elaborate, he describes a violently contradictory movement, from fiery parching thirst that shrinks the limbs to an excessive *fluvidus liquor* that causes the bones to dissolve *minutatim*, "little by little." The language of the body's distinct members (*miseros artus*) under threat from the corrosive power of disease reflects Lucretius' interest in bodily decomposition. Vergil, however, has taken what Lucretius predicted as the eventual condition of the body after death by the plague (*tabes*; Lucr. 6.1201) and made a similar putrid matter, associated with decay, a cause of the disease's transmission.[15] Here Vergil reflects the common conceptual link between rotting flesh

[14] For the correlation, see also Hor. *S*. 2.6.19 (Mynors 1990, 252). Early autumn was of course pestilential throughout the Greco-Roman world (cf. Celsus 2.1.7–8).

[15] As discussed in Chapter 3, Lucretius' reference to *tabum letumque* at 1201 is understood as hysteron-proteron, though the order also implies that rot precedes death, an implication Vergil perhaps develops here. In light of the longstanding but imprecise attribution to rot as a source of disease, there is inevitable slippage in Vergil's use of *tabum*; see above, Chapter 1, p. 26.

and the spread of pestilence. What is difficult to convey with the *tabum*-stained fodder in the *Georgics*, particularly in English that wishes to locate in the word a source of contagion and impose a sequence on its spread,[16] is the etymological link between Vergil's term and its relatives, not only the Lucretian *tabes*, but also the verbs derived from it (like *tabere* and *tabesco*), which designate plague as a cyclical and perhaps interminable process: these cognates refer not only to the origins of disease, but also to the processes of physical wasting as well as the putrid matter and fluids that result from disease (*OLD tabes* 1–3), nuances that will become especially pronounced when Vergil revisits the term at the end of his plague narrative (3.557).[17] The poet's identification of rot as both an origin and culmination of disease grants the Noric plague a cyclical logic, and one impossible to interrupt within the frame of Book 3.

The fluid connoted by *tabum* and the word's association with a collapse of the body's boundaries, moreover, vie with atmospheric changes to figuratively locate the plague's origins in bloodshed. Mynors (1990, 252) points to a close verbal echo of the *Georgics* in Tacitus' *Histories*, where *tabum* refers to the rot that comes from slaughter on the battlefield. During a famously horrific year of Roman civil strife (69 CE), Vitellius returns to the scene of a victory that occurred some forty days earlier and takes in a "foul and atrocious sight" (*foedum atque atrox spectaculum*): *lacera corpora, trunci artus, putres virorum equorumque formae,* infecta tabo humus, *protritis arboribus ac frugibus dira vastitas* (2.70, "mutilated bodies, severed limbs, rotting forms of men and horses, ground stained with gore/decay, grim devastation from toppled trees and crops"). The historian's reference to ground "stained with *tabum*" to describe an oddly georgic scene of battlefield decay is, on the one hand, more in keeping with Vergil's use of the word in the *Aeneid*, where it refers to the gore

[16] West (1979, 71), drawing attention to the odd chronology and difficult logic that governs the passage ("as clinical history, this is not satisfactory"), interprets as "decomposing flesh." Fairclough/Goold (1999, 211) translate *tabum* as "venom"; Wilkinson suppresses the force of the noun behind the verb (*infecit*), rendered as a participle: "it killed, infecting pools, contaminating fodder" (1982, 115); Ferry (2005, 131) adopts a similar strategy: "the lakes were all infected, the pastures poisoned." Lewis (1963, 70) renders as "blight" ("put a blight on their fodder"); cf. Jermyn (1947, 66), who translates, "infecting with disease even the hay."

[17] On Lucretius' use of *tabes* and its relatives to express human anxieties about the transgression of corporeal boundaries, see Segal (1990, 144–52).

and ensuing rot that accompanies violent slaughter on Italian soil (*A.* 8.487; 9.472; cf. 8.197).[18] On the other hand, Tacitus' *Georgic* phrasing and its embedding within an agricultural context interprets Vergil's Noric plague as especially appropriate for connoting the consequences of civil war. Such use, what we might describe as an early reception of *tabum* in the *Georgics*, looks beneath the metaphorical veneer of disease and focuses on the gruesome costs of human conflict it implies.

As fluid and viscous substances, *tabum* and the *fluvidus liquor* it produces in the limbs gesture toward liquefaction as both the cause and the result of the epidemic, though Vergil also emphasizes the violent oppositions that accompany such a process. As Harrison notes (1979, 8), liquefaction is Vergil's innovation, a "fresh horror all his own," and a "clinical paradox" not mentioned by Lucretius as a symptom of the Athenian plague. Where the poet of *De Rerum Natura* couples external signs of the body's decay with language of internal dissolution, as "all the bolts of life did totter" (*omnia tum vero vitae claustra lababant*, 6.1153), Vergil intensifies the liquidity of the organs and their transgression of boundaries (*abundabat*, 3.484) in order to juxtapose these symptoms with parched shriveling (*ignea sitis adduxerat*, 483–4) and create the "paradox" Harrison observes.

Non simplex, then, glosses the contradictory nature of the symptoms of the disease and underscores the conditions of a body at war with itself. The poet offers a more explicit demonstration of self-destruction later in his account of the plague's epidemiology: wine, touted as a remedy for the disease, compels horses to rend their own limbs with their teeth. Putnam observes (1979, 223) how the self-cannibalism inflicted by the sick and maddened steed reflects a "diseased self-destruction of the body politic" that "can readily be understood as an allegory for deadly civil strife in which brother maims brother." Such explicitly self-destructive behavior is an anomaly within the larger description of plague's effects on the animal population, and yet it is an appropriate outward reflection of the internal symptoms, expressed as conflicts, already at work within the bodies of the ill.

[18] *A*.8.487 and 9.472 refer to Mezentius' bizarre practice of binding living and dead bodies together, and the impaled heads of Nisus and Euryalus, respectively; at *A*.8.197 the word describes gore/decay oozing from the faces of men killed by Cacus and posted at the entrance of his cave.

As West notes (1979, 71), the origins, dissemination, and symptoms of Vergil's Noric plague are frustratingly opaque, if poetically evocative. Still, scholars have identified in *Georgics* 3 a standard structure of "narrating the plague" established in medical treatises and also evident in Thucydides and Lucretius (Farrell 1991, 84): thus his aetiology and symptomatology are predictably followed by epidemiology.[19] Vergil spends the majority of his account attending to the impact of the disease on the livestock population, as well as the way in which the suffering of the livestock impinges on the human community: the poet initially describes the failed sacrifice (presumably of a heifer or young bull) that looks forward to further devastation (486–93); he then remarks on generally erratic behavior among the flocks and herds, the malaise of a formerly proud racehorse in particular, and a foolhardy attempt, noted above, to cure the disease by administering wine (495–514); in this section the poet draws an especially poignant portrait of a dying bull (515–30). From here, the poet describes how humans must step in to labor over those religious and agricultural duties formerly performed by animals (531–6). Widespread destruction among animal species continues, even to marine life (537–45); medical efforts, those practiced by well-known mythological healers, resoundingly fail, and the fury Tisiphone is left free reign over Noricum (546–58). It is only in closing that the third *Georgic* looks to the plague's manifestation among the human populace: with startling efficiency, the plague seizes upon those who try on animal skins; in a kind of closure that promises to undo itself, Vergil's plague leaves a *sacer ignis* eating away at human limbs (*artus*, 566), recalling the very *sitis ignea* that wasted the limbs of livestock at the start of the account (482–3).

But before this non-ending, let us return to the beginning of Vergil's epidemiology. The poet's description of a failed sacrifice is the first human response to the plague, one that orients us to view from the perspective of a perplexed *sacerdos*—later referred to as a *vates*, a term

[19] Vergil's variations on the symptoms given in Lucretius indicate that he consulted some medical treatises independently of Lucretius; see Farrell (1991, 85). A similar structure governs plague narratives in contemporary film and novels, though Stephen Soderbergh's film *Contagion* (2011) is noteworthy for positioning revelation of the source of contagion (a strain of birdflu) conspicuously at the end of the film.

with particular literary resonance during the Augustan era[20]—the suffering experienced by a sacrificial calf, from whom only a meager (*ieiuna*) trickle of fluid (*sanies*) stains the sand (3.489–93). For an attempt to divine the will of the gods in a Noric context, the ritual *extispicium* has a peculiarly Roman articulation (Mynors 1990, 251). Where, in Livy's accounts, divine consultation during Rome's early plagues (usually through the Sibylline books, followed by the importation of new cultural practices) results in clear directives, Vergil's sacrifice patently fails to tell his investigator anything of use. As Thomas notes (1988, 132–3), the passage confounds attempts to see a consistently productive alignment between proper religious observance and the success of human *labor*.[21] If a polluted individual dwells among the Noric people, his or her identity and curative function as a scapegoat will not be revealed by traditional divination. Moreover, if we are inclined to see the Augustan poet behind this particular *vates*, the passage speaks to his reticence or even impotence to divine, interpret, and correct the plight of contagion (*nec responsa potest consultus reddere vates*, 3.491).

If the Noric people are guilty of no obvious transgression, it is also true that the moral transgression looming the largest in the poem as a whole is that of civil war, whose stationing of identical arms on the battlefield (*paribus . . . telis*) throws the age into confusion (*everso saeclo*) and invokes the wrath of the gods in Book 1 (1.489, 500). To make sense of the widespread disaster in *Georgics* 3 we might put aside the immediate question of culpability in Noricum and situate the crisis within the poem's implied narrative recounting Rome's early (but already compromised) virtues, its recent calamities, and its post-Actium prospects. Vergil's constant recourse to the myth of the ages as a way of charting the vagaries of Roman development encourages us to recognize similar language in the cattle plague and

[20] On the Augustan resonance of the term and the role of the *vates* in this passage, see Newman (1967, 26–8), who stresses the interpreter's lack of culpability in the disaster.

[21] *Contra* Harrison (1979), who argues that the role of the gods is critical to understanding Vergil's plague. See also Farrell (1991, 94), whose analysis of Vergil's *oppositio in imitando* of Lucretius in the passage suggests a "view of religion . . . as grim and dissatisfied as anything in *De Rerum Natura*"; Liebeschuetz (1965, 75–7) also stresses the absence of any role assigned to the gods in the plague, reflecting their general disinterest in human affairs. Cf. Gale (1991, 424): "in the face of such calamities, no certainty is possible, and all one can do is continue to 'venerate the gods' with no guarantee of success."

orient it in eschatological terms. Readers of *Georgics* 1 observe a teleology of human progress, as *ars* is developed and implicitly limited. In particular, the famous theodicy of Jupiter explains certain threats to human welfare, such as the serpent, that serve to necessitate the progress of civilization (*G*. 1.121–46). Within the course of Book 2, Italy initially assumes a quasi-Golden-Age status (in the famous *laudes Italiae*, 2.136–76), a status that it will by the end of the book reluctantly shed, as the poet reminds readers of transgressions leading to the end of Saturn's rule (532–40). Just prior to the discussion of disease in Book 3, we are reminded of the threat to livestock posed by various types of snakes (3.414–39), a threat invoked again by the serpentine movement of contagion (*serpant*, 3.469) and very much at home in the Iron-Age conditions that introduce the Noric plague.

As disaster spreads and the internal conflicts that riddle the bodies of plague victims gradually play themselves out, however, intimations of a new age emerge. The poet draws a poignant intersection between the lives of farmer and flock, as the *tristis arator* abandons his plough and relinquishes the Iron-Age *labor* imposed by Jupiter. As a composite of the *grandis arator* and *tristis sator* whose perspective on unceasing *labor* frames a world in decline in Book 2 of *DRN* (2.1164–74), Vergil's ploughman signals the epochal evolution witnessed by his predecessors, but that evolution is ironically reversed. Readers of the third *Georgic* behold various *adynata* ("impossibilities"), the marvelous denial of threatening animal behaviors, which suggest that this plague-ridden world has returned to the Golden Age. As birds and sea creatures abandon their natural habitats (541–3; 546–7), predatory animals (wolves and dogs, 537, 540) no longer stalk their accustomed prey (sheep and deer, 537, 539). An eerie peace ensues, though it is a tranquility achieved through death rather than concord. Most strikingly, the snake that metaphorically ushers in contagion will die out, the clearest possible evocation of the Golden Age (Thomas 1988, 142).

Additionally, the suffering of cattle and other infected species is juxtaposed with those markers of abundance and satiety that characterize a primitive Golden-Age existence: *hinc laetis vituli vulgo moriuntur in herbis/et dulcis animas plena ad praesepia reddunt* (3.494–5, "from here calves die everywhere amidst thriving grass and they give up their sweet spirits before full troughs"). Again, evocation of the Golden Age here is problematic—for a feeding trough to be full, some farmer had to fill it. But the bounty of the passage does point to a world that no longer needs *improbus labor.* This kind of plenty is revived after a poignant description of a bull and his *frater* collapsing at the plough: in such circumstances, "shade of lofty groves fails to please, as do soft meadows and cool rivers" (*non umbrae altorum nemorum, non mollia possunt/prata movere animum*, 3.520–1). The world is restored to a condition where the earth seems to provide all things *nullo poscente* ("with no one demanding," 1.128), quite possibly because there is no one left to demand.

As Harrison observes (1979, 20–1), the return to the Golden Age in lines 535–47, signaled primarily through the mollified behavior of traditional predatory animals, rekindles the relationship between the *Georgics* and Horace's *Epodes*: Vergil's language of sheep now free from the threat of wolves and serpents recalls the seventh and the sixteenth *Epodes*, both of which depict the horrors of civil war, epitomized in *Epode* 7 by the slaughter of Remus (7.19–20), as endemic of an Iron-Age existence. In the vision of an alternate, blessed realm in the sixteenth *Epode*, "neither does the evening bear groan and circle around the sheepfold, nor does the ground swell high with vipers" (*nec vespertinus circumgemit ursus ovile/neque intumescit alta viperis humus*, 16.51–2).[22] Harrison reads the intertexuality as one way the *Georgics* poet develops his view of the efficacy of orthodox Roman religious practice, in contrast to the failed ritual observances in Noricum.[23] But the more immediate effect of the references to Horace's adumbrations of the Golden Age within the narrative of the Noric plague is to invoke the conditions of civil war and its central paradox: fiercely contested internal divisions must ultimately yield to a world without divisions, that is, to a pristine condition before the first boundary-line was drawn: *ne signare quidem aut partiri limite campum fas erat*, *G*.1.126–7.

[22] The passage in *Epode* 7, also addressing animals traditionally viewed as threatening, underscores the madness of civil war: at least these animals, unlike Horace's Roman contemporaries, do not turn against each other (*neque hic lupis mos nec fuit leonibus/numquam nisi in dispar feris*, 7.11–12).

[23] For Harrison (1979, 21–8), the verbal echoes between *Epode* 7 and *Georgics* 3 (esp. *sacer*) point to the impiety of the people of Noricum. On the whole, his arguments that the population experiences a plague because they have failed to expiate an offence against the gods are unconvincing, not least because Vergil is so evasive about any crime committed and relatively thorough in depicting their attempts to divine the will of the gods.

Vergil's inversion of the Golden Age thus has the effect of undoing the cultural progress that was achieved in the famous theodicy of Jupiter in Book 1, where the upside of harsh labor was the productivity of human arts. If the original theodicy prompted humankind's gradual distinction from and dominance over the natural world, the plague has the effect—as Gale (1991, 418; cf. 2000, 127–8) and others note—of erasing the hard won boundaries between human and animal.[24] This erasure of distinctions is observed most readily in the description of human devotees of Juno who must pull their own cart to perform worship of the goddess; other humans are reduced to tilling their own fields, scraping the hard earth with their fingernails. The moral implications of this reversion to a Golden-Age existence are problematic; as Perkell notes, "[h]ere, although without technology, man does not attain a new innocence, but a new barbarism . . . The poet has taken up conventional Golden Age features in successive isolation and permutation and finely revealed thereby what is absent—a spark of willed mutuality and illumined purpose" (1989, 123). That sense of collective purpose will emerge later in the *Georgics,* in the aftermath of a similar disaster, in conditions that point to positive recuperation of the Golden Age; but it remains conspicuously absent from Vergil's account of suffering in Book 3. Here, the cumulative effect of Golden-Age imagery is to evoke an atmosphere of devastation.

While any collapse of the existing Iron-Age order might also point to the promise of a fundamental restructuring, of a clean slate upon which a new order might be inscribed, the poet leaves indelible traces of casualties in the process. At the very moment where Vergil's disease in Noricum is undoing the divisions between human and animal *corpora,* the poet also inserts a reminder of the distinctions, here familial and fraternal, that govern human relationships:

> ecce autem duro fumans sub vomere taurus
> concidit et mixtum spumis vomit ore cruorem
> extremosque ciet gemitus. it tristis arator
> maerentem abiungens fraterna morte iuvencum,
> atque opere in medio defixa reliquit aratra.
> (*G.* 3.515–19)

[24] Liebeschuetz (1965) suggests that parallels between humans and animals in Vergil evolve primarily from the poet's observations of their fundamental similarities. Thomas (1988, 141) notes of line 536, "now man takes on the image of the beast."

Behold the bull, seething under the hard plough, falls and spews forth blood mixed with foam and stirs up his final groans. The disheartened farmer, separating the grieving bull from his dying brother, goes and abandons his plough left stuck in the middle of its task.

Amidst universal collapse, readers of the poem encounter the perspective of the individual, defined primarily by grief over the loss of kin. To better understand the concept of the individual that Vergil articulates here in relation to the collective, we can turn to Lucretius, whose second book of *De Rerum Natura* balances the similar properties of all atoms against their variations required to construct recognizable entities.[25] As Farrell has shown (1991, 90–1),[26] Vergil's portrait of the yoke-mates is inspired in part by Lucretius' (famously "anti-Lucretian") illustration of how atomic variations create distinctions among individuals, a sentimental portrait of a mother cow searching for her recently slaughtered *vitulus* ("calf"). Lucretius' account of the bereaved cow juxtaposes the experience of recognition with the grief ensuing from failure to recognize (2.352–70). Where the Epicurean explicitly links the experience of the mother cow mourning the loss of her calf to that of all species, including humans (2.351), Vergil capitalizes on the so-called pathetic fallacy here to suggest a crisis that can be readily converted into human terms (Farrell 1991, 91).

And yet it is significant that Vergil has reformulated a drama of recognition and loss shared between mother and child into one shared between brothers, a revision that again prompts us to convert the sufferings of disease into those of civil war. As Bannon argues in her study of brotherhood in Rome, just as fraternal *pietas* was often viewed as an expression of loyalty to Rome, the inverse was also true: in the civil strife of the late Republic, "fraternal *pietas* took on new metaphorical dimensions. Instead of emphasizing fraternal solidarity, civil war narratives focused on brothers fighting brothers, and dramatic scenes of fratricide came to epitomize the experience of civic strife" (1997, 137). For Bannon, the vignette of the dying bull, phrased in distinctively human terms (*fraterna morte*), expresses the failure of a cooperative spirit that healthy fraternity had come to symbolize;

[25] *Qualia sint et quam longe distantia formis/percipe* 2.334–5, "see (the *primordia*) what kind they are and how much they differ in shape."

[26] Cf. West (1979, 10), who also detects echoes of the Lucretian passage in Vergil's scene of failed sacrifice earlier in the plague narrative.

such a loss in turn "expresses the loss inherent in civil war" (147). Unlike other representations of brotherhood in the poem, however, the sorrow and innocence ascribed to the bulls illuminates rather than negates their mutual *pietas*.

Though the adjective *fraternus* is found only here in the poem, three of the five uses of *frater* in the *Georgics* come at the end of Book 2,[27] where the speaker famously praises the life of the *felix arator*, who lives far from the civil strife that plagues Rome and the "discord driving on faithless brothers" (*flexit et infidos agitans discordia fratres*, 496).[28] The happy farmer does not seek the *Urbs* (Rome), unlike the nameless wretch, *hic*, who betrays country and kinsmen for wealth:

> hic petit excidiis urbem miserosque penates,
> ut gemma bibat et Sarrano dormiat ostro;
> condit opes alius defossoque incubat auro.
> hic stupet attonitus rostris; hunc plausus hiantem
> per cuneos geminatus enim plebisque patrumque
> corripuit; gaudent perfusi sanguine fratrum,
> exsilioque domos et dulcia limina mutant
> atque alio patriam quaerunt sub sole iacentem.
> (*G.* 2.505–12)

This one sets upon his city and his wretched household gods with destruction, in order to drink from a jeweled cup and sleep on Tyrian purple; another stores away wealth and hovers over buried gold. This one is stupefied, thunderstruck at the rostra; doubled applause through the theater—for it comes from both the *plebs* and the *patres*—has seized this one, who is open-mouthed with wonder; those splattered with the blood of brothers rejoice, and they exchange their homes and sweet thresholds for exile and seek a fatherland lying under another sun.

If we have missed Vergil's emphasis on a distinctly fraternal strife that seizes upon (*corripuit*) Rome, just as disease threatens to seize upon the flock in Book 3 (*corripiunt*, 3.472), we will be reminded of just how well-woven civil discord is within the fabric of Roman tradition: happy as those quasi-Golden-Age farmers are at the end of Book 2, their plenitude is bound by Remus and his *frater* who preside over it

[27] *Fratres* in Book 1 (*G.*1.280) refer to the giants of myth who attacked heaven and placed Olympus on top of Ossa and Pelion; and to Phoebus, brother of Luna/Diana (*G.* 1.396).

[28] Mynors (1990,169–70) finds the reference to civil strife misplaced here in light of its recap in line 510, though concedes its possibility and cites parallels for this kind of *discordia* (*E.*1.71; *G.* 2.459, 4.68, and esp. *A.* 6.608, *invisi fratres*).

(*G.* 2.533), the latter of whom is destined to commit Rome's foundational act of civic bloodshed. I offer this digression on the second *Georgic*'s closing vision as evidence that we cannot read the reference to a brother's death in Book 3 without brushing up against the political context in which fraternal bonds have been articulated thus far in the poem. As the foundational slaughter of Remus indicates, brotherhood in the Roman imagination exists as measure of how precarious the claims of the individual are in relation to the greater good of the community, and how rivalry over limited resources and *honores* will constantly assert itself.[29]

As observed earlier with reference to Lucretius' depictions of interfamilial violence,[30] brotherhood bears a special relationship to the plague narrative broadly conceived in the Western tradition. Brothers, as virtual doubles in terms of age, status, gender, and claims to authority, signal at a universal level the strife among equals that, according to Girard, constantly threatens the social order; narratives of contagion and cure are written to address and resolve the proliferation of doubles. Vergil's metaphoric use of pestilence to recapitulate Rome's long history of civil strife would seem to neatly fit the bill that Girard uses to address how plague narratives function to recognize and neutralize reciprocal violence as a means of stabilizing the community (Girard 1974, 836–41). All the same, the Mantuan poet dispenses with facile resolutions to such strife by rewriting brotherhood through the dying *tauri* as an empathetic and harmonious, if ultimately tragic, relationship—and one whose latent frictions are patently not resolved in Book 3 by the expulsion of any individual identified as a scapegoat.

The relationship between the *tauri* constitutes Vergil's final portrait of individual suffering among the livestock, and is punctuated by brief comment on the bull's innocence and the futility of his *labores* in the face of death (3.525). To conclude his epidemiology, the poet addresses those fantastical, Golden-Age inversions of formerly hostile relationships, discussed above, that now define the animal realm. Just as the symptomatology of the plague, initially driven by conflict, resolved itself in a brutal eradication of difference, at level of

[29] For the threat of division (embodied in the figure of the double) as characteristic of Roman foundation narratives, especially in epic poetry, see Hardie (1993, 10), discussed further below; cf. Armstrong (2002, 327).

[30] See above, Chapter 3, pp. 106–7.

epidemiology Noricum experiences a process by which old oppositions are neutralized through morbidity and death rather than concord. The end result of this process is the obliteration of personal identity and interpersonal relationships among heaps of *cadavera*. The conclusion of Book 3 uses a decidedly Lucretian term, *catervatim* (*DRN* 6.1144), for piling up corpses in the stables, an echo of the Lucretian term for breaking things down used earlier, *minutatim* (Thomas 1988, 144), which in conjunction suggest a ruthlessly systematic process of deterioration:

> iamque catervatim dat stragem atque aggerat ipsis
> in stabulis turpi dilapsa cadavera tabo,
> donec humo tegere ac foveis abscondere discunt
> nam neque erat coriis usus, nec viscera quisquam
> aut undis abolere potest aut vincere flamma.
> ne tondere quidem morbo inluvieque peresa
> vellera nec telas possunt attingere putris:
> verum etiam invisos si quis temptarat amictus,
> ardentes papulae atque immundus olentia sudor
> membra sequebatur, nec longo deinde moranti
> tempore contactos artus sacer ignis edebat.
> (*G*.3.556–66)

And now she [Tisiphone] piles up in heaps and even in the stables themselves bodies decayed with foul putrescence, until they learn to cover the corpses with earth and hide them in trenches. For there was no use for the hides, nor was anyone able to destroy or do away with the innards (or "flesh") by water or fire. Indeed they were able neither to shear the fleeces corroded by disease and unwashed nor to touch the rotting warps: but if anyone tried on the accursed garments, burning sores and filthy sweat pursued their pungent limbs, and not long from then did the sacred fire eat away at their contaminated limbs.

Herein lies the only lesson learned by the Noric farmer from the plague, the proper disposal of bodies. It is a trope repeatedly performed in plague dramaturgy: the burial of the dead—abbreviated, along with all those other hallmarks of individualism—is written into accounts of contagion from Thucydides in the fifth century to Camus' account of the dispensaries in plague-besieged Oran, constantly burning and grimly haunted with echoes of Nazi crematoria.

Vergil's closure, hiding bodies under layers of earth, is never complete, but instead issues a new (and yet strangely familiar) narrative of plague's effects on the human community. With "foul putrescence" (*turpi tabo*) we again confront the source of contagion in Noricum that lurked in ponds and feeding troughs (cf. 3.481); moreover, "contaminated limbs" (*contactos artus*), signaling inevitable outbreak in the human community, recalls not only the liquefaction caused by the disease in the limbs (*artus*) of animals (cf. 3.483), but also the caveats introducing the plague. The derivation from *contingo* shared by *contagia* (3.469) and *contactus* summons us back to the preface to plague in Noricum, in which Vergil weighs the *contagia* that threaten the flock against the suffering of a single listless sheep. By invoking the "contagion" of civil unrest that has prompted the wanderings of Meliboeus in the *Eclogues* and Horace's *pia gens* in the *Epodes*, the *Georgics* poet invokes an already scripted eschatology that anticipates a new age to remedy current Iron-Age conditions. At the same time, the book's conclusion observes a repetitive strand of contagion fragmenting without any foreseeable *telos*.[31]

Vergil's artistry, his careful piling up and breaking down of infected bodies, demonstrates what some scholars have identified as a hallmark of the post-apocalyptic narrative, its dramaturgy of interminable piecemeal suffering. Such evocations of suffering bear political implications, and not just in the sense that any writing *after* an apocalyptic event—such as the plague that Vergil positions himself after (*quondam*, 478)—is generated from a diagnostic impulse, a critique of the existing social order (Berger 1999, 7). Gomel links the entropy of the post-apocalyptic narrative to the peculiar conditions of civil war. In its protracted experience of dying together, the body politic coalesces: "Civil war destroys the fragile balance of the body politic and yet at the same time confirms itself as a self-defined entity. The communal body of the plague . . . only comes into its existence at the moment of its impending dissolution" (2000, 417). Vergil will resume disease and its reflections on the fractured body politic in Book 4, forcing coalescence in the aftermath of a *morbus* (*G.* 4.318) that afflicts the apian community in the shape of a new hive born from the *bougonia*; but for the moment we are left lingering, poised for the worst-case scenario. Vergil's plague has dramatized the dissolution of discrete *corpora* and, through imagery that alludes to the unbound satiety of the Golden Age, orchestrated a collapse of those Iron-Age structures in which both civic and individual *corpora* had traditionally found a home.

[31] Precisely what Lucretius has left us with, whether intentionally or not. On the closure of Lucretius' poem, see Chapter 3, pp. 79–81.

4.2. BEES AND THE BODY POLITIC

At the beginning of the fourth *Georgic*, following immediately on the heels of the plague, Vergil introduces his topic, honey and the bees that produce it, a "marvelous spectacle of a tiny world" (*admiranda levium spectacula rerum*, *G*.4.3). The role of Vergil's anthropomorphic bees and their relationship to the Roman people has been thoughtfully discussed;[32] Jasper Griffin (1979) in particular has highlighted certain un-Roman, as well as inhuman qualities of the bees, despite the many advantages of their collective, communal existence (*omnibus una quies operum, labor omnibus unus*, 4.184). Neville Morley notes the tendency of a number of Roman authors (e.g., Pliny the Elder, Columella, Varro) to project Roman conflicts, and that of civil war in particular, onto their observations of the hive, and is especially concerned with how these authors variously explain the problem of conflict resolution—that is, whether they invoke the necessity of a beekeeper to enact a resolution and restore peace. Vergil's demand for a beekeeper to manage an internal crisis has the effect of fracturing the analogy between apian and human communities, which notably lack a beekeeper: "Vergil's account is thus a less realizable model and more an image of unattainable peace and simplicity . . . if only human society could be managed like a beehive" (2007, 464; cf. Miles 1980, 235).

If, however, we press the often-recognized identification between Aristaeus and Augustus, and its attendant implications for leadership in the wake of Actium, we might view Augustus as a bee-keeper for Rome (a formerly superior bee whose ontological status has shifted to *pastor* by the end of the poem; cf. *G*.4.317). Such an identification is corroborated by a simile in the *Aeneid* which will cast the eponymous hero (another doppelgänger for Augustus) as a shepherd (*pastor*, *A*.12.587) who smokes out unwanted bees as they frantically emit a

[32] Herrmann (1931) argued for a specific correspondence between the bees of the fourth *Georgic* and the participants of Actium. Following that lead, Nadeau has interpreted the *bougonia* as a symbol of the brutality and bloodshed of the civil wars leading up to Actium (1984, 67). Other critics have taken a more generalizing approach to the parallels between human beings and Vergil's bees; see, e.g., Otis (1995, reprint of 1964,181–90); Johnston (1980, 90–105); Thomas (1982, 70–92); Ross (1987, 207–14); Habinek (1990, 210–12).

loud buzzing from a rocky enclave (12.586–92). The hive, in turn, represents the citizens of Laurentum, in a state of civil strife (*trepidos inter discordia civis,* 12.583) upon realizing their walls are under assault and uncertain as to the best response. Augustus' power to resolve internal conflicts is predicted by the poet's elevation of his textual analogues from a position as superior within the bee community to figures presiding over it and ridding it of unwanted elements. Beyond the scope of allegorical correspondence, however, we can also draw from the apian community lessons about the relationship between individual desires and collective behaviors, lessons that once again interrupt rather than confirm the identification between Romans and bees. The ancient understanding of industry and devotion to the hive among bees is equivocal, both in the fourth *Georgic* and throughout the tradition of Greco-Roman lore on insect kingdoms. The uniformity of these diminutive creatures exists in distinct tension with some individualizing characteristics, a tension dramatized in Vergil's poem through the conflict that flares up between the superior or "better" (*melior,* 4.92) king of the hive and his rogue adversary (*ille horridus alter,* 4.93). Thus, if uniformity and a collective spirit are the bees' most striking qualities, Vergil tempers those qualities with occasional hints of self-serving individualism. Although the poet upholds bees as divine and worthy of emulation (149–209), Book 4 also finds in their battles (*proelia,* 4.4) a didactic impetus equal to that which compels his instruction on their "customs, pursuits, and peoples" (*mores, studia* and *populi,* 4.5). Vergil's reduction of such battles to those surrounding one resplendent king and his *alter*, moreover, manipulates the process of rivalry and expulsion that, as noted above, from Girard's perspective haunts the metaphoric resonance of plague throughout the Western tradition. The "two leaders" (*ambo ductores,* 4.88) of the hive, though making claim to equal honors, are drawn as foils, whose followers mimic the same antithetical and recognizable qualities, sloth and deformity on one side, as opposed to industriousness and splendor on the other (4.95). The gravity with which *discordia* strikes the *duo reges* (4.67–8), at least from the apian perspective, underscores the problems of evaluating superiority within the Roman social order and resolving the imitative conflicts that had plagued its recent history (cf. Girard 1974, 836).

Despite the mere handful of dust needed to check violence between warring factions, Vergil frequently betrays the tenuous stability of the hive. On the one hand, the apian community shares the rewards of its exceptional *labor*:

> et patriam solae et certos novere penates,
> venturaeque hiemis memores aestate laborem
> experiuntur et in medium quaesita reponunt.
> (4.155–7)

They alone know a fatherland and fixed gods of the hearth (*penates*), and mindful of the coming winter they tend to their work in the summer, and they put aside for the common store what they have gained.

Virtually unique (*solae*) in their collective recognition of household gods and fatherland, the bees assume such Golden-Age harmony that some critics have viewed them as emblematic of a modified, "agriculturally-oriented" Golden Race (cf. *G.* 1.127, *in medium quaerebant*).[33] The better ones gleam with gold (4.91, 99) and devote their lives to production of that Golden-Age staple, honey (1.131), all while sharing a single mind (*una mens*, 4.212) under the guidance of a king. As a response to the perverted Golden Age in Noricum, the poet here summons the conditions of a relatively orthodox *aurea aetas*.

At the same time, when the king of this community is harmed, faith is summarily broken. The bees, moreover, must internally check the loitering of those who resist the battle call, or as drones (4.167–8) idly consume the produce of the hive, while a beekeeper is required to check those bees whose "lingering" in shade (28) might hinder collective efforts. The bees also exhibit an innate "love of gain" (*amor habendi*, *G.* 4.177), the very greed that is coupled with the madness of war in the *Aeneid* and, according to Evander, marks the decline from Saturn's Golden Age in Italy (*A.* 8.327; Perkell 2002, 27; O'Hara 2007, 101). The bees mentioned in the *Aeneid* assume a similarly ambiguous guise: their collective spirit is implicitly praised as reflecting Carthaginian prosperity (*A.*1.430–6), but the role of a

[33] More precisely, Johnston (1980, esp.104–5) views the poet's emphasis on cattle in Book 3 and bees in Book 4 as working together to prescribe a Golden Race (the bees) based on an agricultural existence (symbolized by cattle). As Mynors (1990, 179; cf. Thomas 1988, 176) observes, *solae* exaggerates the unique status of bees, since the ancients were aware of other, if "universally unpopular," species like wasps and hornets. The ant was considered by some to be economically, rather than civically oriented, though Ovid's use of the ant rather than the bee as a model for collective behavior in the aftermath of disease reflects on important similarities between the two species; see Chapter 5, pp. 179–81.

"sudden swarm" (*examen subitum*) as prophetically signaling to Latinus the arrival of the Trojan *agmen* is hardly benign (*A*.7.64–70), at least from the native Italian perspective. If a drive to preserve the "hope of the race" (*spem gentis*, *G*.4.162) defines the collective and ultimately trumps the interests of individual lives of bees (*ipsae*, 206), such a drive is by no means innate, and must be cultivated both internally and externally.

One problem with Vergil's bees as a model for human existence, and for human suffering in the context of plague—a problem made more apparent when their representation is compared with that of dying livestock in *Georgics* 3—is that they lack unique identities. As Vallillee notes (1960, 94), in turning to the event of disease within the hive, Vergil directs us to Lucretius' portrayal of plague in Athens by comparing the apian crisis to *morbus* in humans (*quoniam casus apibus quoque nostros/vita tulit*, 4.251–2) and in using the verb *langueo*, found in *De Rerum Natura* as an indication of the spiritual malaise that afflicts those recently stricken. And yet, where Lucretius uses the verb to shift his focus from individuals succumbing to illness (6.1157) to families entangled in death (6.1254) to groups of farmers languishing in a collective crisis (6.1260), Vergil keeps his eye on the hive. The death of the bees in *Georgics* 4 is rendered with a few poignant details (4.251–9), but we observe them functioning constantly as a unit[34]—even those who linger listlessly (4.257, prompting comparison with the sickly sheep in Book 3), do so as part of a group: Vergil repeatedly uses the third-person plural to describe the activities of sick bees; no individual bees are identified and his epidemiology is capped by similes that confine pathological behavior to single sounds, either that of the south wind or the "troubled sea" or a "devouring flame" (4.260–3). In sickness the beekeeper recognizes symptoms and behaviors collectively, just as in health he observes the activity of the *agmen* (59), *vulgus* (69), or *plebs* (95).

It is precisely this collective portrayal that will give us pause when we weigh the cost of the apian renewal against the slaughter of an individual required to procure it. The miracle of the *bougonia* is presented with some skepticism by the *Georgics* poet after he broaches the topic of the hive's destruction (*G*. 4.281–5; cf. Thomas 1988, 196; Ross 1987, 218). Born originally in exotic Egypt, the practice

[34] With the obvious exception of their king and his adversary, mentioned above.

may be gradually Romanized in the course of the epyllion,[35] but it remains a *monstrum* that relies immediately on the death of a single calf, whose body must maintain a perverse kind of integrity, with its orifices blocked and hide unbroken throughout its destruction (*huic geminae nares et spiritus oris multa reluctanti obstruitur*; *per integram... pellem*, 301–2): the resultant creation is a marvel of striking uniformity, though, as noted at the start of this chapter, its potential remains decidedly ambiguous.

The *bougonia*, described prior to the Aristaeus epyllion, varies significantly from the ritual performed by Aristaeus at the end of the poem in atonement for the deaths of Orpheus and Eurydice. The odd circumstances of the procedure described at the conclusion to Book 4 have been defended by Habinek, who, interpreting them through the lens of a Greek sacrificial model, argues that the poet has created a "unifying and re-creative social phenomenon" (1990, 215). Thomas has challenged his argument, observing not only that such a Greek model bore little if any resonance for contemporary Romans, but also that the only proper sacrifice in the poem is that performed by the people of Noricum in Book 3. More recently, Feeney has questioned the very attempt to identify ritual orthodoxy in a text—that is, textual representation of a ritual faithfully reflecting the "real" context of Roman life: literary evocations of ritual sacrifice exist precisely to prompt readers to question the meaning and nature of sacrifice (2004, 19).

One effect of sacrificial ritual in the *Georgics*, initially observed by Gale (2000, 101–12), but made especially apparent when refracted through Ovid's allusions to Vergil's poem in the *Fasti*, is its unsettling "denaturalisation." For Feeney, Vergilian sacrifice emerges as:

> A token of the loss of the Golden Age, as the life of agriculture involves humans endlessly dominating the land and the animals that share it with us, and endlessly placating certain deities by giving them many varieties of animal life. Human life is denaturalised, and sacrifice must be endlessly repeated in order to stave off the everpresent threat of having to pay the full consequence of that denaturalisation.
>
> (Feeney 2004, 16)

If we opt for this interpretation, the violence and dissolution emphasized by the *Georgics* poet in his depiction of the *bougonia* is precisely

[35] On Vergil's sources for the *bougonia*, see Habinek (1990, 209, 220).

the point, and one whose Iron-Age implications foreclose any possibility of a permanent return to the Golden Age. Pestilence and sacrifice may restore a broken social order temporarily, but humans will require further violence to keep it so: "the sacrificial imperative behind the life of civilization keeps breaking through" (15).

Both procedures as described at the beginning and end of the epyllion victimize the very creature, a bull, albeit at a different stage of development, whose loss of a brother has earned our sympathies in Book 3's Noric plague. Moreover, the process of dissolution that begets the new hive in both descriptions of the practice are strikingly similar. Like the progress of contagion and symptoms in Vergil's plague, the *bougonia* relies on flesh putrefied and liquefied; from this heap a new race is born: *solvuntur viscera, G.*4.302; *liquefacta boum per viscera, G.*4.555.[36] But within its birth already exist the germs of its deterioration, whether those germs materialize in the mimetic violence of the resplendent bee and his *horridus alter*, or, shifting the analogy to the realm of human *Quirites*, in that of Romulus and Remus: as observed, the brothers are poised momentarily within an *aurea vita* at the close of the second *Georgic*, but bound for the impious sacrificial feast that will mark their fall into an Iron-Age existence and the endemic civil war that defines it (2.532–40).

The sickness and hunger that strike Aristaeus' bees do so to the destruction of the entire hive (*amissis . . . apibus morboque fameque*, 4.318), leaving the mythological founder of the custom at a loss and imprecating his divine parent for aid (*G.*4.320–32). After learning Proteus' account of Orpheus' loss of Eurydice and ultimate failure to resurrect her, Cyrene directs her son to undertake the bloodletting of four exceptional bulls and an equal number of heifers (*quattour eximios . . . tauros/totidem . . . iuvencas*, 538–40). Underlying the narrative of desire, death, and atonement, are hints of Girard's sacrificial logic and conflict between mimetic doubles, embodied in the figures of Orpheus and Aristaeus, both of whom are driven by desire for Eurydice. While the contrasts between Orpheus and Aristeus have been well demonstrated,[37] the similar nature of the crises that

[36] Thomas (1988, 200) remarks on the similar phrasing used to describe the effects of plague (3.484–5) and the disintegrating entrails of the calf.

[37] There is a sizeable bibliography on the Orpheus epyllion and its meaning for the relative virtues of the lover-poet and the statesman-*pastor*. I have been especially influenced by Otis (1964, 144–214), Perkell (1978), Nadeau (1984), Segal (1988, 36–53), and Conte (2001, 123–49).

determine their actions in the poem is also worth recognizing. Structural and verbal echoes speak of parallelism and "doubling" between the two heroes: both come to grief over loss, "lamenting much" (*multa querens* 320; cf. 520), undertake katabasis to consult with divine authority (*gressus*, 360; *ingressus*, 469), and do so in order to create new life or restore life lost.

Orpheus' death, mimetically reproduced in the ritual prescribed by Cyrene, temporarily "solves" the problem of disease and the strife it represents. Here we observe the same kind of resolution through violence that Hardie ascribes to the conflict between Aeneas and Turnus in their recurring portrayal as doubles in the *Aeneid* (1993, 21–2).[38] The identification of such an underlying structure in the *Georgics* is to some extent a reductive approach to a tale that, rather than merely replicating antagonists, explores the complex interdependency of two different ways of being in the world. At the same time, interpreting both the Noric plague and the *morbus* that strikes Aristaeus' bees in terms of conflict, contagion, and the possibility of restoration allows us to better comprehend the conditions of uniformity that are both the end result of the disease and its remedy. The Golden Age's distinctive absence of differentiation appropriately signals the brutal destruction of boundaries and homogeneity effected by plague, but the value of that Age, in so far as it is actuated in both dystopic Noricum and Aristaeus' new hive, remains an open question.

The foregoing focus on a Golden-Age collapse of boundaries and a uniformity that depends upon destruction and decay, evident throughout the *Georgics* and drawn in part from late-Republican poetic discourses, has shed light on how Vergil uses plague to reflect on the dynamics of Roman civil war. We have observed possible solutions to the problem of disease as well as their costs, as the poet constantly weighs the interests of the individual against those of the

[38] See also Bandera (1981) for Aeneas and Turnus as doubles: his essay uses Girard's model to explore not only why so many sympathetic characters in the poem are presented as sacrifices to Roman *imperium*, but also to understand why sacrifice is assumed to be necessary in the first place: "why should such a 'terrible price' be paid? How did human suffering ever become something valuable or productive?" (222). Following Bandera, Hardie (1993) invokes Girard's model of a cultural order founded on sacrifice, as developed further in *Violence and the Sacred* (1977). Hardie notes that, while "as a 'historical' account of cultural origins Girard's model is open to serious doubt," it remains, "a productive tool for the analysis of imperial epic. If Girard is in the end a mythologist rather than an anthropologist, his is a mythology that seems to have been shared by Romans of the early Principate" (21).

collective. The birth of indistinguishable bees, devoted to homeland, hearth, and the acquisition of honey, is hardly a satisfactory remedy for the contagion afflicting the people of Noricum, about to be reduced, along with their livestock, to heaps of indistinguishable *cadavera*. Sacrificial logic may provide a quick fix to internal conflict, but the necessity of its repetition speaks to its inadequacy as a way of organizing human life. Interpreted within the Roman historical context, Vergil's corresponding treatments of disease in the *Georgics* address civil war as the result of pathological rivalries among members of the aristocracy in the mid-first century BCE and propose, in the wake of Actium's turbulent waters, caveats as well as alternatives for the process of recovery.

My reading of the Noric plague thus keeps company with approaches to the *Georgics* that have emphasized Vergil's tendency to create ambiguities of meaning or "indeterminacies"; more recently, critics have acknowledged those ambiguities, but reframed them as "problems to be solved" (Nappa 2005, 15). While the poet as *magister* may advertise his role as healer,[39] explicitly of animal *corpora* and implicitly of the Roman civic corpus, it is also characteristically Vergilian to indicate the limits of poetic authority: if the *artes* of legendary healers Chiron and Melampus failed the Noric people, we are given little to suggest the Mantuan poet's *remedia*, offered to the Italian shepherd in the event of a single listless sheep, would have had a similar efficacy in the context of the corrupt atmosphere that seizes Noricum. The reticence of the Noric *vates* in reading the signs before him speaks volumes.

4.3. CODA: THE CRETAN PLAGUE OF *AENEID 3*

If we conceive of the poem as a whole, whose answers to questions concerning the human condition lay at least partly in its linear arrangement of material, then the fourth *Georgic*'s loyal and acquisitive bees are revealed as one solution to the problem of epidemic disease in the third. Aristaeus' bees are not Vergil's final word on the problem of plague, however, for he revisits the topic, lending it more

[39] On Vergil's invocation of poetry's power to heal, drawn from Lucretian as well as Greek Hellenistic models, see Hawkins (2019).

explicit implications for the foundation of Roman *imperium*, in the *Aeneid*. In *Aeneid* 3, the hero narrates an attempted settlement at Crete, one of his many stops along the route from Troy. The Trojans misinterpret an oracle of Apollo at Delos (*A*.3.94–117) and mistakenly identify Crete as a new Pergamum, intending to settle there:

> ergo avidus muros optatae molior urbis
> pergameamque voco, et laetam cognomine gentem
> hortor amare focos arcemque attollere tectis.
> iamque fere sicco subductae litore puppes;
> conubiis arvisque novis operata iuventus;
> iura domosque dabam: subito cum tabida membris,
> corrupto caeli tractu, miserandaque venit
> arboribusque satisque lues et letifer annus.
> linquebant dulcis animas aut aegra trahebant
> corpora; tum sterilis exurere Sirius agros;
> arebant herbae et victum seges aegra negabat.
> (*A*.3.132–42)

Therefore eagerly I construct walls of the longed for city, and I call it Pergamum, and urge my people, happy with the name, to cherish their homes and to raise a citadel high with roofs. And just now were ships drawn up upon the dry shore; and I was giving homes and laws, when suddenly a pitiable pestilence corrosive to the limbs came under a corrupt region of heaven, and with it a deadly season for trees and crops; and [Trojans] were relinquishing their dear lives or dragging about their sickly bodies; then Sirius parched lifeless fields; and grass dried up and the sickly crop denied us sustenance.

The corrosive and pitiable nature of the disease (*tabida*; cf. *tabum* *G*.3.481, 557; *miseranda* *G*.3.478), the "dear lives" of the settlers (cf. *G*.3.495), and the evocation of a Golden Age reverting to Iron, when Dodona "denied her sustenance" (*victum Dodona negaret*, *G*.1.149) return us momentarily to the dystopian realm of the third *Georgic*.[40] Again, in the aetiology of the disease, the poet makes overtures to miasma theory before turning his attention to the possibility of divine displeasure. In the *Aeneid*, the source of the *lues et letifer annus* is more easily found: a nocturnal visit from the Penates soon remedies the confusion, directing the Trojans to find their rightful homes in Hesperia, and Aeneas departs from the island.

[40] For verbal echoes and similar phraseology in the two passages, see Williams (1962, 85–6) and Heyworth and Morwood (2017, 123–4).

Readers of the episode have had difficulty situating the Cretan plague either as part of a larger scheme of the epic hero's wanderings (neither Odysseus nor Jason confronts a similar obstacle) or within the traditional lore concerning Aeneas (the stop is unattested elsewhere).[41] Grimm usefully observes that the episode shares with the poem *in toto* its concern with foundations (1965, 60):[42] thus its occurrence functions as "an important stage in the course of progressive initiation" (*eine wichtige Etappe im Verlauf der progressiven Initiation*), in so far as its occurrence returns the Trojans to the task of founding an empire. Grimm also suggests, however, that another form of disaster (e.g., storm, shipwreck) would have proven equally useful in marking this stage in the hero's progress. So we are left to wonder why Vergil uses a pestilence in particular to signal a significant stumbling block on the way to founding Rome.

Reading Aeneas' momentary misstep from a retrograde rather than teleological perspective, Armstrong has noted more recently that Crete offers a "symbol of misdirection" and thus serves as one of many doubles (rivals to Rome's founding) that emerge throughout the poem, the most notable of which is Carthage (2002, 334).[43] Armstrong, moreover, has drawn attention to the link between Crete and the apian community there that harbored Jupiter from Cronus during his infancy—a link that encourages readers to invoke

[41] Dionysius of Halicarnassus, with whom Vergil concurs on a number of stops, does not mention the episode. Servius, ad *Aeneid* 3.133, notes the founding of a new Pergamum recognized *in libris antiquioribus*. Heinze (1993, 78) interprets Servius' comment on the passage to mean that Vergil was following an established tradition. Lloyd (1957, 395), however, notes the ambiguity of Servius' comments, which by no means refer to a tradition that was established prior to the *Aeneid*; his analysis of Book 3 includes the stop at Crete among four Vergilian innovations in the tradition of Aeneas' wanderings. Servius (ad 3.121) also explains that Idomeneus abandoned his kingdom after he had sacrificed his son in accordance with a vow to the gods; a pestilence was visited upon him and his people as a result of the sacrifice. Horsfall (2006, 134) notes that while the plague on Crete is mentioned in Herodotus, its connection with Idomeneus' sacrifice of his son is probably Servius' invention. Regardless of when the story emerged, it is worth observing that at least one reader felt that the entangling of pestilence and sacrifice on Crete was relevant to the losses experienced by Aeneas in his misguided attempt to found a colony there.

[42] Cf. Heinze, who notes that the unity of Book 3 is found in its concern with the gradual revelation of destiny (1993, 69; cf. Lloyd 1957, 388). Horsfall (2006, 134–5) observes in the episode various features conforming to patterns in colonization stories.

[43] See also Heyworth and Morwood (2017, 124–5), who stress the themes of regression and misdirection in the episode and throughout their recent commentary on Book 3.

the association between Trojans and bees, especially the bees who are fortunate in having "homeland and household gods" (*et patriam solae et certos novere penates*, G. 4.155) but also those less fortunate who suffer from disease in the fourth *Georgic* (2002, 323).

If we are meant to recall the epidemic among the apian community in *Georgics* 4, perhaps we are also meant to take courage in the reassurance offered by Aristaeus' success, plague as an opportunity for a fresh start (or a clean sweep, à la Sontag), and to impress the fourth *Georgic*'s pattern of loss and restoration upon the wandering bee-like Trojans of the *Aeneid*. Aeneas' people do not, of course, experience *discordia* and the emergence of rivalry within—their problem is the incorrect interpretation of the gods' will. In this case the source of contention among (near) equals is the claims of both Dardanus and Teucer as *parentes* of the Trojan people (Williams 1962, 92), a kind of rivalry that requires the foreclosing of one ancestral lineage in order to secure the other as the proper home for the correct founding; Anchises recognizes these competing possibilities in remarking on the "two-fold offspring and twin parentage" of the Trojan people (*agnovit prolem ambiguam geminosque parentes*, A.3.180).

At the same time, verbal echoes of the devastation in Noricum, mentioned above, complicate the promise that the fourth *Georgic* holds for the proto-Romans of the *Aeneid*, who must encounter further trials—in a war identified by many accounts as civil (cf. Hardie 1993, 20)—when they reach their rightful Italian home. An impressionistic blur of decay, pitiable human suffering, and saecular evolution leaves the Cretan settlers poised on a threshold between the dissolution of one age and the inception of another that has yet to be realized. I would suggest that in the *Aeneid*'s Cretan episode Vergil offers two windows on the *Georgics*: one views the apparently irrational and irremediable plague suffered by the people of Noricum, while the other views the rational and remedied disease experienced by Aristaeus' bees. The two images juxtapose the possibilities and limitations of a new order, tempering the promise of a New Jerusalem with protracted scorpion stings punctured in the bodies of plague victims, relinquishing their "dear lives" *in perpetuum*, like the blameless calves of Noricum in *Georgics* 3. As Aeneas' vivid narration of continuous action in the past suggests (*dabam, linquebant, trahebant, negabat*), the slate is hardly ever clean with Vergil: duly advised, Aeneas presses onward and away from the island once called home, but not without a few would-be citizens left behind (*paucisque relictis*, 3.190).

5

Ovid's Origin of the Myrmidons and the New Augustan Order

> When the cries of the last human beings on Aegina had ceased, the ant colonies left their oak, flowed down the trunk like water from a cloudburst, spread out in many veins across the charnel fields, and defeating the superior numbers of the flies, took possession of every empty spot, conquered eye sockets, open mouths, bellies, ear chambers and the eye pits left by plague boils. In troops that grew ever denser, they ran to close ranks in these cavities, clotted to form new twitching muscles, eyes, tongues, and hearts, and where limbs had rotted and were missing, they replaced arms and legs with their own bodies. They *became* arms and legs, and at last, formed facial features, for expression and pantomime . . . they became a wholly new race on Aegina, a people who stood under the sign of the ants.
>
> (Christoph Ransmayr, *The Last World*, trans. J. Woods, 1990, 47–8)

Christoph Ransmayr's novelistic treatment of Ovid's exile follows the intriguing thesis that it was the *Metamorphoses,* rather than the *Ars Amatoria*, that provoked the wrath of Augustus and resulted in the poet's banishment to Tomis.[1] In particular, the poet's reading of a passage from Book 7, an account of a devastating plague and the metamorphosis of ants into new citizens on the island of Aegina, gradually causes such a stir among the Roman populace that the Princeps, prompted by an irate bureaucrat, decides the poet's fate, "without a word, with just an abrupt, curt motion of his hand, hardly more than if he were shaking off a housefly" (1990, 54). Ransmayr is

[1] For an early proponent of the thesis, see Rand (1925, 92); cf. Segal (1969, 261).

not writing history, or even literary history, but his reading of the episode as one that might prove offensive, particularly to the underlings and secretaries swarming throughout the Palatine complex, constructs an Imperial response worth pondering.[2] From the perspective of the novel's Princeps, the correlation between *Quirites* and insect swarms is easy enough to make (as we have just seen, Vergil had done as much with bees and ants throughout the *Aeneid*): but what is it about these ants and this king in Ovid's poem, as well as the former population's experience of suffering, that could, at least in the imaginings of one late-twentieth-century novelist, so irritate Augustus and his administration?

In this chapter I argue that Ovid uses Aeacus' narrative of plague on Aegina to consider changes—many of them instigated by Augustus—between the Roman population of the late Republic and its post-civil war emergence under the new regime. Following the lead of Lucretius and Vergil, the *Metamorphoses* poet exploits the utility of the plague topos for exploring communally experienced norms, crises, and transformations. Vergil had equivocated in determining the value of Aristaeus' hive in the fourth *Georgic*: the hive is first decimated by disease and then replaced after violent sacrifice, leaving readers to ponder both the docile and militant qualities of the bees, as well as their implications for individual loss as the price for communal stability. Ovid's conclusion to the plague that destroys the population of Aegina (*Met.* 7.490–660), the birth of the Myrmidons, may be understood as a commentary on the destruction and restoration that accompany the progress of disease in the *Georgics*. His ant-born men, like his predecessor's bees, are militant and exploitable; yet the extended reach of his narrative foregrounds not only the identities eradicated under the new order, but also the problems of prolonging the utilities and the communal spirit of that order beyond a single generation.

The path of disease in the *Georgics*, guiding Ovid in his own treatment, finds its origin point in corpse-strewn Noricum of Book 3, and is halted only by the ritual that gives birth to a new apian offspring in Book 4. Ovid's narrative combines elements from both books of the *Georgics*: the epoch-changing scale of the disaster and

[2] See Barchiesi (1997b, 1–3) for discussion of Ransmayr's novel as one of three recent fictional accounts of Ovid's exile that bring to light different assumptions about the poet's "anti-Augustan" stance.

sympathetic treatment of individuals, as in Vergil's Noricum, precedes Ovid's focus on the utility and industry of a new race, qualities reminiscent of Aristaeus' new hive. The *Metamorphoses* poet thus brings into closer proximity the two *Georgic* disasters, juxtaposing them in before and after portraits. As such, plague on Aegina underlines the fantastical nature of the *bougonia* as restoration when the connotations of disease among animal populations are transferred to the post-Actian world of Roman citizens in which Vergil and Ovid were writing.[3] The latter poet, who came of age long after the dust at Actium had settled and experienced more of the Augustan reconstruction, implies that the *bougonia*, as a model for recovery from civil war, will not work: the thoughtless homogeneity of the new hive requires people to be something that they are not—beings without prior histories, loyalties, and family entanglements that complicate, but also enrich the human experience.

Ovid's treatment of plague on Aegina exposes complications in the fabric of Roman social life and he is, as Vergil was, attuned to conflicting interests of the individual and the greater community. Like the symptomatology and epidemiology of the Noric plague in the *Georgics*, the metamorphic path of plague on Aegina enacts Golden-Age inversions and initiates processes of decay, culminating in a collapse of discrete *corpora* as grounds for building a *novus ordo*. Aeacus' new order, moreover, orients individuals primarily in relation to the state, rather than within the family units that had traditionally had a critical impact on Roman identity. Such state-oriented identity anticipates by over 1500 years the model for the individual as articulated through various "positive technologies of power" (*technologies positives du pouvoir*)—social controls ranging from training manuals to quarantine procedures to penal institutions—developed primarily in the early modern period.[4] After examining Ovid's treatment of pestilence in *Metamorphoses* 7, I turn to Michel Foucault's account of the origins and effects of these technologies of power in order to clarify the attributes Ovid assigns to his ant-born community

[3] I initially explored the link between Vergil's bees and Aeacus' Myrmidons in Gardner (2014), as well as its implications for the new Augustan order; this chapter is an expansion and development of that argument.

[4] In *Les anormaux*, Foucault (1999, 44) links "the invention of positive technologies of power" (*l'invention des technologies positives de pouvoir*) to recurrent outbreaks of plague in the early modern period; discussed further below, pp. 176–9.

and address the question of why such a population might be useful to the emerging Principate.

Ovid contextualizes and Romanizes his plague narrative by intensifying Aeacus' focus on familial bonds of *pietas*: this focus allows the poet to reflect on a value recently co-opted by the Augustan regime in a way that makes explicit how the Princeps' initiatives would replace personal and familial allegiances with loyalty to the state. While Aeacus' memories of his former citizenry haunt him, the new race granted by Jupiter has no recollection of or attachments to the city's former inhabitants. The Myrmidons, whose uniformity and shared ideals match those of the *Georgic* apian community, function above all as an answer to the call to war issued by the Athenian king Aegeus: by repopulating Aegina with a group of *iuventus* available for military service (*Met.*7.514), Ovid foregrounds the Augustan concern of creating a generation of loyalists in the aftermath of civil war.

There is of course no climate of civil *discordia* pre-existing on Aegina. The citizens there are exceptionally devoted to each other in the face of calamity. Aeacus' account, however, disclosing the intricate entanglements between a citizen and his or her natal home and using a language of putrescence among mounting *corpora*, summons the resonance of civil war echoing throughout both Lucretian and Vergilian accounts of plague. The *Metamorphoses* poet defers explicit internal discord beyond the frame of Aeacus' tale, in an almost passing reference to the fraternal strife among the king's sons (*Met.* 11. 266–82; cf. Hawkins 2019; Carnes 1995, 11). The effect of such a narrative coda is one of blurring the vision of stability and uniformity among the homogeneous ant-born population and implying that even the cleanest of slates, re-inscribed with bodies granted by Jupiter and educated under the most just governance, will not remain so for long.

5.1. NORICUM IN AEGINA: OVID'S *GEORGIC* PLAGUE

The narrative impulse behind Ovid's treatment are two questions posed by Cephalus, who seeks military aid from the Aeginetans led by King Aeacus: why are all these young men of the same age (*tam par aetate iuventus*, 7.514)? And where are all those other fine fellows

I'd met on a previous visit (7.515–16)? In response, Aeacus describes the initial onset of the plague sent by Juno and various failed attempts to treat it through medical arts (523–7); he reports the origins of the disease, muddling divine causation with atmospheric contaminants that taint the water supply (528–35); the georgic section of the plague follows, with Aeacus' account of its effects on livestock and wildlife (536–51). It is only after the disease has afflicted the human population that we are given an account of the symptoms of the plague, along with the modified, if not conventionally deviant, behaviors of those who suffer from it (552–81); Aeacus then offers a more tightly focalized narrative of his own reaction to the plague and his attempts to placate the gods through a botched sacrifice (582–605). The king's lament for the unburied dead is followed by a prayer to his father Jupiter, who sends omens in the form of thunder, a swarm of ants filing up a nearby oak tree, and a dream of ants metamorphosed into young men the following evening (606–42); the next morning Aeacus awakes to find that a new population has miraculously replaced the old one (643–54).

Aeacus' immediate assurance to Cephalus of a happy outcome (*melior fortuna secuta est*, 7.518) alleviates the dramatic tension that characterizes earlier plague narratives and has perhaps influenced some faintly unappreciative readings of the episode, which fault the poet's sacrifice of pathos and humanity at the altar of literary artifice (Galinksy 1975, 117–26). The king frames his testimony, moreover, with a language of memory that advertises the poet's self-conscious invocation of tradition:

> flebile principium melior fortuna secuta est;
> hanc utinam possem vobis memorare sine illo!
> ordine nunc repetam, neu longa ambage morer vos,
> ossa cinisque iacent, memori quos menti requiris,
> et quota pars illi rerum periere mearum.
> (7.519–22)

A better fortune followed a lamentable beginning; would that I could tell you the one without the other! I'll now recall them in order, and lest I delay you with lengthy digressions, the ones you ask about and mindfully recall (lit. recall "with remembering mind"), they lie bones and ash, and such a great part of my realm perished with them!

Through Aeacus' reference to Cephalus' "remembering mind" Ovid signals the many allusions to earlier plague narratives that will follow; but such a nod to tradition warrants further investigation: will Aeacus' tale parrot those of his predecessors or unfold as an act of "creative imitation" (Hinds 1998, 4)?

Ovid makes the trope of remembering his own in part by aligning it with a poetic agenda in the *Metamorphoses* that uses the language of memory as a marker of persistence and continuity in the face of change (Anderson 1963, 5). Our appreciation of the novelty of the Myrmidons will be matched by our desire to locate threads of continuity, not only between ants and Myrmidons, but also between old citizens and new, essential qualities that reflect in some form "the continuity of individuality" (5)—or, in this case, the continuity of the civic body. Aeacus' metapoetically charged reminiscence, rather than merely offering a signpost of poetic virtuosity, is thus thematically integrated into the *Metamorphoses*: as remembering here serves the king's attempts to connect his people's narrative past with present, the act also speaks fundamentally to the difficulty of forgetting, to the challenges of making a break between past and present, remembering the good without the bad (*hanc sine illo*).[5]

Ovidian innovation also extends to deviance from the mythological tradition as established in Hyginus and Apollodorus, who offer various accounts of the Myrmidons' birth to replace the eradicated population of Aegina. Ovid agrees with Hyginus in attributing the cause of the eradication to the wrath of Juno, who sends a snake to poison the water supply, though it is only in Ovid that Juno's snake is multiplied by thousands and triggers a plague.[6] Aeacus casts Juno in a role similar to that she plays in Vergil's *Aeneid*, and refers to the disease sent by the goddess as a *dira lues*: *dira lues ira populis Iunonis iniquae/incidit exosae dictas a paelice terras* ("a grim plague befell the people because of the anger of unjust Juno, who hated the land named for [Jupiter's] mistress," 7.523–4). Juno's interventionist and retributive role is consistent with that of divinity throughout the poem, a role that Lucretius denies to the gods in his account of Athenian plague and Vergil suppresses in the *Georgics* (cf. Delcuve 1936, 207). More importantly, her responsibility for the *lues* ties the foundation, and

[5] Recent work on Roman cultural memory has observed Augustus' interest in manipulating it, calling attention to anecdotes on the Princeps' destruction of writings that concerned the recent civil strife (App. *BC* 5.132; cf. Galinsky 2014, 5). Aeacus' comments here would seem to reflect on the difficulties of forging and imposing a homogenous cultural memory.

[6] Bömer (1976, 331) notes the origins of the story in Hesiod (frag. 205 M.W.); he also cites Strabo, who mentions and discredits the plague variation of the story.

eventual renewal, of Aegina to the settlement of Rome, which was thwarted time and again by the anger of the same goddess.[7] *Dira lues* is high epic diction (contra *morbus* and *pestis* in Vergil's *Georgics*) and Ovid will call attention to his use of it later in *Metamorphoses* 15 (626), as he offers an account of Aesculapius' entrance into Rome after the city suffers its own devastating plague. The rarity of the word in the poem, used only on these two occasions and both times with *dira*, makes its applications to Rome and Aegina, and the resultant link between the two cities, all the more pronounced. The resonance of a new, if floundering, Rome in Ovid's *lues* may be further strengthened by the context of the word in the *Aeneid* (3.139; 7.354): Aeneas and his men suffer a *lues et letifer annus* ("a plague and a death bearing year"), just as the epic hero is trying to lay down roots and establish a settlement, a new Pergamum in Crete.[8] As discussed in the preceding chapter, the Cretan *lues* reviews Vergil's *Georgic* past in a double vision that eyes the devastation of Noricum at the same time that it glances at the role of destruction through brutal sacrifice in the founding of a new order. Ovid follows suit in allowing both Noric calamity and the progeny of the *bougonia* to guide his account of suffering and renewal in Aegina.

In the initial georgic section of the narrative, the poet exploits the serpentine quality of pestilence found in both Lucretius and Vergil: the illness of *De Rerum Natura* creeps serpent-like (*serpere*) among populations who confront "alien/hostile air" (*alienum caelum*, Lucr. 6.1120); so too do *contagia* "creep" (*serpant*) among the *Georgic* poet's unsuspecting flocks (3.469). Ovid literalizes the metaphor by introducing thousands of serpents swarming through the island's uncultivated fields:

> constat et in fontes vitium venisse lacusque,
> miliaque incultos serpentum multa per agros
> errasse atque suis fluvios temerasse venenis.
> (7.533–35)

[7] For Grimm (1965, 67) the implied comparison between the plague that decimates Aegina and the one that interrupts the founding of Rome suggests the triviality of Juno's complaint and the motive (sexual jealousy) behind her actions.

[8] In other words, the catastrophe that interrupts the founding of a new Troy in the *Aeneid* parallels the one that destroys and ultimately restores a settlement of Aeginetans in the *Metamorphoses*. The only other use of *lues* in the *Aeneid* occurs at 7.354, where Allecto's possession of Amata is described as a *lues* (*ac dum prima lues udo sublapsa veneno*).

It's agreed that the *vitium*[9] came into our springs and pools, and that many thousands of serpents wandered through uncultivated (or "deserted") fields and violated our rivers with their poisons.

Since Ovid has staged the first part of his plague, its effects on livestock, in an agricultural landscape, we might ask why he describes these fields—at the very moment the plague is let loose—as *inculti*?[10] Anderson (1972, 300) explains the adjective as the natural result of farmers too sick to till them, an explanation that seems forced in light of the fact that Ovid has not yet depicted the effects of the disease on the human population. *Principio* at line 528, followed by *primo* at 536, confines the initial stages of the disease (designated as a *subitus morbus* 7.537) to the animal kingdom and implies a clear sequence dictating that, as in the *Georgics*, animals fall prey to the disease before humans do. Ovid may wish for us to think sequentially about two conditions (onset of plague, failed cultivation of the fields) described simultaneously. I would argue, however, that, by referring to fields as *inculti*, Aeacus is signaling the same inversion of the natural order that defines the Golden Age. Uncultivated fields are named first and foremost as a condition that Jupiter transforms in Vergil's *Georgic* theodicy (*G.*1.121–5); the absence of cultivation, moreover, distinguishes the renewed Golden Age of Vergil's fourth *Eclogue*, a time when the blushing grape will hang from "uncultivated brambles" (*incultis . . . sentibus*, *E.*4.29); so too is untilled earth characteristic of Ovid's *aurea aetas* in the *Metamorphoses* ([*tellus*] *rastroque intacta nec ullis/saucia vomeribus*, 1.101–2).

And yet because *inculti* refers as often to fields once cultivated, but now neglected as it does to fields never cultivated we are left to ponder, with Anderson, whether these fields were formerly attended and now abandoned. As observed in Livy (3.6–7; cf. 2.34.2), abandoned fields outside of Rome register dysfunction within the city walls, an indication that itself draws on a wider literary tradition linking agricultural squalor to moral decline. In particular, reference to uncultivated fields in Ovid and Livy may look back to the abandoned fields of Catullus 64, which frames its story of Theseus and

9 Bömer (1976, 337) glosses as "poison" ("das Gift"), but remarks that this use, which normally implies a kind of moral or religious failing, is unique in the tradition of plague narratives; cf. Galinsky (1975, 117), "baleful infection." We may wish to view it as analogous to Vergil's *tabum*, though Ovid's term, frequently used to describe defects of procedure or character (*OLD vitium*, s.v. 4–7), has a much stronger moral resonance.

10 Miller (1921, 379) and Lombardo (2010, 191) both translate as "deserted."

Ariadne with an account of the wedding of Peleus and Thetis. The event, a clear indication of the Heroic Age and predecessor to the Iron Age, is such a cause for celebration that farms throughout Thessaly are abandoned to attend it (*nemo rura colit*, 64.38).[11] Thus the literary provenance of *incultus*, beyond merely indicating the physical properties of a rustic landscape, imports contradictory moral implications—Golden-Age bounty as well as squalid neglect—that will re-emerge in evocations of saecular evolution throughout Ovid's account.

As Aeacus continues, the moral resonance of uncultivated fields expands into a larger portrait of failed agricultural productivity, further challenging his audience to locate Aegina in a post-lapsarian world. Aegina's citizens demonstrate exceptional *pietas*, as observed further below, and we have been assured that the cause of the plague is Juno's anger over Jupiter's erotic transgressions. It is with sympathy rather than judgment, then, that we confront the dismay of the unlucky *arator* and suffering of his livestock, within an intensified atmosphere of saecular upheaval:

strage canum primo volucrumque oviumque bovumque
inque feris subiti deprensa potentia morbi.
concidere infelix validos miratur arator
inter opus tauros medioque recumbere sulco;
lanigeris gregibus balatus dantibus aegros
sponte sua lanaeque cadunt et corpora tabent;
acer equus quondam magnaeque in pulvere famae
degenerat palmas veterumque oblitus honorum
ad praesepe gemit leto moriturus inerti;
non aper irasci meminit, non fidere cursu
cerva nec armentis incurrere fortibus ursi.
omnia languor habet: silvisque agrisque viisque
corpora foeda iacent, vitiantur odoribus aurae.
mira loquar: non illa canes avidaeque volucres,
non cani tetigere lupi; dilapsa liquescunt,
adflatuque nocent et agunt contagia late.

(7.536–51)

[11] The Catullan poem offers a matrix for such imagery by linking agricultural squalor in Thessaly with a clearly articulated decline of the ages: the wedding signals the flowering of the Heroic Age, since this son of Aeacus—a paternal connection I shall return to—sired the greatest Homeric hero, Achilles. The marriage, however, also ushers in the Age of Iron, since various forms of impiety (among gods and family) were fated to follow the Trojan War.

At first, in a heap of dogs and birds and sheep and oxen and among the wild beasts, the power of the sudden disease took hold. The unhappy farmer marvels as the strong bull collapses in mid-task and falls backward in the middle of the furrow; from the wool-wearing flocks who give forth mournful bleating the wool falls off of its own accord, and their bodies waste away. The horse once fierce and greatly renowned in the race-course disgraces the victory palm and, forgetful of his old honors, he groans, about to perish in an ignoble death at the stall. The boar does not remember how to rage; nor the stag to trust in his speed, nor the bears to attack the strong herds. Listlessness holds everything. Diseased bodies lie in the woods and fields and roads, the air is poisoned by the stench. Allow me to speak of marvels: neither the dogs nor the greedy birds nor the gray wolves touched them. Bodies decay and dissolve into liquid. They do harm with their stench and spread the contagion far and wide.

Lucretian influence, at a thematic rather than verbal level, frames the passage, as the speaker initially conveys the relentless and chaotic accumulation of bodies (536–7) and ultimately suggests their collapse into liquefied substance (550–1). As bodies are piled on one another in heaps, Ovid also turns insistently to the end of the third *Georgic*, where *stragis* (*G.* 3.556) marked the heaps of rotting corpses that the people of Noricum learn to bury in the single advantage forged from the catastrophe.

As in the Noric plague, we confront the Golden-Age absence of animals (bear and boar; wolves, dogs, and greedy birds) that threaten the farmer and his flocks. Moreover, the *labor* of Ovid's farmer in happier times might be considerably lightened were all sheep able to shear themselves (540–1). The phrase *sua sponte* is not a rarity, but in this agricultural context it echoes the Golden-Age rural life described at the end of *Georgics* 2 (501; Mack 1978, 28), as well as the miraculously color-converted sheep of the fourth *Eclogue* (4.42–5; Van Noorden 2015, 241). The phrase also echoes (in diction as well as prosody) the condition that initially defines Ovid's *aurea aetas*: *aurea prima sata est aetas, quae vindice nullo,/sponte sua, sine lege fidem rectumque colebat* (*Met.*1.89–90, "the first age sown was golden, which of its own accord, and with no need for a defender, kept faith and did the right thing").[12] Like Vergil, Ovid uses Golden-Age imagery

[12] As Van Noorden points out (2015, 237–8), Ovid's use of the *automaton* motif (*sua sponte*), a cornerstone of Greek Golden-Age mythology, initially applies to spontaneous moral rectitude, rather than the earth's productivity. Ovid reassigns spontaneity to the earth in the lines that follow (101–4).

to indicate a fundamental shift in the order of things. These signals can predict a return to Golden-Age pleasance, seriously modified, as in the *Eclogues*, or, as in *Georgics* 3, indicate a complete collapse of humanity's finely orchestrated dominance over nature.

Ovid relies on *Georgic* vocabulary throughout the passage,[13] making his divergences from Vergil in narrating the responses of subjects within the agricultural tableau all the more pronounced. The scene is focalized through an *infelix arator*, recalling similar witnesses to decline and devastation in Lucretius and Vergil. But where the death of a single *taurus* severs a fraternal bond in the *Georgics*, Ovid omits the familial connection sympathetically invoked by Vergil (Mynors 1990, 254), reserving his interest in familial ties for Aeacus' account of the disease's impact on the human community. When Ovid is interested in anthropomorphizing animal behaviors, he hones in on processes of memory and forgetfulness, and the fetters of experience that bind the past to the present. As observed in Chapter 3, Thucydides and Lucretius had both commented on the amnesia suffered by human victims of the plague who later recovered, but no longer knew themselves or their former kin and associates (*atque etiam quosdam cepere oblivia rerum/cunctarum, neque se possent cognoscere ut ipsi*, Lucr. 6.1213–14; cf. Th. 2.49). Both instances address plague's impact on identity, its ability to strip humans of former markers of distinction. Ovid relies on his predecessors' illustrations of contagion as a dehumanizing force, but nuances the trope of forgetting—the break between past and present—to offer a window onto former glories and rivalries, now neutralized in the face of disease. While we might explain the boar's "forgetfulness" of his characteristic rage as periphrasis for lack of enthusiasm (=*non studeo*),[14] Ovid's portrait of a dying racehorse conveys a more complex meditation on the continuity of the self over time. The syntax of lines 542–4 introduces readers to an old, esteemed identity (*acer equus*) transformed as the hexameter proceeds and looks forward to an inglorious, static death (*leto moriturus inerti*) at the conclusion of line 544. The metrical shape of line 542 matches the temporal rupture between past and present, as an initially dactylic *acer equus* slows to a spondaic rhythm, beginning with *quondam* of the second foot.

[13] Cf. *concidere, arator, tauros, opus,* and *medioque*, parallels cited by Vallillee (1960, 109).

[14] As recommended by Bömer (1976, 339).

Ovid's depiction of the once swift, now ailing horse also recalls a similarly despondent steed in the *Georgics* (3.498–502) and strengthens in his Vergilian model the intricate links between victory, glory, defeat, and trampled *dignitas*. Vergil and Ovid both indicate the illustrious career of their respective racehorses: the *Georgics* poet names him *victor*, while his triumphs are signaled in the *Metamorphoses* through a descriptive genitive, *magnae in pulvere famae* ("of great renown in the race-course," *Met.*7.542). Both poets moreover signal a break between past and present instigated by the illness, as each horse loses interest in former pursuits. Vergil describes a general malaise accompanied by forgetfulness of food: *infelix studiorum atque immemor herbae* (*G.* 3.498).[15] Ovid exploits his predecessor's anthropomorphism, heightening the former glory of the horse's career by contrast with his current decrepitude (*degenerat palmas*) and failure to remember old honors (*veterum oblitus honorum*, *Met.*7.543).

Ovid's reference to victory palms (*palmae*) won by the horse may also nod to an earlier passage of the third *Georgic*, which observed the racehorse exulting in triumph or, with equal passion, grieving over defeat: *et quis cuique dolor victo, quae gloria palmae* (3.112, "[you will observe] what grief there is for each one in defeat, what glory there is in victory").[16] By allowing his dying *equus* to forget the past, Ovid revives a *Georgic* context that explains animal behaviors through human psychology, and, in particular, through wounded pride (*dolor*) that seeks to reclaim honor, despite the threat such retaliation poses to the stability of the collective (cf. *G.*3.209–41). Lucretius' account of disease infused the sufferings of plague victims and their kin with ethical language, and language from the vocabulary of Roman political life:[17] that infusion suggested a metaphorical relationship between the futile struggles for self-preservation during pestilence and the equally futile, and often destructive struggle to preserve one's reputation as described elsewhere in *De Rerum Natura*.

[15] Thomas relies on Ovid for his reading of Vergil's line, and takes *immemor* with both *herbae* and *studiorum* (1988, 135).

[16] Commentators stress Vergil's use of similar language in his account of the destructive passions of livestock in the first half of Book 3 and in his narrative of the plague's destruction in the second half (Putnam 1979, 221; Thomas 1988, 135; Mynors 1990, 253); such language invites recall between images of healthy and morbid animals.

[17] See above, Chapter 3, pp. 98–9.

A tinge of sympathy colors portraits of the ailing, former champion racehorse in both Vergil and Ovid, though both reflect, from different angles, Lucretius' demonstration that personal renown can rend the state apart: Ovid's plague materializes within the animal community in a way that recognizes former identities and the rivalries that shape them, then severs ties to the past through forgetfulness, and finally collapses distinctions between individual animals in death.

Commenting on Ovid's interest in rotting corpses, Anderson (1972, 302) remarks, "Lucretius and Thucydides leave the details to our imagination; Ovid's delight in the grotesque encourages us to spell them out." Few would deny that Ovid delights in the grotesque, and the power of a grotesque aesthetic to challenge the stability of a world order promoted through Augustan ideals has been rightly noted (Segal 1988, 71). At the same time, we have observed liquefaction as symptom of plague explicitly in Vergil and implicitly in Lucretius, though Ovid's predecessors shift their gaze (and ours) more often to the internal processes of dissolving *corpora*.[18] In line 541 the decay experienced by the bodies of sheep (*tabent*) gestures toward Lucretius' *tabes letumque* (6.1201) awaited by plague victims, and perhaps even more emphatically toward Vergil's *tabum*, used twice to describe the kind of putrefaction and decomposition that infect the remaining population of livestock (*G.* 3.481, 557). Ovid uses *tabere* only here (Bömer 1976, 338),[19] and in so doing subjects his animal *corpora* to collapse that leaves all remains liquefied (*dilapsa liquescunt*, 7.550). Along with its power to invert the ages and disrupt the continuity between past and present, Ovid finds in Vergil's Noricum the corrosive power of disease most instructive: there carcasses were also left *dilapsa* (*G.* 3.557) after having experienced liquefaction (*fluvidus liquor*, *G.* 3.484). If this is what pestilence

[18] Ovid's interest in liquefaction is of course not confined to the Aegina episode. As Myers (1994, 45) has observed, the *Metamorphoses* consistently demonstrates processes of "cosmogonic flux," and its initial account of the four elements (from Book 1) resurfaces throughout the poem as a reminder that "human physiognomy and the cosmos are intimately related because of their identical constituents" (43)—an observation that again recalls a fundamental philosophical kinship (despite different ideas concerning atomic entities) between Lucretius and Ovid.

[19] Less rare in Ovid, but related to *tabeo*, is *tabesco*, used by the poet in the speech of Pythagoras in *Metamorphoses* 15 to explain how new forms grow from decayed bodies (*nonne vides, quaecumque mora fluidove calore/corpora tabuerint, in parva animalia verti*? 15.362–3). The *bougonia* serves as a primary illustration of this phenomenon (15.365–7).

does to bodies—animal, human, civic—in the Latin epic tradition, it is left for readers of that tradition to ask why: how do such symptoms and effects of contagious disease determine the meaning of the plague metaphor?

Ovid's rotting corpses, and their two-fold implications for the spread of disease, through *contagia* (551) and miasmatic contamination of the atmosphere (*adflatu*, 551), conclude the georgic plague of the *Metamorphoses*. By explicitly signaling a process of transmission through proximity, the poet picks up the threads of those garments made with infected animal hides, whose touch would introduce Noric plague to the region's human inhabitants in Vergil's account (*contactos . . . artus*, G. 3.566).[20] Lucretius and Vergil both conclude their plague narratives with a kind of iterative mortality[21]—as disease continues its tireless march well into the conclusions of *De Rerum Natura* and *Georgics* 3. Ovid, though propelled initially by a similar impulse, seizes upon plague's power to wipe the slate clean and build a New Jerusalem. Having thus far indulged in poetic reminiscence as a way to construct an epoch-changing stage, littered with the collapsed bodies of animal inhabitants, he turns to dramatize the sufferings of Aegina's human citizens, travails that will be neatly relegated to the past by the time of Aeacus' narrative present in *Metamorphoses* 7.

5.2. THE TIES THAT BIND: FAMILIAL BONDS AND THE AEGINETAN PLAGUE

In describing the plague's effects upon the human population within the city walls, the speaker indulges with relative restraint in symptomatology, drawn from accounts of the Athenian plague. Lucretius had adapted and expanded into more than sixty (1145–1214) evocative lines Thucydides' painstaking account of the progress of the disease, from its initial stages causing a feverish headache through its

[20] See Introduction, pp. 27–8, for the etymological nuances of *contingo* and its derivatives.

[21] For the tendency of some plague narratives to resist closure in part by lingering on body counts ("iterative mortality that undermines the teleological progression of the apocalypse"), see Gomel (2000, 410), and above, esp. Chapter 3, p. 95.

final stages resulting in loss of extremities and memory among survivors. Ovid condenses the physical symptoms into six lines, foregrounding the intense heat and thirst of the ill, and describing paradoxical circumstances by which the earth, rather than cooling the bodies of the sick, grows warm from them (7.558–60). Such intense heat allows Ovid to exploit the spectacular value of sufferers crowded around pools and fountains, drinking themselves to death.

While the detail of indulged desires (*indulgent animis*, 566) and "modesty put aside" (*posito pudore*, 567) recognizes the convention of moral collapse in the context of an epidemic, Ovid's epidemiology initially shies away from disclosure of deviant behaviors, and the context of his observations—aberrant behavior as the result of excessive thirst—hardly reflects a moral failing. Thucydides had recognized the moral degeneration that accompanied the twin assaults of war and pestilence in Athens: he notes how rapid changes of fortune encouraged "the indulgence of pleasures previously concealed" and the pursuit of "satisfactions that were quick and pleasurable," amidst a general atmosphere of lawlessness and disrespect for the gods (2.53). As noted earlier, the author of *DRN* primarily confines his observations on Athenian morality to behavior, especially neglect of kin, inspired by an excessive fear of death. For Lucretius, alternating attendance to or neglect of "one's own" sick (*suos ad aegros*, 1239; *populum suorum*, 1247) reflected on the desire to preserve autonomy, as well as on the loyalties and factions driving the engines of strife in the late Roman Republic.

Possibly because Aeacus as narrator makes little pretense of objectivity—these people are his own (*meorum*, 583; *meos*, 618), and their suffering is his to share—he overlooks the hedonism and self-preservation that characterized earlier accounts of the Athenian plague. His account, however, is articulated with distinctively Roman idioms that betray tensions that alternatingly rupture and suture the individual's place within the home. The king observes a correlation between proximity and death: the more dutiful and humane the citizens are in treating the sick, the more rapidly they are felled by the disease, *quo proprior quisque est servitque fidelius aegro,/in partem leti citius venit* ("the nearer each one is, and the more faithfully he serves the sick, the more swiftly he meets his end," 7.563–4). Ovid does not mention the inversion of this dynamic, that those who neglect the sick encounter equal mortality rates, as described in Thucydides and Lucretius (Anderson 1972, 303). Countering the destructive reciprocal fidelity of Aegina's citizens to each other, however, is the individual's fearful alienation from his or her own home:

> corpora devolvunt in humum fugiuntque penates
> quisque suos, sua cuique domus funesta videtur,
> et quia causa latet, locus est in crimine parvus (notus).[22]
> semianimes errare viis, dum stare valebant,
> adspiceres, flentes alios terraque iacentes
> lassaque versantes supremo lumina motu.
>
> (7.574–9)

They roll their bodies onto the earth and each one flees his own household gods, and to each one his own house seems deadly and, because the cause lay hidden, the confined (or "known/recognized") place is held to blame. You would see them wandering half-dead in the roads, while they had the strength to stand, some weeping and lying on the ground and turning their wearied eyes with a final effort.

The flight from one's own *penates*—spirits located in the innermost part of the home and metonymically conjuring household and family lineage—is Ovid's invention, one that hints at divine displeasure (Anderson 1972, 304). Vallillee (1960, 140) suggests a practical motive for the innovation: while overcrowding was an aggravator of disease in Athens and resulted in public demonstration of the plague's impact on the population, Aeacus' people have no obvious reason to die in the streets. Practicality alone, however, cannot explain the specific terms of each citizen's flight. Ovid crafts his public display of suffering in reflexive language that underscores the ties that bind a citizen to a *domus* (*quisque suos, sua . . .*), even as those ties, simultaneously familiar (especially if we read *notus*) and threatening (*in crimine*), are stretched to the breaking point.[23]

[22] Manuscripts are divided between *parvus* and *notus*, with many editors viewing *notus* as a scribal attempt to correct the less comprehensible, but equally plausible, *parvus* (Anderson 1972, 304). Judging from Ovid's love of paradox, on which see especially Tissol's insightful comments (1997, 13–18), *notus* evokes a more characteristically Ovidian condition in which the place that should be most familiar is rendered most alienating.

[23] The *Georgic* reminiscence that has colored Juno's *dira lues* so far might also encourage readers to measure Aeacus' reference to citizens alienated from home and household gods against the corrupt and divided Romans at the end of *Georgics* 2: there Vergil used the betrayal of city and "wretched household gods" (*miseros penates*, 2.505), as well as the forsaking of "homes and sweet thresholds" (*domos et dulcia limina*) for exile in a foreign *patria* to define the conditions of fraternal discord (510–12).

In light of the very Roman, Augustan (*Met.* 1.174, 15.864) nature of the household deities mentioned at 7.574, it is moreover rather odd to find them lurking in an otherwise Greek context. Ovid's first reference to *penates* in the poem comes in an ekphrasis of the dwelling of an explicitly Augustan Jupiter on "heaven's Palatine" (*Palatia caeli*, 174–6); his final mention celebrates the goddess Vesta's placement "among Caesar's household gods" (15.864). Certainly, Ovid uses *penates* to signify hearth and home in Greek contexts elsewhere in the poem (e.g., 1.231, 1.773, 3.539). His innovative terminology conjuring Roman discourses of family and interfamilial relations, however, reflects Aeacus' larger interest in how this plague impacts each citizen's relation to his natal home, and alerts readers to a contrast between the familial ties that anchored the old population and the unfettered condition of the new Myrmidons.

As the very homes that shape human identity are considered suspect (*in crimine*), the plague marches relentlessly among the populace and increases its dehumanizing effects. Aeacus' concern for how individual citizens responded to each other and within their own *domus*, his expression of identification with his people, and his insistence on sharing their suffering (*cuperem pars esse meorum*, *Met.* 7.583) are interrupted by a vision of the citizen body as a relatively homogeneous group. After encouraging his interlocutors to imagine gazing upon the disease stricken (*adspiceres*, 578), he describes his own path of vision, a gesture of surveillance over his people that re-emerges later in the account in the advent of an entirely new citizenry. Here, however, Aeacus' vision is dismal, conveyed through a simile that reduces people to apples and acorns fallen from shaken branches:

> quo se cumque acies oculorum flexerat, illic
> vulgus erat stratum, veluti cum putria motis
> poma cadunt ramis agitataque ilice glandes.
> (7.584–6)

Wherever I bent my line of vision, there the crowd was scattered in heaps, just as when rotten fruit falls from disturbed branches, or acorns fall from the shaken ilex.

While Ovid has reserved graphic decomposition for the afflicted livestock, his sense of the grotesque impinges here on human bodies now likened to rotting fruit (*putria poma*) and recalling the rotting warps (*putris telas*) that threaten the people of Noricum at the end of the third *Georgic*. Bömer detects Homeric resonance and the influence of the simile used by Glaucus, who famously compares human generations to those of withering leaves to explain his lineage after being challenged by Diomedes in the *Iliad* (6.143–50; 1976, 348). In its context, Glaucus' comparison distinguishes the evanescence and insignificance attributed to a single human life from the Homeric warrior's desire to outlive his own mortality through his reputation or *kleos*. The Metamorphic simile, as an implicit rebuttal to that desire, likens citizen bodies to rotting fruit in a way that insists on death and anonymity as the essential conditions of plague, explicitly foreclosing the possibility of a glorious death-defying reputation won on the battlefield.

While the putrescence of the apples alone would convey the physical condition of the bodies littered throughout the streets of Aegina, Ovid adds another term to the comparison, acorns scattered from the shaken ilex. *Glandes* exist as a slippery place marker in Vergil's *Georgics*, since they provided a sufficient diet for the inhabitants of the Golden Age (*G*.1.147–8), but are also what the hungry Iron-Age dweller will seek, shaking them from the oak tree, in the absence of a productive farm (*G*.1.159). Ovid's invocation of acorns here amidst the rapidly decomposing population of Aegina evokes both the pleasance and corporal unanimity of the Golden Age and the harsh reality of its end.[24] As with his use of similar epochal language in the georgic segment of Aeacus' account, the poet's aim is not to mark the Aeginetans as the inhabitants of an unambiguously pristine or corrupt age. Rather, he (like Vergil before him) invokes language of the Gold and Iron Ages, almost interchangeably, to indicate a world on the brink of saecular evolution, and prepares his audience for a new phase in the cycle, with its attendant questions surrounding moral and social renewal.[25]

[24] Vergil's theodicy scatters acorns from a *quercus* (*G*.1.159), linked with the woods of Dodona, sacred to Jupiter (*G*.1.8, 1.149). In Ovid's own Golden Age in the *Metamorphosis*, *glandes* are produced from the "tree of Iove" (*Met*. 1.106), but the poet caps his vision of the *aurea aetas*' spontaneously generative earth with the verdant ilex—this time a source of honey (*Met*. 1.112), that other Golden-Age staple (*flavaque de viridi stillabant ilice mella*).

[25] That is, Ovid's references to saecular evolution, less pronounced here than, e.g., in Book 1, prompt his readers to reconsider what essential characteristics make—or would make, in light of its present Augustan return—an age worthily described as "golden." On this point I am influenced by Perkell (2002, 11), who argues that ambivalence surrounding Vergil's Golden Age throughout his oeuvre performs a

Aeacus' account soon turns away from the homogenizing and dehumanizing description of corpses and lapses back into observation of discrete, living bodies. He recalls family members acting on each other's behalf, reciprocal gestures within the sacred context of Jupiter's temple, made more pronounced by comparison with accounts of the Athenian plague. Ovidian irony stages their deaths while they pray for the lives of their kin, what Anderson describes as "a supreme moment of *pietas*" (1972, 305):

> templa vides contra gradibus sublimia longis:
> Iuppiter illa tenet. quis non altaribus illis
> inrita tura dedit? quotiens pro coniuge coniunx,
> pro gnato genitor dum verba precantia dicit,
> non exoratis animam finivit in aris,
> inque manu turis pars inconsumpta reperta est!
> (7. 587–92)

You see across the way a temple raised high by a long flight of steps. Jupiter is worshiped there. Who did not burn incense in vain on those altars? How often did a husband die while praying on behalf of his wife, or a father on behalf of his child, upon altars unable to be won over, and part of the incense was found unburned in his hand.

Such conjugal and parental affection, whose failure marked the advent of Ovid's Iron Age, when "*pietas* lay conquered" (*victa iacet pietas*, 1.149), acquits the citizens of Aegina, not only of the usual deviance characterizing a plague-stricken populace, but also of the moral *crimina* that characterize a fallen race. Observations on family members expiring mid-ritual both evoke and depart from the unsettling convention established in Thucydides (2.52), and echoed in Lucretius (6.1272–9), by which the bodies of plague victims are left to rot in sacred spaces. But neither account of the Athenian plague describes any ritual activities occurring in the city's temples, only the neglect of bodies of citizens who had fallen ill after taking refuge there. Descriptions of bodies in various stages of decomposition within the sacred space of a temple allowed Ovid's predecessors to

similar interrogative function, and that the questions it prompts (e.g., what makes an age "golden"?), "tend to cluster around moral values centrally implicated in Augustan imperial ideology"; see Chapter 4, p. 115–16. O'Hara makes a related point concerning Jupiter's relationship to the Golden Age in Vergil: "If allusions to Gigantomachy sometimes make it unclear who is on Jupiter's side, allusions to the Golden Age make uncertain what it means to be on Jupiter's side" (2007, 101).

dramatize a collapse of physical boundaries within the city, one that mirrored the collapse of social boundaries. Lucretius in particular directs our gaze to Athens' polluted sacred spaces (*sancta deum delubra, caelestum templa*, 1272–4) largely to highlight the failure of *religio* (*nec iam religio*, 1276). The *Metamorphoses* poet forestalls this stage of plague dramaturgy, lingering over reciprocal devotions of Aegina's citizens; his depiction of mutual respect among family members in the temple of the city's tutelary deity thus distinguishes the *pietas* of Aegina's citizens from their Athenian counterparts. While readers (as well as Aeacus' audience) of the episode may sense the futility of their gestures, heightened by the death of family members in mid-devotion, the island's population clearly resisted yielding to such cynicism.

5.3. THE OLD *PIETAS* OF AEGINA AND THE AUGUSTAN PRINCIPATE

Before observing the failure of Aegina's familial devotions, we now pause to consider how such demonstrations of family-oriented *pietas* might resonate with those ideals being promoted in the emerging Principate. Civil war in particular was viewed as a threat to *pietas* and is held responsible for the destruction of the Roman family in late-Republican and early-Imperial sources (Jal 1963, 391–401). Richard Saller's survey of legal and literary sources on *pietas*, drawn largely from the *exempla* of Valerius Maximus as well as notices in Cicero and Pliny the Elder, challenges the view, often supported with reference to *pius Aeneas* of Vergil's epic, that *pietas* was throughout Roman history narrowly conceived of as obedience to gods, country, and family (1994, 105–14; cf. Lee 1979, 22–3). For Saller, *pietas* implied from fairly early on in the Republic reciprocal affection and responsibility among family members, attested as strongly for parents acting on behalf of their children as for children responding to harsh paternal dictates.[26]

[26] He specifically counters views that see the affectionate and reciprocal aspects of *pietas* as emerging initially in the Augustan period (1994, 112); see further below, pp. 169–70. Contra Hellegouarc'h, who cites Cicero as evidence for *pietas* in the Republic as primarily one-directional (from children towards parents) rather than reciprocal (1963, 277).

It is precisely this kind of mutual concern that the Western plague narrative since Thucydides has problematized in varying degrees: mysteries surrounding the processes of contagion force a conflict between the desire to minister to kin and the drive for self-preservation.[27] Ovid, however, responds to Roman cultural norms in articulating this tension, answering the flight of some citizens from their *domus* and *penates* with careful attendance to family members in the home of the city's tutelary deity. A kind of reciprocally affectionate *pietas*, extending beyond the boundaries of a son's obedience to his father, enacted between spouses (*pro coniuge coniunx*) and by a father on behalf of his child (*pro gnato genitor*), occurs amidst the devastation on Aegina. The *Metamorphoses* poet here may be inspired by Lucretius' introduction of familial entanglements in death outside the walls of Athens.[28] If so, he has revised physical entanglement among parents and children as affectionate devotion played out in a context woven with signifiers of Roman ritual and social life.

Saller cites a number of illustrations of *pietas*, also drawn from Valerius Maximus, where duty to or affection for family members clashes with obedience to the state (1994, 109; Valerius Maximus, 5.4.3; 5.4.6).[29] Such *exempla* and the splintering of loyalties they illustrate underscore the urgency, at least from the perspective of a newly emerging Principate, of streamlining and redirecting the affective feelings traditionally encompassed in the virtue of *pietas*. While Galinsky has stressed the cooperative effort and social responsibility conveyed by Augustan *pietas*, in contrast to other relatively "competitive" Roman virtues (1996, 85–6), demonstrations of *pietas* could also widen divisions within the body politic by recognizing a

[27] Well known, relatively early examples include Boccaccio's *Decameron*, where the narrator observes entire families carted out on funeral biers as well as how, "fathers and mothers refused to nurse and assist their own children, as though they did not belong to them" (1972, 54, G.H. McWilliam, trans.); these tensions and the strain they place on the family unit are exacerbated under the pressures of quarantine in Defoe's London in *Journal of the Plague Year* (2001, 43–44, 55–6), and have persisted well into the contagion narratives of modern and contemporary eras; see esp. below, Chapter 7, pp. 257–8.

[28] See 6.1256–8, also discussed above, Chapter 3, pp. 102–3.

[29] In the first example, Manlius Torquatus is charged (*inter alia*) with extending the term of his military *imperium* beyond the legal limit. His son adamantly refuses to testify against him, and even threatens the life of the prosecuting tribune. In the second, the tribune of the *plebs* C. Flaminius tries to pass a popular measure for redistributing Gallic territory against the wishes of the senate. Respect for his father's wishes restrain his efforts.

distinction between familial and civic devotion, the very distinction and resultant divisions that we have observed Lucretius wrestling with in his account of the social pathologies that afflict the Athenian citizen body during the plague.

Scholarship on Augustan values has frequently observed how Augustus appropriated *pietas* and positioned himself, in his role as *pater patriae*, as the predominant object of its devotions. We should contextualize this process within the gradual erosion of boundaries between public and private life, well documented in monographs by Severy (2003) and Milnor (2005), who demonstrate how family life in the Augustan period became increasingly subject to state intervention.[30] An honorary shield (*clipeus virtutis*), among the tokens bestowed on Augustus during the (so-called) great settlement of 27 BCE, promoted four attributes characteristic of a noble ruler (Zanker 1990, 95–6): *virtus*, *clementia*, *iustitia*, and *pietas erga deos patriamque*. The bestowal significantly limits the range of *pietas* "to gods and fatherland," rather than granting its traditional relevance to familial relationships, a reasonable modification in light of the senate's wish to encourage the new ruler's devotion to the state, but one enthusiastically adopted by the Princeps in his display of copies of the *clipeus* throughout Italy as well as his reference to its display inside the Curia Iulia in his *Res Gestae* (34.2).[31] Ovid's dramatization of *pietas*, in a context that has already evoked the sanctity of the Roman *domus* and its *penates*, reclaims for the value the interfamilial,

[30] For Milnor, various discourses of the first Principate promoting "traditional Roman domestic values" (2005, 11) collude in forging new ideals of femininity; such ideals were conceptually located within a "private" sphere that was increasingly made the object of public scrutiny. She is thus more interested in representations of Augustan women than their real-life counterparts. Severy's (2003) monograph charts the political maneuvers of the Princeps to promote his own family as an instrument of the state and gradually create conditions accommodating dynastic succession. While she is thus more focused on the agency of Augustus in the process of shoring up his political dynasty, her study shines light on how constructions of family life and gender among the greater Roman populace were also transformed in the process. With regard to the changing value of *pietas* in the period, she observes that, as the *domus Augusta* emerged as crucial to the stability of Rome, "*pietas*, a term for familial and religious devotion, came to be used to describe loyalty to it" (2003, 6).

[31] The omission of familial *pietas* is made more apparent by comparison with late-Republican definitions of the term, e.g., that of Cicero, *Inv.* II.66: *pietatem (appellant) quae erga patriam aut parentes aut alios sanguine coniunctos officium conservare moneat.* The passage and its relationship to political and familial life are discussed in Hellegouarc'h (1963, 276).

and relatively "private" territory excluded by one especially iconic Augustan monument.

Those scholars shifting their focus from *pietas* as an Augustan value to its particular articulation in Ovid's Augustan poem have stressed its use in paradox, as characters such as Myrrha and Byblis mask criminal desires with the name of *pietas*, and ultimately seek to avoid its obligations (Anderson 1963, 14–17; Tissol 1997, 14–15). Ovidian *pietas* can also heighten discrepancies between public and private obligations, reflecting the very tensions observed in Valerius Maximus' anecdotes, as illustrated in the *Metamorphoses* through Agamemnon's decision to honor his role as *rex* over that of *pater* in the sacrifice of Iphigenia (12.29–31). Focusing on the relationship between fathers and daughters, Meredith Prince (2011) has recently observed how Ovid's treatment of *pietas* frequently exposes its frailty when subject to conflicting claims. *Pietas* often demonstrates paternal weakness, when the authority of fathers like Pandion and Ligdus is undermined in the narrative outcome.[32] Myrrha's dilemma insistently problematizes the term as she and her story's narrator, Orpheus, obsessively examine the proprieties and improprieties of love among family members (10.321, 324, 334, 366; cf. 345, 354, 366, 431, 451, 469). Manson has in fact suggested that among Latin poets it is in the *Metamorphoses* that we first encounter a notion of *pietas* as reciprocal affection between parents of both sexes and their children (1975, 26).[33] While Saller rightly cautions against views that deny *pietas* from earlier periods a reciprocal dimension, Manson offers evidence for a distinction between the concept articulated in the *Aeneid*, where *pius* and *pietas* rarely convey reciprocity or affection, and the multivalent expressions of *pietas* in Ovid's epic—at precisely the historical moment when Augustus attempted to circumscribe the virtue with reference to gods and *patria* alone.

[32] Pandion's daughter Philomela is raped, and Ligdus' child is brought up against his wishes; fathers in the *Metamorphoses* also frequently prove blatantly undeserving of filial devotion (e.g., Erysicthon).

[33] Manson cites in particular Philomela's feelings of *pietas* toward Itys (*Met.* 6.629), ultimately overwhelmed by her desire to exact vengeance from Tereus. He observes how such use opened up the semantic possibilities of the term, allowing it to express "affection et tendresse entre les membres de la famille et ensuite la bienveillance et la compassion envers les autres hommes" (1975, 26).

While we are reminded early in the epic that Augustus should be the premier object of *pietas*, as *pater patriae*,[34] *pietas* re-emerges in various familial contexts throughout the *Metamorphoses*, heightening the tension between private interests and civic duty and interrogating the nature of a father's authority: the poem's persistent interest in what makes a father worthy of reverence and what sort of children are likely to bestow that reverence reflects upon the newly structured familial relationship between Romans as children and their paternal emperor (Prince 2011, 65; cf. Severy 2003, 56). Embedded within the poem's sustained interest in *pietas*, Aeacus' narrative thus prompts readers to ask what kind of father to his people Aeacus has been, or, more pertinently to the island's current crisis, what kind of father is Jupiter?

5.4. TOWARD A NEW KIND OF *PIETAS*

The pressures of the plague ultimately incite the Aeginetans to abandon their acts of *pietas*, and anger at the god's indifference eventually spurs utter impiety: corpses are hurled before temple doors, strewn upon the earth unburied, tossed upon pyres without funeral rites, and left to burn with stolen flames, those kindled by "others" rather than family members, *alienis ignibus* (*Met.* 7.602–10). Ovid borrows from Lucretius to heighten the sense of lawlessness, summing up his exposé of transgressions with the comment that "no longer is there any reverence" (*et iam reverentia nulla est*, 609), an allusion to Lucretius' pithy expression of the failure of *religio* in plague-stricken Athens (*nec iam religio,* Lucr. 6.1276). But Ovid holds up before and after sketches for comparative evaluation:[35] it is only after repeated acts of devotion that we observe the ineffectual nature of *pietas*, and witness its inversion, failed *reverentia.* In one sketch, we observe family members tending to each other in illness and supplicating Jupiter on each

[34] Cf. Book 1's account of the response of the Olympians to Jupiter's desire to punish Lycaon: *nec tibi grata minus pietas, Auguste, tuorum/quam fuit illa Iovi* (1.204–5, "nor was the *pietas* of your people less pleasing to you, than that *pietas* [of the gods] was pleasing to Jupiter").

[35] As discussed above (Chapter 3, pp. 103–6), Lucretius acknowledges the attempts of some family members to bury their kin, though the practice is viewed as violently destructive to the social order. Ovid's narrative artistry offers a clearer demarcation between initial attempts to sustain *pietas* and their eventual, utter failure.

other's behalf, dramatizing the reciprocal devotions that Roman *pietas* entailed. In another sketch, we find a surfeit of neglected bodies, and a city unable to accommodate the funeral rites that should be their due (cf. 607). Shades of the dead wander unlamented by kin:

> qui lacriment, desunt, indefletaeque vagantur
> natorumque virumque animae iuvenumque senumque,
> nec locus in tumulos, nec sufficit arbor in ignes.
> (7.611–13)

Those who would mourn are absent, and the spirits of sons and husbands and of young men and old men wander about unwept; there is neither enough space in the tombs, nor enough trees for fire.

Line 612 has been contested, partly on the basis of its reference to strictly masculine gender identities. Adherence to the manuscripts allows the poet to represent four ages of man (Anderson 1972, 307–8), one of which we have already observed as the object of parental devotions in Jupiter's temple (*pro gnato genitor*, 590). At this stage in the development of Aegina's catastrophe, however, the same sons are "unwept" by loved ones—an Ovidian coinage (Bömer 1976, 355)—and wander untethered to any space (be it home or *tumulus*) or familial identification.

If we have doubts about the power of the family-oriented *pietas* practiced by the former inhabitants of Aegina, Aeacus' inauspicious sacrifice would appear to confirm its failure. In a passage evoking the efforts of the *vates* in Vergil's Noric plague (*G.* 3.486–93), the king describes his attempted sacrifice on behalf of himself, his sons, and his *patria*:[36]

> ipse ego sacra Iovi pro me patriaque tribusque
> cum facerem natis, mugitus victima diros
> edidit et subito conlapsa sine ictibus ullis
> exiguo tinxit subiectos sanguine cultros.
> exta quoque aegra notas veri monitusque deorum
> perdiderant: tristes penetrant ad viscera morbi.
> (7.596–601)

While I myself was making a sacrifice on behalf of myself, my country, and my three sons, the victim gave forth grim bellowing, and, having suddenly

[36] For the reminiscence of *G.*3.486–93 here, see esp. Anderson (1972, 306) and Vallillee (1960, 113–15).

collapsed before a blow was struck, stained the knife I'd thrust up under him with a meager trickle of blood. The diseased entrails had also lost the marks of truth and warnings of the gods; the gloomy pestilence penetrates to the innards.

Vergil, who is ostensibly more interested in the diseased condition of the sacrificial animals than the plight of the priest performing the rites, leaves the beneficiaries of the sacrifice implicit, presumably the people of Noricum. Aeacus makes prayers explicitly for himself, his country, and his sons, mirroring, in his use of *pro* with the ablative to indicate a beneficiary (589–90, cf. *OLD* 3b), the familial devotions staged earlier in Jupiter's temple. Judging from the corrupted entrails, efforts of both citizens and king prove equally unsuccessful, restating the inadequacy of family-oriented *pietas* and the need for more effective bonds to stabilize the community. Significantly, Aeacus does expand the beneficiaries of *pietas* beyond kin to encompass fatherland (*patria*), a move predictable in light of his status as king, but also one that elides his role as *pater* to both sons (*natis*) and citizens. Still, it is only after the king transfers his supplications outside the shared space of the temple and appeals to the familial bond he shares exclusively with Jupiter that his prayers are answered. As such an initial parallel between the *pietas* observed by the king and his subjects eventually yields to a divide between the successful outcome of his later prayers and the inefficacy of the citizens' efforts. In fact, Aeacus, *patria*, and sons *will* survive, an outcome that distinguishes one family's dynastic continuity from the failed continuity of the Aeginetan people.

In exploring the mythic origins of Aeacus as reflected in Pindar's Aeginetan Odes (esp. *Nemean* 5.12–19), Jeffrey Carnes (1995, 12–14) has emphasized how the king and his family are freighted with a history of internally destructive episodes, particularly civil war, as suggested by the sons of Aeacus, a characteristic frequently defining peoples claiming autochthonous status. Pausanias, moreover, records a number of details concerning the problems faced by the king in finding a successor (2.29.2), a problem with uncomfortable resonance for Romans aware of challenges faced by Augustus in securing dynastic continuity. In *Metamorphoses* 11, Ovid will address the fratricide of Phocus by Peleus, who is named explicitly through his patronymic as a "son of Aeacus" (*Aeacide*, 11.250, 275) and who found asylum in Trachinia only after being driven from Aegina, the "home of his father" (*domo patria*), as a criminal stained by his brother's blood: *fraterno sanguine sontem/expulsumque domo patria Trachinia tellus/accipit* (11.268–70). Such a narrative coda to the experience of plague and its aftermath on Aegina, in mirroring the imperatives and challenges of the early Principate, implicates Augustus and his methods of promulgating a new dynasty within a questionable model of authoritarian power. Aeacus' family becomes the sole object of *pietas* because his population has been eradicated and will be replaced by a population that knows no other parental object of devotion. Augustus, with his promotion of a *domus Augusta*, offers a surrogate family, one whose foibles and vulnerabilities would become all too apparent, to Romans already entangled with the families of their birth.

The passage describing Aeacus' prayers and sacrifice on behalf of his country and his family encourages us to take up interpretive threads that lead to a less than sanguine image of dynastic promulgation, with a detour that also prompts reflection on the poet's role in the production of that image. As noted, lines 593–601 remind us of the *sacerdos-vates* figure who fails to interpret and resolve the problem of disease that has beset the Noric people in *Georgics* 3, resolution deferred until the recovery of the hive from liquefied entrails of oxen (*liquefacta boum per viscera*) in *Georgics* 4, with its speculations on the possibilities of a new order under Octavian. Where Vergil resists explicit comment on the entrails heaped on the sacrificial altar in Noricum (*impositis . . . fibris*, 3.490), Aeacus as *sacerdos* observes the plague's corrosive effect on the innards (*exta . . . viscera*) of a bull, which makes it impossible to interpret the *notae* and *monitus deorum* (*Met.* 7.600, "the marks and warnings of the gods"). Ovid, by expanding on the inscrutable nature of the entrails, replicates Vergil's resistance to assign a discernible cause for (or resolution to) the Noric plague. And yet, by having the *notae* denied here soon restored in a sign from Jupiter, the *Metamorphoses* poet rewrites his predecessor's deferred solution to plague, forcing the bee-like ants into uncomfortable proximity to the actual human community that has fallen victim to the plague.

A few lines after the cryptically failed examination of entrails, the god inspires Aeacus' confidence by offering him one of the very *notae* denied earlier in the sacrifice (*ille notam fulgore dedit*, as well as *felicia signa*, 7.620–1). Aeacus initially expresses a wish to have his own people (*meos*) restored or to join them in death (7.618). The king, however, changes his request for the restoration of an old population after observing orderly, in fact militant (*agmen*), troops of ants filing up Jupiter's sacred *quercus* (7.622–6), the very swarms multiplied with such flourish in Ransmayr's reception of the episode. Rather than conduct an ongoing lament for departed individuals, friends, and family, Aeacus demands a fresh supply of loyalists to equal the number of ants he spies: *totidem, pater optime, . . . tu mihi da cives et inania moenia supple*! (7.627–8, "Give me, highest father, just as many citizens and fill up my empty walls!"). Where Vergil's Noric plague effectively blurs the line between humans and animals as it reverses human cultural progress, Ovid's *dira lues* ingeniously wipes the slate clean, filling emptied walls with citizen bodies miraculously elevated from the insect population.

5.5. ANTS AS CITIZENS: ANTICIPATING ANOTHER DREAM OF PLAGUE

> They arose, silent, left the slopes of Mount Oros en masse, and moved forward only en masse in the future as well. They were docile and asked no questions and followed their leaders, who were of the same descent, into the triumph and miseries of time—without complaint, through the ice of the Alps, across seas and through deserts, into war, even into fire, a conquering army. They were a strong people of few wants, who became an army of workers wherever ditches were to be dug, walls razed, or bridges built. In times of war, they were a nation of warriors. In times of defeat, they were slaves, and in victory, masters. And yet through all these transformations, they proved more tractable than any other race.
>
> (Ransmayr 1990, 48)

As Ransmayr's expansion on the uncomfortably Roman qualities of Ovid's Myrmidons suggests (at least from the irritable perspective of the Princeps), the ant-born citizens of Aegina are usefully similar in their habits. Reporting his first encounter with the Myrmidons, Aeacus emphasizes their *corpora* and *mores*, as well as the process by which a new population has replaced the old:

... egredior, qualesque in imagine somni
visus eram vidisse viros, ex ordine tales
adspicio noscoque: adeunt regemque salutant.
vota Iovi solvo populisque recentibus urbem
partior et vacuos priscis cultoribus agros
Myrmidonasque voco nec origine nomina fraudo.
corpora vidisti: mores, quos ante gerebant,
nunc quoque habent; parcum genus est patiensque laborum
quaesitique tenax et quod quaesita reservet.
hi te ad bella pares annis animisque sequentur.

(7.650–8)

I go outside and I look upon and recognize in order men such as those I had seen in my dream: they approach and greet their king. I pay my vows to Jupiter and divide the city and the fields left empty by the former inhabitants among the new population, and I call them Myrmidons; nor do I lie about their origins from the name. You've seen their bodies. They have the same habits as those they carried on before: they're a thrifty sort and enduring of hard work and they cling to gain, storing away for keeps what they've gained. These fellows, equal in years and courage, will follow you to war.

Ovid's focus on the bodies of the Myrmidons (*corpora vidisti*) recalls and challenges Lucretius' spectacular reduction of individual Athenians to material *corpora*, implying that it is largely the materiality of the new race, their corporeal nature, that will prove serviceable to the state. Aeacus for his part readily assumes an authoritative and administrative role, promptly partitioning the city and the lands left vacant by their old inhabitants among the new citizens. While redistributing lands is a practical measure, the act also constitutes another point in the narrative in which Aeacus summons the specter of Augustus, this time in the Princeps' earlier role as the triumvir Octavian, attempting to settle the legions after Philippi.[37] Appian's account of the process, which had excluded Antony, much to the dismay of Antony's supporters, emphasizes the loyalty of the soldiers won by the distributor Octavian (5.2.12–15). At the same time, the resettlements had provoked resentment throughout Italy, from citizens who, unlike Aeacus' former people, were still alive, resentment famously reflected in Vergil's first *Eclogue*, as Meliboeus laments his own displacement by an *impius miles* (*E.* 1.70). In this

[37] Thanks to Megan Drinkwater for suggesting the parallel between Aeacus and Octavian in their roles as land redistributors (*per litteras*).

post-plague Metamorphic context, the unmooring of citizen from familial *domus*, as well as the spatial confusion in which the process culminates, has been reversed: city and fields are now carefully allocated among the new inhabitants.

These inhabitants are above all thrifty, hardworking, and productive, if a tad eager to hold on to what they have produced. Industry and acquisitiveness are of course two salient qualities of Vergil's apian community. Yet the bee's *amor habendi*, as we observed earlier, assumes a negative valence, at least from Evander's perspective, in its application to those Italian people whose greed (*amor habendi, A.* 8.327) and war-mongering marked their decline from Saturn's Golden Age. Ovid too includes greed among the vices that mark the Iron Age (*amor sceleratus habendi*, 1.131). Aeacus and his interlocutors, however, view the acquisitive productivity of this new population with approval. In recognizing the equality of the young men, Aeacus closes a tidy ring structuring the episode and brings us back to Cephalus' original comments on the equality and pulchritude that define the youth of Aegina (*adveniens equidem modo gaudia cepi,/ cum tam pulchra mihi, tam par aetate iuventus/obvia processit*, 513–15; Anderson 1972, 311). Ovid, again reveling in paradox, has taken the disturbing resemblance that defines soldiers on the battlefield in representations of Roman civil war (e.g., *G.*1.489, *paribus telis*) and transformed it into a virtue, the most salient feature of this new post-plague citizenry. Where the Vergilian *vates* fails to divine a remedy for the Noric plague in *Georgics* 3, Ovid's Aeacus is granted one that reflects on the loyal and acquisitive insect population born from the *bougonia*, both its practical value (new population of single-minded citizens), as well as its possibilities and limitations as a model for human existence.

What Ovid shows us in this reflection—and what has the potentially irritating effect of speaking truth to power—is a useful, and in fact exploitable, society. The Myrmidons evoke that other dream of a society born from plague, envisioned by Foucault, who chronicles the technologies of power facilitating finely calibrated divisions within the population, generated partly from the waves of bubonic plague that swept Europe from the fourteenth through the eighteenth centuries. After describing the "literary dream of plague" (*le rêve littéraire de la peste*)[38] in which old identities are abandoned and the law is forgotten, he proposes a different vision:

[38] Foucault (1999, 43), from Gallimard's edition of *Les anormaux.*

> But you can see that there was another dream of the plague: a political dream in which plague is rather that marvelous moment when political power is exercised to the full. Plague is the moment when the spatial partitioning and subdivision (*quadrillage*) of a population is taken to its extreme point, where dangerous communications, disorderly communities, and forbidden contacts can no longer appear. The moment of the plague is one of exhaustive sectioning (*quadrillage*) of the population by political power, the capillary ramifications of which constantly reach the grain of individuals themselves, their time, habitat, localization, and bodies. (2003, 47)

Aeacus, of course, has not yet subjected his new race to the exhaustive sectioning Foucault refers to here, where he documents various inclusive responses to plague:[39] such responses, primarily forms of surveillance over and organization of the population, offered a template for "normalization" (*normalisation*) of sexual behaviors, and ultimately, a model of political control.[40] All the same, the distribution of Myrmidon *corpora* among the homes of former citizens surely anticipates the process of *quadrillage*. Moreover, the king's observations of those very qualities that make such bodies serviceable to the state bear witness to how the plague on Aegina might also prove useful in building those technologies of power that would shore up the fledgling new regime. Augustus' attempts to engineer a population more compliant with the needs of the state (i.e., more conducive to stabilizing the Principate he had initiated), especially through marriage legislation, are well documented in ancient sources. Such attempts undeniably impacted Ovid, whose epic had just begun circulating in Rome in 8 CE upon the poet's exile, in part for verses in ill accord with such legislation. Scholars have also demonstrated Augustus' interest in curbing the license of young men and cultivating their support, partly to replenish military resources drained through protracted civil war.[41] Might Ovid, or even Augustus, have found the faces

[39] "Inclusive" as opposed to the more exclusive measures of relegating the sick outside the city's purview, as with leper colonies (2003, 43–4).

[40] "The reaction to plague is a positive reaction; it is a reaction of inclusion, observation, the formation of knowledge, the multiplication of effects of power on the basis of the accumulation of observations and knowledge. We pass from a technology of power that drives out... to a fundamentally positive power that fashions, observes, knows, and multiplies itself on the basis of its own effects" (2003, 48).

[41] For Augustus' attempts to pass moral and marital legislation as well as evidence for the reception of such legislation among the Roman populace, see esp. Suet. *DA* 34 and Cassius Dio 54.16, 56.1 ff.; cf. Prop. 2.7; Ovid *Ars* 1.31–34, 3.57–8. The secondary literature on the topic is vast: Csillag (1976) is fairly comprehensive; Galinsky (1981)

of young Romans reflected in the faces of these uniformly loyal and martially inclined young men?

In *Discipline and Punish*, Foucault further charts the relationship between state hegemony and social controls, exploring various discourses of training emerging in France in response to commercial evolution, military expansion, and (often) the accidents of disease that accompany them.[42] His observations on the wide range of directives that reflect the state's investment in individual bodies (e.g., practical advice to the soldier on posture, dress, and exercise) further clarify the utility of the new ant-born race and its relationship to both the mythological *rex* in Ovid's poem and the historical Princeps (1995, 144). Such discourses, which Foucault traces in part to the model of the historical Roman *castra* (1995, 146), had a coercive impact, creating by *quadrillage* an easily controlled collective out of confused masses: "each individual has his own place and each place its individual. Avoid distribution in groups; break up collective dispositions (*les implantations collectives*); analyse confused, massive or transient pluralities. Disciplinary space tends to be divided into as many sections as there are bodies or elements to be distributed" (143; French from Foucault 1975, 168).

Within the context of late Republican Rome, *pietas*, as a show of due respect to family members, was one way an individual articulated his or her place in the social order; that is to say, individual identity was expressed largely through kinship networks, which registered roles both in the family (as mother, father, child, sibling, etc.) and in the civic body (e.g., as being from a patrician or plebeian family). Such familial identities and the allegiances they fostered might, with many centuries of hindsight, be viewed as the kind of "collective dispositions" that resist seamless incorporation within Foucault's early modern state. After the *pietas* structuring the citizen body on

speculates on the motives behind the legislation; see also Wallace-Hadrill (1985) for poetic responses to the laws. The laws also incentivized marriage at a younger age and indicate the Princeps' interest in the Roman youth; see Gardner (2013, 33–44). Yavetz (1984) considers how the Princeps' initiatives directed at the youth bolstered his own public image; cf. Fear (2005, 25). See also Eyben (1993, 112–14) for Augustus' youth-oriented policies.

[42] Cf. Foucault (1995, 144): "The medical supervision of diseases and contagions is inseparable from a whole series of other controls: the military control over deserters, fiscal control over commodities, administrative control over remedies, rations, disappearances, cures, deaths, simulations."

Aegina collapses, Aeacus is left with little raw material, aside from his own three sons, for building a new social order. A troubling prospect initially, but one that cleans the slate for a new population, without former markers of identity, and one that might be easily shaped—coerced according to the needs of the state and loyal to the king alone. The disciplinary tactics described by Foucault work to individuate members of a community according to the function each performs, or will perform, since individuals can graduate under supervision from one function to another, and his/her position relative to other members can evolve. At the same time, the goal of such individuation is a perfect taxis, a well organized collectivity, responsive to the dictates of authority: for members of one religious order, The Brothers of the Common Life, "the striving of the whole community towards salvation became the collective permanent competition of individuals being classified in relation to one another" creating a model for "individually characterized, but collectively useful aptitudes" (1995, 161–2).

Ovid's Myrmidons are defined partly through their former identity as ants, the eu-social and collectively motivated species *par excellence*. Ancient accounts of insect communities regularly highlight the industry and collective purpose of these creatures (Pliny *Nat.*11.36; cf. Morley 2007, 462–3). While Ovid borrows from mythological tradition in locating the origin of the Myrmidons in the ant community, he innovates in stressing here, as he does throughout the poem (Anderson 1963, 4–5), the continuity between former and current identities (*mores, quos ante gerebant/nunc quoque habent*, 655–6). *Ante* not only returns to a general ancient notion of how ants behave collectively, but also to the specific image of how these ants behaved when Aeacus originally glimpsed them:

> hic nos frugilegas adspeximus agmine longo
> grande onus exiguo formicas ore gerentes
> rugosoque suum servantes cortice callem.
> (7.624–6)

Here we spied in a long (battle) line fruit/grain-gathering ants, carrying a large burden with their small mouths and sticking to their own track in the wrinkly bark.

Ovid draws attention to the industry of the ants, coining the adjective *frugilegus* and distancing it from the noun (*formicas*) it modifies. The poet will coin a similar term for use later in the poem, in his own rendering of the bees born from the *bougonia*, as explained by

Pythagoras (Hill 2000, 214): there, *florilegae* (15.366) describes the industrious apian collective (*quae more parentum/rura colunt operique favent in spemque laborant*, 15.366–7), underscoring the almost interchangeable (and equally exploitable) properties of the two insect communities. *Agmine longo*, moreover, frequently applies to Roman military formations, leaving audiences to wonder—before finally arriving at *formicas* in line 625—whether these will be humans or ants under the king's observation (Anderson 1972, 309). Aeacus implicitly asks his listeners to transfer such productive and militant qualities, combined with the orderly, single-minded nature of their effort (*servantes callem*), to their impressions of the post-metamorphic young men.

The metaphoric shaking of branches (*motis ... ramis*, 585–6) to indicate the deterioration of a plague-stricken populace earlier in Aeacus' account has been answered by a sign from Jupiter (*ramis ... motis*, 629), an oneiric vision of ants shaken from Jupiter's oak and presaging the new order on Aegina. Indeed, the Romans lacked the surveillance mechanisms and prescriptive controls that Foucault identifies as emerging in the early-modern state. Yet the biopolitics that are born to subtend such mechanisms and controls offer an apt analogy for the strategies of population management executed by those attempting to rebuild post-civil war Rome.[43] That analogy, as refracted through the lens of Ovid's strikingly industrious and uniform Myrmidons, can instruct us in the motives behind (and to a lesser degree, the effects of) the Princeps' attempts to manage birth rates and office holding as well as social and familial interactions.

5.6. NO ONE WANTS A PLAGUE, OF COURSE: A CHANCE TO BEGIN AGAIN

Aeacus' experience of devastating disease, followed by prayers to his divine parent and restoration of an insect-born race, is enough to suggest that Ovid is thinking of Aristaeus' *Georgic* plight and recovery

[43] While biopolitics have been variously defined, Foucault uses the term in "The Birth of Biopolitics" to refer to attempts, "to rationalize the problems presented to governmental practice by the phenonomena characteristic of a group of living human beings constituted as a population: health, sanitation, birthrate, longevity, race" (1997, 73). Thus, for Foucault, biopolitics shore up governmental authority by managing populations rather than territories and national boundaries.

in his account of the Myrmidons. The *Metamorphoses* poet's substitution of ants for bees, moreover, should not surprise readers of Vergil's *Aeneid*, which, as observed at the start of this chapter, likens proto-Romans alternatingly to rapacious ants, as they industriously prepare to depart from the shores of Carthage (4.401–7), and then to bees, whose gentle summer buzzing describes those souls about to be born into the stream of Roman history (6.706–9). It is hardly presumptuous to suggest that Ovid's ants resonate with a poetics in the *Aeneid* that links Romans to insect communities, a link whose fullest implications are only felt by tracing those communities to the disease-stricken hives of *Georgics* 4.[44]

As one *vates* interpreting the evolution of Vergil's bees in the *Georgics* and *Aeneid*, Ovid recognizes the fraught nature of the equation between an apian community and a new Roman population, however acquisitive, loyal, and homogenous that population may be: these are the qualities that above all define his Myrmidons, a new citizen body posed as one solution to the crisis that afflicts Aegina. At the same time, such qualities, in human beings at least, could emerge only from a population created *de novo*, without a past and without those familial identities that give us loyalties, affiliations, and occasionally enemies. Vergil, pondering various steps forward after Actium had left much of the aristocracy dead or contaminated with loyalty to the losing side, offers the symbolic potential of plague and *bougonia* as one way of addressing recovery and reconstitution of stabilized government: the liquefied remains of a calf replicate the deteriorative processes of contagion while suggesting that, from the resultant uniformity, a solution to the problem of civil war might be gleaned, and that rivalries might be redirected toward a common goal.

Ovid observes with the vantage of hindsight how a new citizenry was emerging under the Augustan Principate: his doubtful comment on this population in the *Metamorphoses* is best expressed through the perfunctory manner in which the lingering (post-) apocalyptic vision that marks the third *Georgic* is corrected and given forced

[44] It is also worth noting that, in contrast to the Golden-Age characteristics observed in Vergil's bees (see esp. Johnston 1980, 90–105; cf. Chapter 4, p. 137), the Myrmidons, considered in some mythological traditions to be the first sailors, may import a distinctly Iron-Age valence. Cf. the scholiast on Pindar, *Nem.* 3.21, who comments on Hesiod's reference to the Myrmidons in his *Catalogues of Women* as, "the first who fitted with thwarts ships with curved sides, and the first who used sails, the wings of a sea-going ship" (=53, Evelyn-White, trans.).

closure. As pestilence reaches the citizens of Aegina, it functions to define the community and its boundaries in the process of destroying them. Acts of *pietas* allow citizens to assert their own identities as well as their relationships to each other, and the performance of such acts within the public space of Jupiter's temple suggests that familial devotions are not essentially incompatible with the state authority. All the same, if we consider more carefully the resonance of civil war in Aeacus' tale, we might view *pietas* as a cause of as well as a response to contagion: the same family members who flock to Jupiter's temple also find in their own homes a source of blame (*in crimine*). *Pietas* and its implications for interfamilial loyalties thus emerge as a significant impetus behind the spread of the disease and a value that would need recalibrating in the aftermath of plague on Aegina.

5.7. CODA: *METAMORPHOSES* 15

When yet another *dira lues* strikes in the *Metamorphoses* (15.626), an account of the plague in 293/2 BCE that prompted the importation of the cult of Aesculapius, it again has the effect of evaluating Augustan measures to restore a sick city, this time against historically documented alternatives. The poet tersely recounts the excess of funerals and the exhausting of human and medical resources (*Met.* 15.626–30), exchanging extended epidemiology for an extended account of how the Romans initially consult Apollo at Delphi, apparently an Ovidian innovation, as no such incident is described in Livy or Valerius Maximus.[45] From Delphi, the Roman embassy is redirected to Epidaurus, prompting Aesculapius' eventual arrival at his new home on the Tiber Island, as a "health-giver for the city" (*salutifer urbi*, 15.744). Ovid then shifts abruptly (*tamen*) to the contrastingly native status of Julius Caesar (cf. Solodow 1988, 26), a god in his own city, and the glorious achievement of fathering Augustus.

Much ink has been spilt over the tone of the Augustan climax, and how the Aesculapian episode contributes to (or detracts from) the

[45] Liv. 10.47; cf. Per. 11; Val. Max. 1.8.2; on Ovid's inclusion of Apollo's oracle, see Miller (2009, 364); Williams (2009, 81).

emperor's encomium.[46] For our purposes, it is worth stressing that Augustus emerges in Book 15 as but one of Rome's saviors, put in direct competition with Cipus, who refused monarchy and endured permanent exile just beyond the city walls, as well as with Apollo's twice reborn son. As Gareth Williams has demonstrated, the emperor's cultivation of the god Apollo does very little in Ovid's hands to bolster his identity as a successful healer, in so far as the god's failure to rely on his own medical arts is demonstrated throughout the *Metamorphoses.* In fact, Williams suggests that the redirection of the Romans away from Apollo to the healing power of his son might be read as a challenge to Aesculapius' marginalized status in the early Principate, as Augustus fostered his own connection with Apollo Medicus and discouraged foreign cultic practices (cf. Miller 2009, 366): "if Aesculapius' success in cleansing Rome of plague indirectly underscores Apollo's catalogue of medical misadventures earlier in the poem, does the harmonious succession from Apollo to Aesculapius at 15.637–40 effectively amount to a concession of Apolline inferiority?" (Williams 2009, 84).[47] If we answer this question in the affirmative, might the failure of Apollonian/Augustan medical arts in Book 15 also inform Ovid's treatment of that other *dira lues*, whose victims on Aegina are never cured, only replaced by a startlingly tractable new population? Jupiter, rather than Apollo, is entrusted with restoring health in that community, but the two gods share in their roles as avatars of Augustus and reflections of the Princeps' status as *communis salus* (salvation) for his people.

Where the episode on Aegina allowed us to view old familially determined identities in juxtaposition with new Myrmidon bodies

[46] For instance, see Segal (1969); Williams (2009, 79); La Penna (1988, esp. 286–7) stresses the correlation, rather than contrast between Augustus and Aesculapius, suggesting that for Ovid both figures have a role to play as Rome's saviors; cf. Barchiesi, who observes: "[t]he strange and untraditional juxtaposition of Asclepius and the emperor is not the way to show they are the same... but the juxtaposition produces a bifurcation, a redoubling of the conclusion that requires a choice" (1997a, 193). See also Barchiesi (1997b, 213). O'Hara (2007, 128–30) suggests that the tonal shifts and inconsistencies in the poem's conclusion underscore the difficulties of arriving at any certainties about Ovid's alignment of Augustus with Apollo (or Jupiter, as frequently in the poem).

[47] See also Miller (2009, 365–7), who makes a useful generalization concerning the displacement of Apollo by his son in the poem: "Aesculapius' virtual supplanting of Apollo as the curative divinity in the course of the *Metamorphoses* seems to remake an aspect of imperial ideology" (366).

determined by utility to the state and loyalty to the king, the sequence of Aesculapian and Augustan episodes in Book 15 offers two strikingly different notions of Roman governance. As Feeney notes (1991, 209–10), the decision to import Aesculapius is portrayed as a collective effort: third-person plural verbs are used in reference to the embassy throughout, though no individuals are named, and we are assured of the senate's role in securing the god's aid, with the explicit support and participation of the Roman people (15.641, 729–30). The immediately following apotheosis of Julius Caesar is described as the effort of a single man, suppressing the role of the senate and people in the process, a stark revelation of "the appropriation of the corporate by the individual" (Feeney 1991, 213). Plague-stricken Aegina, overseen by a single dynast, and plague-stricken Rome, seeking salvation under the senate and people, both offer opportunities for the poet to explore the optimal functioning of the civic body. Ovid's goal in using a *dira lues* to prompt comparison between two civic bodies in recovery is not to pronounce judgment, but his artistry has the impact of exposing the rupture between Republican governance and that of the *novus ordo*, rather than any continuity between the two. The solution to pestilence on Aegina, humans born from ants, while acknowledging the power of plague to eradicate distinction and rivalries through contagion and death, privileges a collective purpose among inhabitants. Such a purpose, however, is designed primarily to support the regime that oversaw its birth, echoing the very Augustan social controls that were buttressing the early Principate. These controls were exercised not only in the form of explicitly encoded legislative measures, but also through the regime's unique brand of *pietas*, and its ideological realignment of the individual's relationship to family and state.

Part III

Transmitting Roman Plague

6

Imperial Receptions

Lucan, Seneca, and Silius Italicus

. . . omne mortalium genus vis pestilentiae depopulabatur, nulla caeli intemperie quae occurreret oculis. sed domus corporibus exanimis, itinera funeribus complebantur; non sexus, non aetas periculo vacua; servitia perinde et ingenua plebes raptim extingui, inter coniugum et liberorum lamenta, qui dum adsident, dum deflent, saepe eodem rogo cremabantur. equitum senatorumque interitus quamvis promisci minus flebiles erant, tamquam communi mortalitate saevitiam principis praevenirent. (Tac. *Ann.* 16.13)

The force of the pestilence was destroying every kind of human being, without apparent corruption from the atmosphere. But the homes were filled with lifeless bodies, the roads with funerals. No sex, no age was free from danger; the slaves and the freeborn plebeians died off equally quickly, among lamenting of wives and children, who, (infected) while they attended the sick and while they wept, were often being burnt on the same pyre. The deaths of equestrians and senators, though common, were less often wept over, as if through their shared death they were anticipating the savagery of the Princeps.

In his discussion of conjecture, Quintilian distinguishes questions of fact from those of intent and cites disputes over the origins of plague as a question of fact (*Inst.* 7.2.3).[1] He offers four different options used to explain the causes of epidemic disease in ancient Rome: the

[1] *Quaeritur et unde quid ortum, ut pestilentia ira deum an intemperie caeli an corruptis aquis an noxio terrae halitu* ("We also inquire about the origins of something, for instance, whether a plague is due to the anger of the gods or the intemperance of the climate, or a corrupt water supply, or from poisonous vapors of the earth.")

anger of the gods, corrupt sky or water, and noxious exhalations from the earth. His offerings evoke a history of the literary topos, adding to the impression of its flourishing, indeed its excesses, in the early Imperial period. While we need not indict the historian for excess, Tacitus too seems struck by the contagion of plague discourse, reporting in this chapter's epigraph on a pestilence that erupted in Campania during Nero's reign (65 CE) and using language familiar from history, epic, and, as we shall see, drama. After naming a litany of exiles and executions ordered by Nero, beginning with the emperor's wife, Poppaea Sabina (*Ann.*16.6), the historian observes the disastrous impact of *pestilentia* not far from Rome, along with its traditional leveling of the populace (*omne mortalium genus; non sexus, non aetas periculo vacua*). Nevertheless, two classes stand out whose mortality rates were less remarkable, or literally less "wept over": for the senators and equestrians, death in Campania was merely an extension of the *saevitia principis* already begun. Tacitus is not merely using the grim details of pestilence for colorful effect, but instead relies on its ferocity and unchecked movement through all social *ordines* to characterize the operations of the Principate. Plague does not so much suggest civil war as it explicitly demonstrates what Romans were left with in war's aftermath.

In the first two sections of this monograph, I hope to have demonstrated why writers of the late-Republican and Augustan periods found pestilence such an effective (and affective) metaphor for discord within the body politic; we have also observed precisely what these writers added to that metaphor, the distinctively Latin idioms used to describe the deteriorating physical corpus as well as the social pathologies that reflect on distinctively Roman values, under pressure. What remains to be seen is how and why—after civic discord had been, at least for a time, resolved under the Julio-Claudian dynasty—the language of pestilence and its implications for civil war and the end of the Republic continued to proliferate. Equally important is an exploration of how post-Augustan writers, by exaggerating, distorting, or even muting characteristic features of the Latin plague narrative, clarify the efficacy of that narrative in its original context of internal strife (Lucretius) and the immediate aftermath of civil war (Vergil and Ovid).[2] When Lucan uses the

[2] Cf. Martindale's strong and weak theses in *Redeeming the Text* (1993, 7–8), cited in the introduction to this project (p. 13 n. 16): imitations of later poets reveal and clarify meanings embedded in the works of their predecessors; and further, it is

language of epidemic disease to show us heaps of *cadavera* left in the wake of Marius' and Sulla's consecutive bloodbaths in the city (2.134–43), he magnifies the glimpses of civil war hiding beneath inherited plague texts (for instance, Lucretius' own aggregations of flesh in Athens). Lucan's recycling of such language in a new context also revives the original tensions in the Roman social order—tensions generated from rivalries for supremacy—that made the plague metaphor, with its usual *telos* in undifferentiated masses of the dead, such a useful tool for diagnosing morbidity in the body politic.

In this chapter I examine three Imperial poets, Lucan, Seneca, and Silius Italicus, who adapt the pestilence motif in ways that pick at threads in the seams of what should be a metonymic relationship between the individual hero and the Roman collective he represents. As Philip Hardie has observed (1993, 7–10), the singularity of the epic hero and his ability to stand alone as one for many is a fundamental preoccupation of epic poetry, though Roman ventures in epic, especially after Vergil, constantly throw up doubles to confound the power of an individual—no longer "superlative" if he is rivaled—to represent the whole.[3] While Seneca's treatment of the plague narrative in the *Oedipus* is a generic outlier in the group, the dramatist's depiction of a hero who is obsessed with his unique power to save a plague-stricken population finds kinship with the concerns of Lucan's *Bellum Civile* and Silius' *Punica*, which also use pestilence to contemplate the possibility of heroism that does not provoke rivalry within the civic corpus. Seneca's desire to import such epic features into his tragedy not only puts pressure on the limits of generic definitions, but also confirms contemporary interest in reassessing a monarchical government as the outcome of fiercely two-headed civil war, a government imagined as a singular head in charge of the body politic.

6.1. LUCAN AND THE *RABIES* OF CIVIL WAR

Historically and poetically speaking, the origin of Lucan's plague, narrated in Book 6 of *Bellum Civile*, is nebulous: the poet, in keeping

impossible to read the plague narratives of Lucretius, Vergil, and Ovid stripped of the meanings assigned to them (or revealed in them) by later poets.

[3] For rivalry and doubling in the *Aeneid*, see also Bandera (1981) and the discussion above, Chapter 4, p. 141.

with a general skepticism concerning the role of the gods in human affairs,[4] avoids divine causation and gestures vaguely toward the decomposing flesh of horses fed on foreign grain. Lucan relies to some extent on Ovid, whose rotting animal carcasses, while not the ultimate cause of disease, spread plague to the human inhabitants of Aegina (*Met.* 7.550–1, Vallillee 1960, 146). Lucan's intertextual reach may also extend to Vergil's *Eclogues*, where foreign grain was paired with *contagium* as twin threats posed by an Italian landscape suffering the upheavals of civil *discordia* (1.49–50). The episode at Dyrrachium is, moreover, drawn partly from remarks in Caesar's commentary on conditions in Pompey's camp, though Caesar only mentions general ill health (*valetudine non bona*) arising from difficult conditions, the odor of rotting corpses, and a lack of water (*Civ.* 3.49).[5]

Lucan thus concocts a pastiche of sources for his *contagium*, perhaps under pressures from epic conventions, and especially Homeric tradition (Sklenář 2003, 45–6). As much as the episode owes to epic tradition writ large, however, it is specifically indebted to the tradition of using pestilence as a tool for dramatizing the dissolution of the body politic in civil war. Amidst the prophecies on the eve of war that conclude Book 1, Figulus describes the impending calamity as both a *matura lues* (645) and a *pestis* (649) devised by the gods, references that heighten our sensitivities to the way that pestilence and civil war will reciprocally inform each other throughout the poem. In the following discussion I focus initially on two areas of Lucan's engagement with Latin traditions of narrating pestilence: the poet's use of *rabies* to describe the spread of contagion and clarify the psychological dimension of plague as civil war, and his abbreviated symptomatology, which reflects on various distortions of the Roman body politic. In concluding, I consider closure: the closure to Lucan's plague is startlingly abrupt, in a way that at first glance denies the potential of Vergil's Noric and Lucretius' Athenian

[4] Cf. Ahl (1976, esp. 280–3); Sklenář (2003, esp. 5–12) finds in Lucan systematic opposition to Stoic principles, in particular, the belief in divine providential guidance. For an overview of Stoic elements in Lucan, see Roche (2009, 30–6); Johnson is skeptical of Lucan's commitment to Stoic principles, which rely on a rational and divinely guided universe, and finds more evidence for "the blatant absence of any design" reflected in the poem (1987, 8).

[5] As Sklenář (2003, 46 n. 54) observes, though Grimm (1965, 73) stresses the possible influence of Livy's non-extant account.

epidemics to repeat themselves, ad infinitum. Yet by closing the narrative frame of literal pestilence in Book 6, Lucan allows the reciprocally metaphoric relationship of plague and civil war to infect preceding and subsequent books. Drawing on Vallillee's notion of "quasi-plague" in Lucan,[6] I examine key passages that aggressively contaminate battlefield narratives with the language of pestilence, arguing that the poet rejects the purifying, clean-slate potential of pestilence and instead opts for a post-apocalyptic model of aftermaths and remainders. Pestilence motifs persist well beyond the first hundred lines of Book 6, mimicking the interminable nature of Roman civil war and supplementing the poet's strategies to resist the narrative closure that would seal the fate of the Republic.[7]

Treatments of BC within the last half century have drawn attention to Lucan's interest in bodies, announced in the poem's opening lines that posit a suicidal body politic turning weapons against its own innards (*populumque potentem/in sua victrici conversum viscera dextra*, 1.2–3). Lucan foregrounds early on the metaphoric role of the human corpus as civic body (2.21–8) by describing the *res publica* as a corpse in a house of mourning before it has been laid out for burial rituals and lamentations. Scholars have focused on the vulnerabilities of Lucan's bodies as well as their figurative potential for the poem's concept of Roman history ("fractured and amorphous"), and their implications for Lucan's poetic architecture ("deliberately fragmentary" and depicting a "world out of joint"; Quint 1993, 147). Bartsch (1997) turns to Kristeva's notion of the abject to account for Lucan's violation of bodies and the processes of putrefaction that force what was formerly contained to be exposed: the constant failures of the human body to contain the self ("is the self merely guts in a bag of skin?" 20) dramatizes the disturbance of subject–object relations that recognition of the abject activates. This disturbance is rampant at the level of form—in Lucan's syntax logical grammatical subjects become

[6] Vallillee gathers examples of plague motifs outside the plague narrative proper and observes, "Lucan frequently shows a flair for horror-fraught description that includes many ideas already met with in the plague tradition" (1960, 145).

[7] On the poem's use of repetition, delay, and deferral to resist narrative closure, see especially Masters (1992), who argues that the poem's inconclusive ending is a deliberate reflection of Roman civil war as an uncontained, ongoing phenomenon; Tracy (2011) defends BC's abrupt ending on the basis of internal evidence, a similarly inconclusive digression on the Nile in Book 10; for an overview of scholarship on the poem's complete or incomplete status, see esp. Masters (1992, 216–59).

objects—as well as content (e.g., soldiers use their throats as weapons, rather than having their throats cut by weapons).[8] Such a theorization of Lucan's bodies points to the poem's fundamental concern with boundary transgression and confirms a kinship between the bodily violations that exist throughout *BC* and those violations that we first observed in Lucretius' account of putrefaction, the tottering barriers of life within the body of the individual complementing the viscous atmosphere of decay permeating Athenian society. Lucan's plague also foregrounds the signifying potential of the human corpus, but does so in ways that more directly address the body politic transformed under the imperatives of the Principate.

Book 6 of Lucan's epic opens with Pompey's decision to pitch camp at Dyrrachium. Caesar responds to his opponent's attempt to defer battle by surrounding him with entrenchments and fortifications, as majestic as the walls surrounding Troy (*Iliacos . . . muros*, 6.48). Within this confined space, a narrow strip of sand resonant with Homeric tradition, the "madness of civil war seethes" (*aestuat angusta rabies civilis harena*, 6.63). The phrasing imports the context of Roman gladiatorial combat, which lends the episode a spectacular quality as well as calling attention to the nature of participants in this engagement. Unlike the combatants in Roman *munera*, who were usually outfitted to represent enemy nations, the soldiers of civil war have been defined as equals (*pares aquilas et pila minantia pilis*, 1.7; Ahl 1976, 87–8)[9]—parity that was a source of horror coloring the sketches of civil war at the end of the first *Georgic* (489), a marvel reborn in the brave new world of Ovid's equally youthful and courageous Myrmidons in Aegina (*pares annis animisque*, *Met.* 7.658). As Saylor notes, equality among opposing forces is redoubled as both Pompey and Caesar will experience a kind of siege: *circumdatus* describes Pompey at 44, and Caesar's camp is "besieged" (again *circumdatus*, 108–9) by a famine whose dehumanizing effects match

[8] In addition to the more extended treatments of Lucan's bodies in Quint and Bartsch, see also the comments of Narducci (1979, 47–52), who addresses the violation of Lucan's bodies in light of (esp.) Vergilian precedents. Mebane (2016, discussed further below) offers a recent treatment of the relationship between Lucan's bodies and the Roman body politic.

[9] Cf. also Masters (1992, 35), who sees the language of parity as illustrating civil war's paradox of "unified disunity or disunified unity"; see also Roche (2009, 108), on the language of matched standards and weapons as an evocation of Vergil's depiction of civil war at the end of the first *Georgic*.

those of pestilence, forcing men to grasp at food not fit for human consumption (6.116–17). Plague and famine thus conspire in a "mutuality of destruction . . . marked in the symmetrical quality of the afflictions in both camps . . . and underscored by the paradox of besieger besieged. With famine the Caesarians become no different from those they have enclosed" (Saylor 1978, 249).

Such identification between opposing forces justifies Lucan's account of events there as a form of narrowly enclosed "madness." Of the twenty uses of *rabies* in Lucan's poem, the large majority refer to the "madness" of civil war, either directly or in similes describing behavior of the war's participants.[10] Book 6 is the only instance where Lucan doubles down on the implications of civil strife in *rabies* with the adjective *civilis*, and it will be followed shortly after with a metaphor used to describe the pestilential atmosphere that afflicts Pompey's men. The echo in close proximity not only strengthens the conceptual alignment of plague and civil war, but also accentuates the psychological "madness" of *rabies* over and above the physical condition associated with the disease.[11] Following Homer's use of *lyssa*, the Greek term for rabies, to describe Hector's fury at Troy, Latin poets use *rabies* to connote savage possession on the battlefield, or a generally bloodthirsty condition (e.g., Aeneas' description of Trojans fighting in *Aeneid* 2, as if wolves driven by *rabies*, 357). After employing the term with its familiar military implications throughout the first five books of *BC*, Lucan uses it to describe the quality of the air that will afflict Pompey's soldiers, once the horses, sick from foreign fodder, have died and begun the process of decomposition:[12]

> maior cura duces miscendis abstrahit armis:
> Pompeium exhaustae praebenda ad gramina terrae,

[10] E.g., as in the simile at 4.240, which describes the bloodthirsty response of Petreius' men after he has implored them to resume hostilities against Caesar. Of the 20 uses of *rabies* in the poem, the only ones without direct application to civil strife are references to the prophetess Phemonoe's "madness" (5.190, 210), references to weather phenomena (5.603, 9.454), and the *rabies* used to explain the spread of plague in Pompey's camp.

[11] For literary precedents, Vergil *G*.3.496 is perhaps the most pertinent, though the term is used there in a relatively clinical sense to explain the Noric plague's manifestation in dogs (see below, p. 195); cf. Ovid *Met.* 11.369–70 and Hippolytus' horses at *Met.*15.521. Wasik and Murphy (2012, 22–36) discuss accounts of the disease in the medical writers Soranus and Celsus (e.g., *De Medicina* 5.27) as well as treatments for rabies in Pliny the Elder.

[12] The text is Housman's, used with minor alterations in Duff (1928).

> quae currens obtriuit eques, gradibusque citatis
> ungula frondentem discussit cornea campum.
> belliger attonsis sonipes defessus in aruis,
> aduectos cum plena ferant praesepia culmos,
> ore nouas poscens moribundus labitur herbas
> et tremulo medios abrumpit poplite gyros.
> corpora dum soluit tabes et digerit artus,
> traxit iners caelum fluuidae contagia pestis
> obscuram in nubem. tali spiramine Nesis
> emittit Stygium nebulosis aera saxis
> antraque letiferi rabiem Typhonis anhelant.
> (6.80–92)

A greater concern keeps the leaders from engaging in battle: the exhausted earth kept Pompey from providing grain, which the horses had run over and trampled down, as their horny hooves struck the grassy field with quickened paces. The noisy warhorse grew weary in the close cropped fields, although full troughs offered imported grain, and demanding fresh grass with his mouth, he totters, about to die, and breaks off from the middle of his circling on trembling haunches. While rot dissolved their bodies and drove apart their limbs, the stagnant sky drew up the contagion of the fluid/melting pestilence into a murky cloud. With such a blowing does Nesis send forth Stygian air from cloud-covered rocks and (with such blowing) do the caves of deadly Typhon exhale madness (*rabies*).

By couching his *rabies* in the context of epidemic disease, Lucan activates the word's medical meaning, a contagious condition recognized by medical writers as resulting in desperate thirst along with fear of water, confusion, and unpredictable rage.[13] That rage could transform a loved one into an enemy, a conversion reflected in the duality that structures human relationships with those animals predominantly associated with rabies, canines—identified as loyal helpmates as well as vicious threats. Thus the poet's reference to *rabies* imports a distinct psychological dimension to the outbreak at Dyrrachium, as a complement to its physiological properties: "[rabies] was rare, terrifying: violent, and animalistically destructive of others; ultimately (and pathetically) destructive of self. It made creatures maim and kill those closest to them. It hollowed out reason and left nothing but frenzy" (Wasik and Murphy 2012, 17). Where earlier

[13] For *rabies* in medical texts, see above, n. 11.

plague treatments suggest the nearly lifeless (*semianimes*, cf. Lucr. 6.1268, Ovid *Met.* 7.577) condition of its victims, Lucan hones in on the peculiar manifestation of the Noric plague in Vergil's dogs (*G.*3.496), and uses it to imply active aggression more suited to the battlefield than the infirmary. At the same time, his modification is an appropriate response to earlier poets who used pestilence to problematize interfamilial relationships, a reflection of civil war's power to provoke hostilities among relatives formerly deemed nearest and dearest. For Lucan, the peculiar pathologies of civil war, as a condition that prompts Romans to turn on their kin, makes *rabies* the most precise rendering of the contagion that afflicts the not-yet-warring camps in Book 6 and throughout the epic.

Rot (*tabes*) spreads disease from one species to the next, from horses to humans. Lucan's use here conforms to the traditions of the Latin plague narrative in signaling the permeability of the human form and dramatizing the decomposition of individuals. Lucretius brings decay (*tabes*, 6.1201) and homogeneity center stage in his Athenian tragedy, and the same processes logically precede the heaps of indistinguishable *corpora* filling the streets, public spaces, and temples at the end of his narrative. Lucan has pushed the process of rot further back in his plague dramaturgy: the limb-loosening *tabes* among dead horses, indicated as the outcome of disease for the equine community, becomes a source of *contagia* for humans. And yet, as with Vergil's framing of the Noric plague between *tabum*-stained fodder at the initial outbreak (3.481) and *tabum*-riddled bodies at Book 3's closure (557), the sequential confusion that allows "rot" to function as both the source and the outcome of disease mimics the cyclical nature of the plague as civil war: *tabes* will emerge forcefully and repeatedly on the battlefield after slaughter at Pharsalia (see esp. 7.808–9, 822–46), marking the end of one battle but anticipating the renewed fighting that would spring forth from the festering soil of Thessaly, in (nearly) the same battlefield.[14]

Latin writers use language of liquefaction to indicate the failure of the body's structural integrity under the pressure of epidemic disease, and Lucan nods to that convention by describing the pestilence as

[14] On the insistent confusion between Pharsalus and Philippi among Latin poets, see Roche (2009, 385); cf. Mynors (1990, 94–5) on a similar identification of the two battlefields in Vergil's *Georgics*.

fluvidus. Such a property also facilitates the transmission of disease from the equine community to the human one:

> inde labant populi, caeloque paratior unda
> omne pati uirus durauit uiscera caeno.
> iam riget arta cutis distentaque lumina rumpit,
> igneaque in uoltus et sacro feruida morbo
> pestis abit, fessumque caput se ferre recusat.
> iam magis atque magis praeceps agit omnia fatum,
> nec medii dirimunt morbi uitamque necemque,
> sed languor cum morte uenit; turbaque cadentum
> aucta lues, dum mixta iacent incondita uiuis
> corpora; nam miseros ultra tentoria ciues
> spargere funus erat. tamen hos minuere labores
> a tergo pelagus pulsusque Aquilonibus aer
> litoraque et plenae peregrina messe carinae.
> (6.93–105)

From there, the men begin to fall; the water, more ready than the sky to take in all the poison, hardened the innards with filth. Now the taut skin grows stiff and bursts the straining eyes, and the plague, fiery and seething with the sacred disease, spreads to the face, and the (victim's) weary head refuses to hold itself up. Now more and more does headlong fate drive everything, nor do intermittent stages of the disease separate life from death, but with weakness comes death. The crowd of those fallen transmits the disease further, while unburied bodies lay about, mingled with the living. For scattering the bodies of wretched citizens just outside the tents sufficed for a funeral. Still, the sea at their backs and the air struck by the North Wind, as well as the shore and ships filled with foreign corn, lessened their hardships.

Vallillee (1960, 148–9) has usefully catalogued Lucan's borrowings from his predecessors in the realm of symptomatology and epidemiology, borrowings that amount at first glance to an unsystematic composite of familiar imagery ("apparently casual reminiscence"). Certain echoes, however, bring into focus Lucan's specific concern of reflecting on a body politic at war with itself, a body whose morbidity culminates in dissolution. The pathogen in *BC*, much like the *pestis* in Vergil's Noricum, operates by triggering internal oppositions:[15] as we

[15] With varying degrees of nuance and qualification, scholarship on the intertextual relationship between Vergil and Lucan has focused overwhelmingly on the latter's polemical response to the *Aeneid* (Narducci 1979; Thompson and Bruère 2010; cf. Masters 1992, esp. 118–33 on Lucan's challenges to Vergil's narrative strategies in the *Aeneid*); yet the *Georgics*, composed in the wake of Actium and imminently

observed in Chapter 4, in the *Georgic* poet's account, parching thirst first shrivels the limbs (*adduxerat artus*, 483), then swells the body with "a watery humor" (*abundabat fluidus liquor*), an opposition (or "paradox") identified as Vergilian innovation in the tradition of symptomatology.[16] Lucan's *fluvida pestis* reshuffles Vergil's symptoms within the camp, initially confining the liquefying power of the Noric plague to the horses at Dyrrachium whose rotting bodies contaminate the soldiers' quarters. Pompey's soldiers experience, by contrast, various forms of stiffening and rigidity, symptoms introduced paradoxically though a liquid form (*unda*, 93). Imbibed "water" hardens the entrails, as skin grows stiff and eyes grow taught, stretched to the point of rupturing. The skin's rigidity, of course, may also harken back to Lucretius' own account of the tightening dermis experienced in the Athenian plague—there such stiffening was balanced, in the case of those who survived past the ninth day, by subsequent liquefaction and near complete evacuation of the self (*huc hominis totae vires corpusque fluebat*, Lucr. 6.1194–1204).

Lucan does not attempt clinical accuracy, or even a smattering of realistic details, but instead relies on paradox and contrast to stave off the homogeneity that is the plague's inevitable conclusion. Once the division between life and death is rendered meaningless (*medii dirimunt morbi vitamque necemque*, 99), however, other distinctions collapse and the bodies of Pompey's men are reduced to indistinguishable matter, similar to that condition defining the animal *corpora* earlier (6.88). But one symptom is worth dwelling on, since, in its elaboration of the body politic metaphor, it addresses the nature of rivalry, the culmination of rivalry in monarchy, and the powerlessness of Romans to avert either. The rapid confusion of life and death is preceded by the head's refusal to bear itself up (*caput se ferre recusat*), a sign that an end in death would from hereon determine the course of events (*praecaps agit omnia fatum*). Such language returns us to Book 1's sketch of a morbid Roman empire, unable to bear its own weight and bound by fate for destruction. To explain the

concerned with the renewal of strife, offers a rich repository of language for articulating civil *discordia*. Casali (2011, 85 and passim), while concerned primarily with the *Aeneid*, stresses Lucan's engagement with Vergil's depiction of civil war at the end of *Georgics* 1; cf. Narducci (1979, 35).

[16] See Harrison (1979, 8), discussed above, Chapter 4, p. 124, though I argue that Vergil's innovation is influenced by the language of flux and fluidity throughout Lucretius' treatment of Athenian plague.

cause of civil war (*causas tantarum . . . rerum,* 1.67), the poet cites elements of Rome's instability within the greater *discors machina*:[17]

> invida fatorum series summisque negatum
> stare diu nimioque graves sub pondere lapsus
> *nec se Roma ferens. . . .*
>
> (1.70–2)

It was the envious chain of destiny, impossibility of the very high standing long, huge collapses under too much weight, Rome's inability to bear herself... (trans. Braund 1992, 5)

The passage's continuation, which describes the world's dissolution (*compage soluta*), culminates in a pithy refrain of the culprit in Lucan's explication of Rome's ruin (size matters!): *in se magna ruunt* (81). In his haphazard sketch of plague symptoms in Book 6, the poet's recycling of language from Book 1 aligns the head of victims with an empire overburdened by its greatness, a Rome elsewhere likened to the very "head of the world" (*caput mundi,* 2.655, 2.136). The tottering heads of Pompey's men, moreover, invoke Caesar's signature "headstrong" impatience to move all things to conclusion: *Caesar in omnia praeceps* (2.656; cf. Quint 1993, 148). Just as the head, overburdened by pestilence, conspires with "headlong fate" to drive everything toward death (*praeceps agit omnia fatum,* 6.98), Caesar *praeceps* hurries along the demise of the Republic. Where Lucretius (following Thucydides) begins with effects of illness on the head (6.1145)—passing over altogether its unbearable weight—and follows the progress of the disease into the lower parts of the body, Lucan's tottering heads mark the final moment before death. The deviation from his predecessor's symptomatology reconfigures the metaphoric implications of illness in a way that addresses the collapse of a Roman empire upheld by Republican liberties and Caesar's role in hastening that collapse.

Examining how violated bodies address the integrity or corruption of the body politic in Lucan's poem, Julia Mebane (2016) argues that Roman variations on the body politic metaphor are evaluated through Pompey's decapitation in Book 7: these variations range from a Republican model that privileged the belly as a central locus of authority, famous from Menenius Agrippa's parable in Livy,[18] to a

[17] For the *discors machina* as driving the destruction of Rome and (ultimately) the universe, as well as its rather un-Stoical implications, see Johnson (1987, 16–17).

[18] See above, Chapter 2, pp. 50–1.

model in the Principate that locates power in the human *caput*. For Mebane, the severing of the head from the body ultimately reclaims for Pompey the nobility denied him, and the body politic of Rome, when he vied for position as "head" of the state. Moreover, her larger point, that Lucan uses the figure of decapitation to indict the authoritarianism of the Principate, reminds us of the poet's keen awareness of the power of the physical corpus to register changes in the body politic. In light of this awareness, plague and its ultimate leveling of victims in death in Lucan's *BC* are overdetermined registers of the perverse equality—emphasized through language of doubling—that defines a citizen body at war with itself. By focusing on the weight of the head just prior to the plague victim's death and incorporation within the larger crowd of unburied soldiers, the poet rehearses the contention among equals that eventually yields to supremacy (monarchy), but also predicts the collapse of the one, a single governing agent, and subsequent renewal of the same frustrating parity. An empire founded on contention among twins can only temporarily resolve itself in one-man rule, before head(s) roll and the pattern reasserts itself (cf. Hardie 1993, 10). Lucan's plague thus dramatizes the same illogical contention for distinction and for hegemony among citizens deemed equals that had destabilized Rome since its very foundation.

Failed or half-hearted burial rites constitute the whole of Lucan's section on the epidemiology of the Dyrrachian plague, a momentary crisis resolved through a change of winds and a new supply of fodder for the horses—again foreign grain, though apparently uncorrupted. The *telos* of the epidemic at Dyrrachium thus refuses those forms of closure wrought by other poets, who dwell on post-apocalyptic conditions of piecemeal deterioration (*Georgics* 3, *DRN* 6) or predict renewal through a sacrificial scapegoat (Orpheus of *Georgics* 4). The poet also resists revelations of a New Jerusalem with its purified, singularly loyal population (Aegina's Myrmidons). Lucan's soldiers pick themselves up, brush themselves off, and get on with the fighting in a way that all too casually entangles the ending of pestilence with resumption of civil war, issuing a kind of closural challenge to all three of his predecessors in the Latin epic tradition.[19] This challenge evolves primarily through quasi-plague language infecting sections of the poem that do not address epidemic

[19] Cf. n. 7 above; Mebane (2016, 205–8), relying on Masters (1992), Henderson (1998), and Quint (1993), also stresses how the narrative's development consistently points toward the interminable nature of Roman civic strife.

disease, but do address the plague-instigated pathological behaviors we have observed in Lucan's predecessors.

6.2. QUASI-PLAGUE AND FAILED CLOSURE IN *BELLUM CIVILE*

The tendency of the plague narrative to reduce human identity to so much flesh and blood, with one body indistinguishable from the next, emerges in counterpoint to the epic tradition's self-conscious preoccupation with kings, heroism on the battlefield, and foundation stories. While Lucan's protagonists enact their own distinction-granting *aristeiai*, plague is endemic in the text, insofar as the violence of civil war results in body counts that, like the mortality rates of pestilence, defy the poet's commemorative abilities. In describing conditions where "unburied bodies lay about mingled with the living" (*mixta iacent incondita vivis/corpora*, 6.101–2) Lucan not only revisits Lucretian (6.1215–16) and Ovidian (*Met.* 7.606–9) demonstrations of human identities subsumed in the totality of contagion; he also recalls the specters of contagion and boundary violation from earlier passages in *BC* describing the civil strife between Marius and Sulla. As an old man narrates Sulla's brutal vengeance after Marius has invaded Rome and slaughtered its citizens, he singles out as especially atrocious the tombs and the interfamilial bloodshed that fills them:

> . . . nati maduere paterno
> sanguine; certatum est, cui cervix caesa parentis
> cederet; in fratrum ceciderunt praemia fratres.
> *busta repleta fuga, permixtaque viva sepultis/*
> *corpora*, nec populum latebrae cepere ferarum.
> (2.149–53)

Sons grew wet with the blood of their fathers; they struggled over who would win the neck of a slain parent; brothers killed brothers for a reward. Tombs were filled with fugitives, and living bodies mingled with buried corpses, nor could the hiding places of beasts contain (so many) people.

In addition to stressing the internal echo linking the Dyrrachian plague to Sullan slaughter, Fantham (1992, 108) notes Lucretian parallels in the surrounding description of bloodshed, for instance, the general atmosphere of impiety in which sons rival (*certatum est*) each other to commit murder of a parent. Perhaps more pertinent are subsequent remarks in the old man's account of excessive fear of death, in some cases leading to suicide, owing much to both Lucretian and Ovidian comments on drastic measures taken during the plagues at Athens and Aegina (Lucr. 6.1207–11, *Met.* 7.604–5). The story of Sulla's mass executions among the Roman populace is, of course, not a plague narrative, but, by allusively binding it to the disease suffered at Dyrrachium as well as other literary epidemics, Lucan allows the social pathologies of pestilence identified by his predecessors to emerge with greater precision. Through his emphasis on rivalry and impious, interfamilial slaughter as premier perversions within a quasi-plague description, Lucan revisits Lucretius' own indictment of familial discord and contention for honors: in *DRN* such perversions are threaded throughout the symptomatology and epidemiology of the Athenian plague.[20] We might detect a natural sympathy between the two authors, as Lucretius glances in foresight and Lucan in hindsight at the excessive desire for honors that gives birth to the *monstrum* of civil war (*honorum caeca cupido*, Lucr. 3.59; *nimia cupidine caeci*, Luc.1.87).

Both civil war and pestilence render the most fundamental distinctions, in this case that between the quick and the dead, meaningless. Lucan's plague proper allows no opportunity for burial. In other segments of *BC*, however, where burial rites are attempted and some effort is made to restore the boundary between life and death as well as commemorate the life of an individual, the poet (again) turns to Lucretius' plague. Book 3 concludes with a graphic and bloody sea battle between Caesar's forces, led by his admiral Decimus Brutus, and the Massilians. In their defeat and mourning, described in the book's closing lines, the Massilians attempt to gather and bury the dead:

> . . . quis in urbe parentum
> fletus erat! quanti matrum per litora planctus!
> coniunx saepe sui confusis voltibus unda
> credidit ora viri Romanum amplexa cadaver,
> accensisque rogis miseri de corpore trunco
> certavere patres. at Brutus in aequore victor
> primus Caesareis pelagi decus addidit armis.
> (3.756–62)

What weeping of parents there was in the city! What great wailing of mothers was there throughout the shores! Often a wife, having embraced a Roman corpse, believed it was the face of her own husband, since the face had been

[20] See above, Chapter 3, p. 107, for discussion of Lucr. 3.68–73 and its relationship to the Athenian plague of Book 6.

disfigured by the sea, and wretched fathers contended with each other for a headless trunk over burning pyres. But Brutus as victor on the water first gave the glory of the sea to Caesar's forces.

The situational parallels (burning funeral pyres, citizens struggling over bodies of kin) that tie the closure of Book 3 to the final lines of *DRN* are stronger than any explicit verbal allusion. In Lucretius, the episode reflects on the last-ditch efforts to preserve familial identity amidst the swelling numbers of anonymous dead in the face of plague: citizens brawling (*rixantes*) in *DRN* offered a refrain to those struggling (*certantes*) to bury the dead earlier in the plague narrative.[21] Lucan has answered his predecessor's demonstration of the futile attempts to acknowledge familial relationships during outbreaks of civic discord with exaggerated futility, since the bodies of the dead (rendered unrecognizable after the naval battle) that the bereft attempt to preserve are not even their own kin: Lucan transforms desperate attempts to recognize and preserve kinship in *DRN* into a farcical travesty of misrecognition.[22]

Recognition in fact becomes a trope that Lucan regularly exploits in his battlefield narratives, and especially the battle of Pharsalia, where fathers and sons deliberately mark each other for death, enacting constant perversions of *pietas* (e.g., 7.463–9, 550). The irony of such claims to kinship, and their drive to destruction rather than familial preservation, is heightened against the background of growing heaps of *cadavera* and against the poem's push towards unrecognizability. As Quint observes (1993, 146), most scenes of violence culminate in the loss of identity, rather than (as so often in earlier epic) heightened distinction. Lucan constantly manipulates the status-leveling effects of a civil war whose death toll is explicitly likened to plague (*aera pestiferum tractu morbosque fluentes*, 7.412) and renders

[21] Some editors would transpose 6.1247–51 to follow 1286: *inque aliis alium, populum sepelire suorum/certantes; lacrimis lassi luctuque redibant* (1247–8). This move would bind the struggling (from *certo*) over burials more closely to the brawling around the pyres; see above, Chapter 3, p. 81 n. 6. Lucan's characterization of fighting over the dead as acts of contention (*certavere*) may lend support to Lucretius' use of the verb in the final lines of his own poem.

[22] See also 2.166–8, where "rot" (*tabes*) renders faces unrecognizable. This passage generates a similar tension between the perverse equality (more specifically, in-distinguishability) that defines participants of civil war and the distinction that family members (although prevented here and elsewhere in Lucan) were traditionally allowed to convey upon death.

nearly impossible the celebration of any single warrior's glory-gaining death (7.617–18, *singula fata*; cf. 7.630–1).

Amidst so much slaughter Caesar bids his men to spare the *plebs* and mark the senatorial class for destruction. The result is another "quasi-plague" passage used to describe a heap of corpses that, on the one hand, draws from the plague's language of unstructured accumulation, first glimpsed in Lucretius and refined in Vergil (cf. *aggerat*, 3.556).[23] On the other hand, the poet temporarily resists the collapsing of social distinctions: *hic patriae perit omne decus: iacet aggere magno/patricium campis non mixta plebe cadaver* (7.597–8, "here all the glory of the country perished: patrician corpses lay in a great heap without a plebeian mixed among them"; cf. 7.581–3). The singular *patricium cadaver* points to the notion of a unified body politic, but one from which its other members, the plebeian class in particular, have been severed. *Non mixta* responds to the Roman historiographic tradition, as we observed in Livy, who acknowledged the plague's power to collapse class distinctions and effect occasionally salubrious redistributions of power within the body politic (cf. 4.25, 5.13).[24] The mingling that Lucan denies here, however, will soon be accomplished, again through Caesar's command, as he orders his men to loot Pompey's camp:

> . . . capit inpia plebes
> caespite patricio somnos, stratumque cubile
> regibus infandus miles perit, inque parentum
> inque toris fratrum posuerunt membra nocentes.
> (7.760–3)

The wicked plebeians sleep on patrician turf, and the sinful soldiers press upon couches spread for kings, and the guilty have placed their limbs on the bedding of their brothers and fathers.

The poet elides one type of transgression (plebeian incursion into patrician turf) with another (family members turning against one

[23] See Masters (1992, 145) on the "motif of the heap" as a Lucanian leitmotif; he offers a list of relevant passages. For language of heaping and accumulation, see also the poet's description of Caesar, who after battle wades through corpses piled high (*tu, Caesar, in alto/caedis adhuc cumulo patriae per viscera vadis*, 7.721–2), and will later feast his eyes on the mounds of dead beginning to deteriorate the day following the battle (*excelsos cumulis aequantia colles/corpora, sidentes in tabem spectat acervos*, 7.790–1).

[24] For depictions of class intermingling during the plague in *AUC*, see above, Chapter 2, esp. pp. 58–63.

another), transgressions that mutually exclude each other, since kin within the same *familia* will logically reside in the same class. Presumably the poet is thinking of those plebeians who did fight on Pompey's side as the fathers and brothers whose bedding (presumably segregated from the *patricio caespite*) is abused by Caesar's men, but the cumulative effect of such infractions is a buzzing failure of logic, a demonstration of how civil war, again like the plague, renders all categorical distinctions meaningless.[25]

Compared with other natural disasters in Lucan (e.g., the storm that hinders Caesar's departure from Brundisium in Book 5) or with other depictions of plague in Latin, pestilence at Dyrrachium never gains the kind of game-changing momentum that demands divine intervention or heroic measures. As I hope to have suggested here, that is largely because the plague simply replays the wider epidemic of *discordia* that is the poet's primary concern throughout the poem. We find no Aristaeus consulting Cyrene, or Aeneas enjoying visitation by his Penates on Crete, no Aeacus calling on Jupiter in despair. If Lucan's plague holds a mirror to the epidemic's implications of civil war in preceding epic poetry, it also reflects on the nature of heroism in the genre. The question of whether or not Lucan's epic has a hero has continued to vex readers.[26] Where Bartsch argues for Pompey as Lucan's answer to our need for a hero, for instance, only one of two in some ways antithetical Pompeys is allowed to embody Republican *virtus* and perhaps win our favor (7.207–13; 1997, 8).

Hardie sees heroism—in so far as it is constructed as the power of the individual to stand for a collective (*unus/omnes*)—as struggling to gain currency in Lucan through the economy of sacrifice. But the death of Cato, who is, as the staunchest defender of Republican values, an obvious candidate for sacrifice, never occurs in the text, and the manner of his death defies the logic of sacrifice that resolves Girard's antagonism between rivals:[27] "[his suicide] rules out absolutely any possibility of resolution to the sacrificial crisis; turning his

[25] My treatment of quasi-plague here is by no means exhaustive, but meant to emphasize those episodes that resonate with and clarify the implications of civil strife in earlier treatments of pestilence discussed in section 6.2. For other passages in which Lucan draws upon the language of the plague tradition, see Vallillee (1960, 150–6).

[26] See esp. Johnson (1987) on how heroism is problematic for all three major protagonists (Cato, Pompey, Caesar) in Lucan's poem.

[27] For Girard's sacrificial economy as it operates in Latin plague narratives, see Chapter 1, pp. 37–40.

hand on himself, acting out the roles of both sacrificer and sacrificed in one person, he confounded utterly the distinction between killer and killed on which the logic of Girardian victimization rests" (1993, 31). The relatively unquestioned singularity of heroism in previous Latin plague narratives, in which a king, or culture hero, or founder of the Roman race, with help from the gods, can cure and expurgate a stricken population finds no place in either Dyrrachium or in the more pervasive epidemic of civil war. In other words, Lucan's manipulations of the plague narrative demonstrate how the sacrificial process fails—and will continue to fail—to restore the Roman social order.

If there is no expurgation and initiation of a New Jerusalem, neither is there ostensibly a post-apocalyptic lingering on aftermaths and remainders, two options for concluding pestilence observed throughout this project (see above and Gomel 2000, 410). But, as I hope to have demonstrated here, the prosaic quality of this plague is precisely the point—the repetitive operations of contagion mirror and semantically extend to the numbing, if grotesque repetitions of the larger civil war that is the topic of Lucan's poem. As Masters has observed (1992, 3–4), Lucan's poem constantly throws up obstacles to its own progress, often through illogical narrative repetition. While structurally integral to the poem's narrative, these obstacles also have deep seated ideological implications, insistently putting off the closure that would historically define the Principate as an inevitable, unalterable political configuration (Quint 1993, 147). If the plague itself lacks the remainders, or "leftovers" in contemporary parlance, that define post-apocalyptic literature, the ten books of civil war in which it is contextualized furnish those lingering threats, the seeds of perpetual fragmentation and contagion.

And in fact *BC* has a curious kinship with the post-apocalyptic discourses proliferating in the late-twentieth century. Like modern texts that grapple with the century's greatest cataclysms (e.g., the Holocaust), the poem is post-apocalyptic in its position *after the fact* and its desire to replay historical trauma: pestilence motifs, by clarifying the scale and pervasive nature of the disaster of civil war as well as the impact of both on interpersonal relations, and on the body politic, facilitate Lucan's narrative re-presentation of a historical disaster. In suggestively post-apocalyptic fashion, Lucan writes from the other side of a cataclysm—from beyond "the ruptures, pivots, fulcrums separating what came before from what came after," rewriting and attempting to relive the events that have generated a new understanding of the world (Berger 5, 1999). But to conclude his poem, to remedy the plague of civil war, would crystallize both the new understanding of the world and the *novus ordo* in it, something the author, much like his own prophet Figulus in Book 1, cannot fathom: *et superos quid prodest poscere finem*? (1.669, "What good will it do for the gods to put an end to all this?").

6.3. SENECA'S *OEDIPUS*

In his reading of Sophocles' *Oedipus Tyrannus*, Girard follows Artaud by upholding that plague purifies the population it afflicts and isolates the king in his function as scapegoat: Oedipus' expulsion from Thebes completes the purification process by allowing a community to transfer its propensity for mimetic, reciprocal violence upon a single individual. Thus for Girard, Sophocles' Oedipus emerges as φαρμακός, both infected carrier of plague and savior to the Theban civic body (1974, 844), and the king's tragedy, his ruin and subsequent expulsion, illustrates the process by which a given social order disguises and minimizes its potential for internal violence (845). The status of Sophocles' *Oedipus* as a plague text is incontestable. As Mitchell-Boyask argues in his study of nosological patterns in the drama, the playwright's introduction of a λοιμός (*OT* 28) that afflicts Thebes,[28] at a time when Athenians were still reeling from casualties of their own plague, may have negatively impacted the *OT*'s initial reception (2008, 65). At the same time, the tragedy's account of plague's effects on the population is abbreviated and evocative rather than explicit: combined accounts of the priest and the chorus total about thirty lines, without mention of symptoms or epidemiological observations, aside from the countless dead and constant supplication at the altars of the gods.[29]

[28] Sophocles introduces the plague using a term (λοιμός) that, according to Mitchell-Boyask (2008, 59), may have been under stricture; νόσος and related forms are used elsewhere (e.g., 60–1, 150, 169, etc.). For the Theban plague as a Sophoclean innovation, see especially Knox (1956). The original production date is uncertain, though strong evidence places it between 426 and 424 BCE; see Mitchell-Boyask (2008, 57).

[29] For the countless dead and supplication at altars, see *OT* 20–34, the priest's account of the plague; 168–88, two strophes of the first choral ode, also include epidemiological features.

Seneca, writing about 500 years later and in a different cultural context, explodes the smattering of details in Sophocles and fuels the drama of his own project with language of plague in Lucretius, Vergil, and Ovid. As one critic has put it, plague operates in the *Oedipus* as a "textually transmitted disease" (Slaney 2009, 58; cf. Trinacty 2014, 138). The expansion of plague dramaturgy that accompanies the transference of the Oedipal myth from a Greek context to a Latin one demonstrates the peculiar fixation on the topos in the Latin epic tradition,[30] and, moreover, brings into better focus how competing claims of individuality and collectivity have shaped that tradition. Seneca's Oedipus regularly draws attention to his singular status and its uncomfortably superlative relationship to the Theban civic body (cf. *Oed.* 30, 76). Thebes, moreover, is drawn as a template for civil war, as audiences are reminded of the impending conflict between Oedipus' sons (e.g., 738–50). By addressing the communal effects of pestilence within a text that questions the efficacy of Roman law and depicts the isolation that accompanies autocratic power (Boyle 2011 lxxx), Seneca secures the role of contagion as a tool for examining the health of the new order born under the accession of Augustus and grown to maturity under the Julio-Claudian emperors. Using language of plague gleaned from earlier Latin poets, Seneca explores peculiarly Roman concerns over the impact of civil war—e.g., disturbances of *pietas*, the potential of a new *saeculum*—echoed within the tragedy by the war to be fought among Oedipus' successors in the not-too-distant future. Crisis afflicting Thebes is only apparently resolved with the abatement of plague, which is closely identified with the king himself (*atra Pestis et rabidus Dolor/mecum ite, mecum*, 1060–1; cf. Trinacty 2014, 139).

[30] For Ahl (2008, 126–32), the expanded detail points to the play's interest in contemporary plagues that struck Rome. Deeming the Campanian plague of 65 CE too late for Seneca the Younger to have responded to it in the *Oedipus*, he tentatively suggests moving the composition date up, closer to 22 BCE, when a plague struck Rome early in the Augustan Principate and assigning composition to Seneca the Elder. Ahl's solution to the problem of plague in Seneca's version has merit, correlating the prominence of the Sphinx with Augustus' victory over Egypt and use of a sphinx on his signet ring. But he undermines his own arguments with comments aptly situating the play within the traditions of later Imperial literature and its more firmly ingrained practices of self-censorship that did not have the same impact on works composed early in the Augustan Principate, e.g., 22: "the strength of the Senecan *Oedipus* is the concentrated power of its frustrated political and moral energy compressed into poetry."

Audiences are well aware that the same internecine strife, endemic in Thebes (cf. *civile nefas*, 748) and the cause of the current plague, is bound to repeat itself.

In the following discussion, I focus initially on how the playwright has adapted the language of epochal evolution that we have observed in late-Republican and Augustan poets. Plague transforms Thebes into a dystopia: at the opening of the tragedy the king ponders his survival amidst "ruins of his city . . . pitiable funerals and the slaughter of a nation" (*inter ruinas urbis et semper novis/deflenda lacrimis funera ac populi struem/incolumis asto*, 32–6); his portrait of the kingdom, drawn with further depth in the first choral ode, both mimics and inverts the Golden Age in significant details. How pointedly dystopian Thebes reflects conditions of Rome under the emperor Nero, during whose reign some scholars have tried to contextualize the drama,[31] remains an unanswered question, though imagery of a perverted *aurea aetas* may respond to the promotion of Nero's reign as a restored Golden Age.[32]

Oedipus is uniquely poised to resolve the saecular upheaval that has afflicted Thebes, and it is his role as the play's duplicitous hero/scapegoat that will be the focus of the second part of my discussion. Seneca uses the plague to reflect on the relationship between the community and those charged with governing it. This is already a contentious issue in the Oedipal drama Seneca inherited from Greece (Mitchell-Boyask 2008, 64)—though as commentators have emphasized, the originally democratic context of the drama has been replaced with a newly monarchical one in the Julio-Claudian Principate (Ahl 2008, 11; cf. Boyle 2011, xxxiii–xxxiv). As Trinacty (2014) has recently shown, the playwright was an astute reader and

[31] For the composition of the *Oedipus*, see Boyle (2011, xviii–xix), who tentatively suggests a Claudian date in light of the relative hostility of Tiberius and Caligula to theatrical productions. Atkinson (1981) and Bishop (1978) both situate the drama within Nero's Principate; Bishop interprets language in the tragedy as a "code" directing astute audiences to identify Nero with Oedipus; Atkinson is more cautious about the date of the play but interprets Seneca's depiction of the king's rage in the closing scene as a response to imperial tactics of fear and violence.

[32] While Golden-Age rhetoric circulated around the accession of many emperors, it was especially pronounced during the reign of Nero, and Seneca helped develop the emperor's role in presiding over a new *saeculum*; cf. *De Clementia* 2.1.3–4; *Apoc.* 4. Cf. also, e.g., comments in Tacitus (16.1–2) and the *Eclogues* of Calpurnius Siculus; see Evans (2008, 168–9).

interpreter of Augustan poetry.[33] I argue that Seneca expands his account of plague with such detail in part because of his awareness of how the Augustan writers developed plague motifs for reflecting on proprieties and transgressions of familial relationships, and their embedding within the larger community. Plague corrupts family relationships throughout Thebes in ways that not only reflect the perversions in Oedipus' own family, but also reiterate the tendency of Lucretius, Vergil, and Ovid to entangle familial relationships with the pathologies of civil war. By pulling on the strings of pestilence in his predecessors, Seneca tightens the knots of familial dysfunction and civil strife that lay at the center of their original contexts; he also elongates threads for spinning his own drama of a family whose morbidity has become indistinguishable from that of the state it purports to govern.

6.4. REFRACTIONS OF A NEW ORDER

The plague-riddled landscape surrounding Thebes forcefully denies the amenities of the literary *locus amoenus*, while also fostering conditions recalling poetic conventions of saecular decline:[34]

> non aura gelido lenis afflatu fovet
> anhela flammis corda, non *Zephyri* leves
> spirant, sed ignes auget aestiferi Canis
> Titan, leonis terga Nemeaei premens.
> deseruit amnes umor atque herbas color . . .
> nullum serenis noctibus sidus micat,
> sed gravis et ater incubat terris vapor.
> obtexit arces caelitum ac summas domos
> inferna facies. *denegat fructum Ceres*
> adulta, et *altis flava cum spicis tremat*,
> arente culmo sterilis emoritur seges.
> (*Oed.* 37–51)

[33] Trinacty's evaluation of Seneca's references in his *Epistulae Morales* to the process of literary borrowing and on the creative possibilities inherent in certain topoi is especially useful and (to my mind) helps confirm the identification of Seneca the Younger as the author of the tragedies transmitted in the corpus (2014, esp. 6–16); see also Littlewood (2004, 6–7).

[34] Text is that of Boyle (2011).

The chilly gust of no mild breeze nourishes our hearts, gasping with flames; nor do gentle Zephyrs blow upon us, but instead the Titan, pressing on the back of the Nemean lion, increases the fires of the heat-bearing Dogstar. Water has deserted the rivers, vibrant color has left the grass . . . no star shines in the calm nights, but a heavy, black mist settles upon the land. A hellish appearance covers over the citadels of the gods and their elevated homes. Ripened Ceres denies her produce, and although golden she trembles with lofty ears, a lifeless crop dies with its stems parched.

Oedipus' description of the pestilential atmosphere, while summoning ancient theories of miasma and Seneca's own *Quaestiones Naturales* (6.27–8, esp. 6.27.2), intermingles Golden- and Iron-Age indices drawn from Vergil and Ovid. As Littlewood has observed of Seneca's engagement with Augustan saecular rhetoric, the playwright relies especially on *Metamorphoses* 1 and the criminal behaviors of the Iron Age to complicate moral evaluations of his characters (2004, 10). But Seneca's fixation on the myth of the ages is not only anchored with details from Ovid, and, within the context of plague, the myth does more than inform audience response to a given character. Saecular rhetoric participates, at least on some level, in a broader discourse of the new order founded in the Principate, one that relied on a Golden Age (and its inverse) for legitimacy.

Predominant in Oedipus' account is Vergil's theodicy of *Georgics* 1, where Ceres is named as the goddess who first taught humans to till the soil after Dodona had "denied" her abundant acorns:

> prima *Ceres* ferro mortalis vertere *terram*
> instituit, cum iam glandes atque arbuta sacrae
> deficerent silvae et victum *Dodona negaret.*
> (*G.* 1.147–9)

Ceres first trained humans to turn the earth with iron, after the sacred forests failed the acorns and arbutus fruits, and Dodona denied her sustenance.

In Seneca's tragedy, the process described by Vergil, who has Ceres compensate for the lack of sustenance after Dodona has withheld it, is implicitly reversed, as now Ceres assumes Dodona's role in withholding her bounty. The playwright thus further tarnishes an Iron Age whose few consolations included the ability to grow crops, now desiccated in the Theban fields. Reminiscence of Vergil's fourth *Eclogue* also disturbs the landscape drawn in the *Oedipus*. In Vergil's poem the "fields will grow yellow with soft corn" (*molli paulatim flavescet campus arista*, 4.28), signaling the return of a Golden Age contingent upon the maturity of the poem's unidentified child, who must learn the heroism of prior generations. Theban fields possess the same tawny hue of their Golden-Age counterpart (*flava*, 50) in the *Eclogues*, but are worthless, signaling the land's barren condition rather than bounty. Allusions to other Augustan texts press the epochal evolution further: Ovid's account of saecular decline in *Metamorphoses* 1 had added winds to the amenities of the *aurea aetas*, in particular the "gentle Zephyrs" coaxing flowers from the earth with their warm breezes (*placidique tepentibus auris/mulcebant zephyri natos sine semine flores*, 1.107–8). Seneca evokes this feature (*non Zephyri leves spirant*) only to deny it in his dystopic Thebes (38).[35]

In muddling conditions of Iron and Golden Ages, Seneca echoes the epochal confusion found in the pestilence narratives of Vergil and Ovid, for whom widespread devastation brings with it conditions that might otherwise be considered idyllic. As when encountering such alchemy in Seneca's predecessors, we should again consider how various elements of the metallic myth address the optimum conditions of human existence. In addition to advertising a prosperity that begs to be qualified (for whom? what defines having enough?), the rhetoric of *aurea aetas* champions the eradication of hostilities.[36] In their entry song, the chorus of Thebans locates the origins of the disease among animals who exhibit pronounced *Georgic* behaviors: listless sheep (133) and a tottering racehorse (142–4) refrain their original roles from Vergil's poem (3.498–502).[37] The chorus describes a world in which certain fears are dissipated, a world where the stag does not fear the wolf, lions no longer roar, bears lose their ferocity, and snakes lose their venom. The Iron-Age challenges introduced by Jupiter in the first *Georgic* (predatory wolves and poisonous snakes, 1.129–30) are no longer a threat,

[35] Similar conditions, effectively creating a virtual *locus in-amoenus* are described in the first choral ode sung by citizens of Thebes, where again emphatic negatives deny the environment the same gentle breezes, rich soil, and full harvests associated with some evocations of the Golden Age (Sen. *Oed.* 154–9).

[36] As Evans observes, lack of conflict, while a defining component of the Golden Age, is also problematic. Golden Ages leave no room for narrative development, but instead are, "fixed, inert, unable to change—because change would result in a degree less of perfection" (2008, 6).

[37] And to a lesser extent from Ovid's *Metamorphoses* (7.542–4). See Chapter 5, p. 158.

and we observe the same neutralization of hostilities between species that Vergil and Ovid had used to anticipate the collapse of boundaries performed by contagion in Noricum and Aegina:

> incubant agris pecudes relictae.
> taurus armento pereunte marcet;
> deficit pastor grege deminuto
> tabidos inter moriens iuvencos.
> non lupos cervi metuunt rapaces,
> cessat irati fremitus leonis,
> nulla villosis feritas in ursis.
> perdidit pestem latebrosa serpens;
> aret et sicco moritur veneno.
> (*Oed.*145–53)

The flocks lie abandoned in the fields. The bull flags as the herd falls dead. The shepherd fails, with his herd diminished, and dies among rotting steers. The stags don't fear the rapacious wolves, the roar of the angry lion ceases, no ferocity remains in the shaggy bears. The lurking snake has lost its venom; it is parched and dies with its poison dry.

For Boyle, the plague's Golden-Age hues, especially those drawn from Vergil's *Eclogues*, verge on parody, a parody already evident in the plague of Vergil's third *Georgic* (2011, 150–1). Indeed, as Vallillee's catalogue of Seneca's verbal echoes of *Georgics* 3 (537–40) and *Metamorphoses* 7 demonstrates (545–6; 1960, 136–7), Seneca effectively combines the adynata from both texts in what amounts to an amplification of Golden-Age conditions attending the Theban plague. By engaging with the fourth *Eclogue*, however, the playwright does more than merely exaggerate the devastation in Thebes. He also directs us to reconsider the source behind the impossibilities made possible within the more obvious geopoetic predecessors, Noricum and Aegina.[38] In *Eclogue* 4, Vergil predicts a world where flocks need not fear the lions (*nec magnos metuent armenta leones*, 22) and the serpent has perished (*occidet et serpens*, 24). But the socio-historic

[38] Hinds (2011, 10) borrows the term "geopoetic" from Barchiesi's 2001 Gray lectures at Cambridge to describe the presence of Ovidian (Theban) landscapes in Seneca's dramas. While Noricum and Aegina lack the political and colonial resonance of those locations discussed, e.g., in Barchiesi's (2017) study of geopoetics in Vergil's *Aeneid*, the term appropriately addresses the layering of poetic landscapes through allusive language, and the enhancement of meaning that results from such layering. Thanks to Micah Myers for helping clarify the term's usage.

context for the *Eclogue* was a very different Rome.[39] We might ask why Seneca has infused the Theban landscape with the same ambiguity that colored the landscapes of Noricum and Aegina, but ultimately derived from poetry of the triumviral period. To conjure the Golden Age's peace and erasure of opposition long after the *pax Augusta*, and to summon a literary history that converts the utopia of the fourth *Eclogue* into a dystopic Noric landscape, amounts to a subtle interrogation of the cost at which such peace has been achieved.

6.5. *PRO MISERA PIETAS!*

The language of pestilence in Seneca's drama, with its intertextually provocative fusion of the ages, articulates a concern over the prerogatives of a new order, and over the sacrifices of the civil war that gave birth to that order. The *Oedipus* expresses an equally fervent interest in the quality of leadership in the Principate, and in clarifying the relationship between a leader and the community he governs. In Sophocles' tragedy, Oedipus articulates his leadership in Thebes in comparably intimate terms that stress identification between ruler and subjects: "I know you are all sick, yet there is not one of you, sick though you are, that is as sick as myself."[40] Tragic ironies of the statement aside, Oedipus indicates that he has assumed the suffering of the entire Theban populace, in contrast with the private citizen, who has only individual sufferings to endure. Such comments, along with an opening dialogue shared between Oedipus, the priest, and eventually Kreon, embed the king of Sophocles' play within his community.

Seneca parts company with his predecessor by dwelling on the distance between the *rex* and his subjects. As Albini observes in light of the Greek tragedy, Seneca's version isolates the king, whose opening words, now performed as a monologue, betray "solitudine, l' angosciata sfiducia, il dilemma senza speranza" (1995, 428). For Sophocles, Oedipus' opening query about why citizens sit as

[39] Boyle (2011, 151) also observes the influence of Horace's Golden-Age musings in the sixteenth *Epode*, another response to the upheavals of the triumviral period.

[40] *Εὖ γὰρ οἶδ'ὅτι/νοσεῖτε πάντες, καὶ νοσοῦντες ὡς ἐγὼ/οὐκ ἔστιν ὑμῶν ὅστις ἐξ ἴσου νοσεῖ* (59–61, Dawe's text 1982).

suppliants before the palace and throughout the city (*OT* 1–5) is quickly answered by the priest, who speaks of a λοιμὸς and πορφόρος θεὸς that have struck the land (27–8). For Seneca, Oedipus himself names the plague (as *lues*, 28 and *pestis*, 24), and questions his well-being in light of widespread destruction, fearing that he has been reserved for a greater calamity: *nam quid rear quod ista Cadmeae lues/infesta genti tam late edita/mihi parcit uni* ("what (else) should I think when that pestilence spread far and wide stains the Cadmean race, but spares me alone," 29–31). Amidst the widespread suffering of his people, the king's self-interest is striking, and restated at the close of his exposition in comments emphasizing his singular status, *negatur uni nempe in hoc populo mihi* ("[a ready death] is denied to me alone among this people of mine," 76). While initially a source of vulnerability—and later a cause for outright dismay (*in uno Oedipoda*, 943)—Oedipus' singularity is also a point of pride, emerging in Thebes from his unique ability to solve the riddle of the Sphinx (*soli . . . Oedipodae*, 216). By contrast, the citizens of Thebes, standing in the shadows of Oedipus' towering stature (*imperia excelsa Fortunae*, 11), are rendered with increasing anonymity, again through Latin traditions of narrating pestilence that emphasize accumulation, erasure of identity, and boundary dissolution.

In his opening monologue, Oedipus announces his concern with *pietas* (19), a quintessentially Roman value that was, as we have observed, reoriented in the Augustan period: while *pietas* continued to be defined in terms of mutual respect among family members, it gained new resonance in the early Principate as Augustus worked to realign the relationship between Roman subjects and himself in his relatively novel role as leading citizen and *pater patriae*.[41] While Oedipus fears chiefly his own transgressions of *misera pietas*,[42] the plague he describes has placed pressure on the *pietas* practiced by Theban citizens, in such a way that reverberates uncomfortably with the perversions of interfamilial devotion about to be disclosed onstage. The drama of Theban *lues* recalls the same tightening and dissolution of familial bonds we have observed throughout this project, but especially in Ovid, whose incense-burning relatives in

[41] For revisions of *pietas* as an ideal during the Augustan Principate, see above, Chapter 5, pp. 168–70.

[42] As Boyle notes, the modifier *misera* is a striking inversion of the more common *sancta* (2011, 115).

Jupiter's temple foreground a specifically Roman inflection of inter-familial relationships. The citizens of Thebes will (as the Aeginetans did) eventually reject the familial respect associated with *pietas*, but not before making a concerted effort to uphold it:

> nec ulla pars immunis exitio vacat,
> sed omnis aetas pariter et sexus ruit,
> iuvenesque senibus iungit et natis patres
> funesta pestis, una fax thalamos cremat,
> fletuque acerbo funera et questu carent.
> quin ipsa tanti pervicax clades mali
> siccavit oculos, quodque in extremis solet,
> periere lacrimae. portat hunc aeger parens
> supremum ad ignem, mater hunc amens gerit
> properatque ut alium repetat in eundem rogum.
> quin luctu in ipso luctus exoritur novus,
> suaeque circa funus exequiae cadunt.
> tum propria flammis corpora alienis cremant;
> diripitur ignis. nullus est miseris pudor.
> non ossa tumuli sancta discreti tegunt;
> arsisse satis est—pars quota in cineres abit?
> (*Oed.* 52–67)

Nor is any part of the city exempt, free from destruction. But every age and sex equally comes to ruin; the deadly plague joins young men to old, fathers to sons, a single torch cremates (husbands and wives in) the wedding chamber. Death lacks bitter wailing and laments. Indeed the very dogged destruction of so great an evil has dried our eyes and, as often occurs in extreme circumstances, our tears have perished. A sick father carries a son to his final fire, a mother, mad with grief, carries another son and hurries along so that she might collect yet another son for the same pyre. Mourners at funeral fall dead around the body, with the result that fresh grief arises amidst grief itself. Next, citizens burn the bodies of their own kin with flames not their own; fire is stolen. There is no sense of shame among the wretched. Nor do separate tombs cover hallowed bones. It is enough to have burned them—how great (or "little") a part[43] turns to ash!

Plague eventually destroys all familial identities, along all categories of age and sex, an outcome emerging with special emphasis in Latin plague narratives of the early Principate; such destruction also

[43] See Vallillee (1960, 141) on the translation "how great, how much," rather than "how little," as most translators suggest; I feel that V. argues rightly that "how great" captures the original Ovidian source of the passage.

anticipates the status leveling that Tacitus notes during the Campanian plague, in which children and wives of slaves and freeborn plebeians were all incinerated in a single pyre (*eodem rogo*).[44] The familial and relational identities destroyed are included here with thematic resonance, since the destruction of categorical distinctions among the plague-stricken populace mirrors the incest, as an erosion of familial distinctions *par excellence*, within Oedipus' family (Bettini 1983, 148–9; cf. Boyle 2011, 125; Busch 2007, 258).

Before the erosion of these identities, however, Oedipus' language redefines them, and does so consistently with Seneca's tendency to capitalize on the rhetorical potential of kinship terms throughout the play (Frank 1995, 124). Such terms within the context of the plague's epidemiology evoke both Lucretian visual iconography of intertwined bodies (6.1254–8) and the reciprocities of familial *pietas* in Ovid's Aegina. Where the *DRN* poet has the *corpora* of devoted fathers, mothers, and children arranged to inspire both fear and admiration, Seneca's king speaks of the plague "joining" fathers to sons, young to old, husbands to wives, creating an artful combination of antithetical pairs—pairs ironically linking the roles that have become confused in the figure of Oedipus (cf. Trinacty 2014, 139). With similar effect the passage evokes Ovid's pairings of husbands and wives, parents and children, fathers and sons, both supplicating the gods on each other's behalf in the final throes of illness (7.587–92) and as shades wandering unwept in Aegina (7.611–13; Jakobi 1988, 91).

Family members labor to fulfill duties as mothers and fathers and respect the identities of their children, as the homogenizing force of disease, propelled by insistent, repetitive demonstratives, pulls all into a single pyre (*hunc . . . . hunc . . . alium . . . in eundem rogem*, 59–61).[45] But the grief and familial responsibilities that initially burden the citizens of Thebes give way to failed *pudor* and a categorical failure of

[44] Tacitus' Latin is open to interpretation. While *qui* (line 4 of passage cited at the opening of this chapter) grammatically refers to women and children, the syntax indicates that the mingling of the two groups, as a subset of the *servitia* and *ingenua plebes*, is an extension of the mingling already experienced by slaves and freeborn Romans.

[45] As Trinacty observes (2014, 140), language describing the failure of mourning (*fletuque acerbo funera et questu carent*, *Oed.* 56) recalls features of (esp. Vergil's) underworld, a presence that looms large throughout the Theban landscape (Jakobi 1988, 91).

familial distinctions, signaled in the material conditions of death: in an echo of the stolen pyres that provoked fighting in Lucretius' Athens (6.1283–6) and similar contention in Aegina (*Met.* 7.610), Seneca's plague drives citizens to abandon their own (*propria*) kin to another's flames (*alienis*). At the same time, the noisy brawling over corpses (evident, if less pronounced in Aegina, *de rogis pugnant*) that Lucretius introduced to punctuate the collapse of the social order at the end of his poem is muted in Thebes, where citizens, already propelled beyond conventional expressions of grief (*periere lacrimae*, 59), abandon bodies in silent resignation.[46] As graves no longer distinguish one individual's remains from the next (*non ossa tumuli sancta discreti tegunt*, 66), the Theban citizenry fades into colorless dystopia and serves increasingly as a backdrop for the exceptional nature of its ruler.

The end of Oedipus' opening account turns from melancholy observation on the great part of the city already subsumed in flames (*pars quota in cineres abit*?) to his own invocations of the gods (71, *adfusus aris supplices tendo manus*), two details that harken back to another mythological monarch faced with a similar crisis, Ovid's Aeacus.[47] Vallillee notes that Ovid's influence on Seneca's plague is especially pronounced, but little other than temporal proximity is offered to account for that influence (1960, 139). I would suggest that narratological and mythological parallels allowed Seneca to find in Ovid's Aeacus a suitable source of expressions for communicating Oedipus' Theban dilemma: both kings act as narrator in their respective accounts of a plague that they are responsible for curing. All the same, tragic lack of foresight for Oedipus and the reassurance of hindsight for Aeacus create stark, but telling discrepancies in the tone of each narrative. Both kings are asked to interpret signs (cf. *Met.*7.600–1, 620–1), and Aeacus' initial failure but eventual success will cast in

[46] Manilius' relatively concise account of Athenian plague (1.880–91) may also have influenced Seneca (Jakobi 1988, 92). Like Seneca, the poet of the *Astronomica* follows Thucydides, rather than Lucretius, in omitting reference to brawls over bodies and funeral pyres.

[47] The second Ovidian parallel, *tendo* in *Oed.* 71 and *tendunt* at *Met.* 7.580, offered by Vallillee (1960, 142), is less compelling, since it is the dying Aeginetans rather than Aeacus who stretch their hands to the heavens; though the Metamorphic context, in which Aeacus immediately voices his own prayers after observing those of his people, suggests that Seneca has Ovid in mind here. Jakobi (1988, 94, following Vallillee) also cites Ovid's passage as a possible influence.

sharper relief the devastating blindness Seneca's king experiences when it comes to the circumstances in which he is entangled.[48]

Oedipus' remarks on the bones and ash of his people rephrase the comments of Aeacus, who, in responding to Cephalus' request that he disclose a painful memory, laments the bond he shared with his former people, now reduced to "bones and ash" (*ossa cinisque iacent, memori quos mente requires/et quota pars illi rerum periere mearum*, 7.521–2). While the Aeginetan king will eventually embrace his new population of Myrmidons, his remarks here are consistent with other comments in his tale that reflect on his identification with his former people and desire to share their sufferings (7.583, 618).[49] Precise echoes of Aeacus' words from *Metamorphoses* 7 within Seneca's *Oedipus* construct a template for governance and, in particular, for how a king should respond to the hardships of his people—a template to which Oedipus' own response cannot quite conform. Oedipus may express a willingness to experience the plague, but such expressions have the effect of heightening the distinction between ruler and subjects: Oedipus' desire not to be the "last" to fall (74) asserts the king's role as protector of his people, but does so using superlative terms, "after all" as well as "finally" (*neve* post omnis *cadam/fiamque regni funus* extremum *mei*, 73–4), echoing an emphasis on the unique status he has claimed elsewhere in the play.

In light of such verbal and situational parallels, as well as the different embodiments of monarchical authority these parallels reveal, can we say that Oedipus, like other characters in Seneca's dramas who use Ovidian language (cf. Trinacty 2014, 227), is an interpreter of the Ovidian character he evokes? And if so, what is this Oedipus saying about his predecessor, Aeacus? If both are figures who bear some relationship to political authority as it existed in the extra-textual Roman world, how might Aeacus as played by Oedipus comment on the establishment and evolution of the Principate? As Hinds (2011, 13) observes, *Oedipus* is staged in a "post-Ovidian" Thebes, a setting that allows characters from Ovid's Theban

[48] On Oedipus' role as an interpreter of signs and the Ovidian allusions used to emphasize the problems characters in Senecan drama face in making sense of the world, see Trinacty (2014, 229).

[49] Jakobi (1988, 94) observes a further parallel between each king's desire to share the fate of his people (*Oed.* 71; *Met.* 7.580), though, as I hope to demonstrate, Oedipus' desire is less clearly expressed and at odds with the language he uses to reiterate his exceptional status.

landscapes (e.g., Actaeon) to elucidate Oedipus' doomed struggle for self-knowledge. By designing a parallel relationship between Aeacus and Oedipus, Seneca shifts the interrogation from matters of self-knowledge to the nature of a sovereign in relation to the people he governs throughout a crisis and its resolution, though of course the two lines of inquiry frequently intersect.

Frederick Ahl observes that Seneca's *Oedipus* is distinguished from its Greek predecessor through its focus on the hero's sustained "self-examination from beginning to end" (2008, 20). The king's nearly solipsistic reflections on his own predicament initially deny him any relation to his people, though his contact with and contamination of the Theban civic body is gradually revealed: under Oedipus' leadership, the one cannot stand for the many without noxious consequences. Hints throughout the drama that Oedipus himself is the source of plague (e.g. 857–9) culminate in words of departure that explicitly identify the king with the *pestis* and its attendant calamities (Trinacty 2014, 139):

> mortifera mecum vitia terrarum extraho.
> violenta Fata et horridus Morbi tremor
> Maciesque et atra Pestis et rabidus Dolor,
> mecum ite, mecum. ducibus his uti libet.
> (*Oed.* 1058–61)

I drag away with myself deadly stains/infections of the earth. Brutal Fates, the terrifying trembling of Disease, and Wasting, and black Pestilence, and maddening Pain: come with me, with me. It is pleasing to use these as my guides.

If Aeacus presents a model of wish fulfillment, of the Principate operating in optimal condition, and with a citizenry uniquely (if implausibly and only temporarily) situated to accommodate a single ruler, Seneca's Oedipus will continue to dwell among ashes and bones. As Littlewood observes, any optimism in the play's conclusion is tempered by the dismal cast of characters who accompany the king: "Oedipus is not so much resolving and internalizing [the plague] as taking it elsewhere" (2004, 89).[50] Certainly Oedipus' expulsion at the end of the play should make him the scapegoat that restores a healthy civic body—

[50] See also Busch (2007), who argues that the play's ending challenges the Stoic notion that a rational divine order governs the operations of nature, and instead opens up the possibility of nature's perversions repeating themselves.

and yet the play constantly looks forward to the renewal of disease as civil war (*Oed.* 236–8, 359–60, 645–6, 747).[51] The *extispicium* scene in particular, with its split flame (*in duas partes*, 321) and liver bulging with two heads (*capita paribus bina . . . toris*, 360) anticipates war between Polynices and Eteocles, and does so in a way that clearly impacted Lucan's predictions of Roman civil war, through the *vates* Arruns (Boyle 2011, 197).[52]

Like Lucan's offering of Cato as a questionable sacrifice in the *BC*, Seneca's Oedipus, as sacrificial scapegoat in Thebes, will complicate Girard's model of crisis resolution. The king's self-mutilation and extended treatment of Jocasta's suicide define the outcome of his struggle for power with Creon, an outcome on which, in turn, the cure of plague depends. Although within the Greek drama too Oedipus is complicit in his own removal from the community, Sophocles leaves Kreon clearly in charge of Thebes in the final lines of the play. Seneca, by contrast, has Creon imprisoned two-thirds into the drama, and he is not heard from in the final three acts. Thus, when compared with Kreon's clear emergence as ruler in Sophocles' Thebes, no such tidy resolution, or clear model of leadership, defines the ending of Seneca's drama. While the opening remarks of Oedipus and the chorus set a scene that dramatizes the epoch-changing potential of an epidemic, pestilence cannot ultimately play, or play *well*, its expurgatory role. Guided by Sophoclean tradition, we might be satisfied with Oedipus' self-imposed departure as a remedy for the civic body, but that same tradition has been contaminated by a language of Augustan pestilence, language that has already exposed the operations of internecine strife, the interminable cycle of mimetic violence demanding that one head of state be rapidly, almost perfunctorily, challenged by another.

[51] Ahl argues that Oedipus as scapegoat aligns well with Roman traditions of *devotio* (2008, 127), a sacrificial role that others have assigned to various Republican leaders depicted in Imperial literature; see especially Marks (2016) on *devotio* in Silius Italicus. If the parallel works on a surface level, it is less stable when confronted with the repeated references to impending civil war within the tragedy, rendering the *devotio* ultimately ineffective. As scholars of *devotio* observe, moreover, the *devotus* cannot take his own life (or by extension, inflict harm upon himself, as Oedipus does), which must be taken by the enemy (Marks 2016, 427, citing Versnel 1981).

[52] See *BC* 1.616–29, where Arruns similarly observes in the liver the "mass of another head" (*molem/alterius capitis*).

6.6. PLAGUE, INDIVIDUALISM, AND EXEMPLARY BEHAVIOR IN SILIUS ITALICUS' *PUNICA*

For Lucan and Seneca physical contagion holds a mirror to the dysfunction of a community at odds with itself, a dysfunction born in part from a crisis in leadership, as competing heads of state emerge from "blind desire for distinction" rather than from consensus and *virtus*. Silius Italicus draws on the dynamics of internal conflict that shaped preceding plague narratives, but restructures the equation between plague and civil strife in his treatment of the pestilence that afflicts both the Carthaginian and Roman camps during the siege of Syracuse (14.580–640), a critical operation in the context of the Second Punic War. While Silius' pestilence initially conjures tropes that reflect civil strife, the *inimica pestis* (also described as an *importuna lues*, 14.582) emerges as more broadly indicative of the kinds of productive challenges that promote cohesion within the *populus Romanus*. In this function of plague we may glean the historiographical influence of Livy, who bequeathed to Silius certain narratological patterns as well as a wealth of historical detail.[53] This is not to underestimate the resonance of civil strife in Book 14. Recent scholarship on the *Punica* has demonstrated how civil war, as both a literary and historical phenomenon, is felt throughout the epic,[54] and internal divisions surely cripple Roman efforts in the war at various moments in the poem. Silius, however, uses plague to explore how an individual can achieve distinction that does not result in destructive rivalries. This use is remarkable in light of his epic forerunners, but also of particular concern to a writer who had lived through the tumultuous year of the four emperors that preceded the Flavian dynasty.[55]

In contrast to treatments of plague that tend to erase distinctions within masses of unburied, anonymous dead, Silius' treatment of the

[53] As Pomeroy has stressed (2010, 31–2).

[54] See esp. Marks (2010) on Silius' strategic use of Lucan to characterize self-destructive acts among the Romans in the early part of the poem; in the final books (11–17) allusions to Lucan allow the poet to identify the Carthaginians as wracked (like Pompey) by delay and indecision. Mezzanotte (2016, 435–9) emphasizes how incidents from the civil wars of 69 CE are alluded to in the *Punica*. See also Pomeroy (2016, 342), and especially McGuire (1997), who demonstrates the concerns of *civile nefas* evident in all three Flavian epicists.

[55] For Silius' political life during the difficult transition from Nero's reign to the establishment of the Flavian Dynasty, see Augoustakis (2010, 1–23).

Syracusan plague articulates the heroic identity of a single general, Marcellus, under whose leadership the threat of inglorious death is staunchly countered. Where Lucan's Caesar and Seneca's Oedipus suggest that heroism in relation to autocracy deforms the body politic, Silius explores exemplarity in a Republican context, with perhaps the notion that the Principate might also usefully tolerate exceptional individuals (Marks 2010, 152).[56] Although the historical setting of the *Punica* imports the same, if incipient, rivalries that would gradually erode Rome's aristocratic governance,[57] Silius' epic rejects the notion of a singular hero guiding Rome's future (Tipping 2010a, 11, relying on Hardie 1993). The dramatic stage of the Second Punic War, in Lucanian fashion, accommodates a multiplicity of heroes—though in many cases they lack the drive to self-destruction that hounds the players in the *Bellum Civile*.

Through his portrait of Marcellus' leadership, Silius borrows from Livy's account of the Syracusan plague in *Ab Urbe Condita*; though, unlike the historian, he emphasizes that both Carthaginian and Roman camps suffer equally from the disease. Silius' account is sensitive to the kind of contagion dramatized in literary precedents—contagious rivalry over *gloria* defined as a limited resource that leads eventually to annihilation of military and civic *corpora*. But plague for Silius reflects even more intently on the ameliorative transmission of ideals, especially that of cooperative behavior under sound leadership, more productive for stabilizing Roman *imperium*. In the following, I demonstrate how Silius has refashioned Livy's account in order to augment Marcellus' heroism, while also clarifying its utility to the collective *Aeneades*. "The same image of death" (*eadem leti . . . imago*) that defines plague in the *Punica*, with its emphasis on brutal equality (*par . . . parem*, 14.615–16), works on a literal level to suggest a grim parallelism defining the relationship between Roman and Carthaginian camps. Such equality also identifies the circumstances of plague at

[56] Cf. McGuire (1997, xiii), who detects in Flavian epic the sentiment that, "a monarchic system such as the Principate necessarily entails the potential for further strife." While such potential may be inscribed in the *Punica*, it does not necessarily preclude the poet's interest in models of behavior that might mitigate strife under monarchy.

[57] See especially McGuire (1997, 101–2), Pomeroy (2016, 341–2), and Tipping (2010a, 13) on the uneasy balance of individualism and concessions to the commonwealth that characterizes Scipio Africanus. Tipping (2010b) explores further evidence in the text for the problematic nature of Scipio, especially his exchange with Alexander the Great (205–8), and the parallels that emerge from that interaction.

Syracuse with the jarring equality that defined the conditions of pestilence for Pompey and famine for Caesar at Dyrrachium in Lucan's *Bellum Civile*. *Eadem leti imago* thus signals at a metatextual level the mirroring that Silius establishes with his forerunner in narrating pestilence as an extension of civil war. By the plague's abatement, however, mirroring yields to innovation as the poet of the *Punica* casts plague as another Roman *labor*—a crucible in which Roman *virtus* is forged.[58]

Silius' primary source for the episode, Livy's third decade (212 BCE), situates the conflict between Rome and Carthage at Syracuse, where Marcellus, the Roman general, leads the siege of Achradina. *Pestilentia* (a *commune malum*, 25.26.7) interrupts the designs of both Roman and Carthaginian armies and functions as a diversion from war. The role played by the closely knit social fabric of the Roman *castra* in spreading disease is poignantly acknowledged, though contagion soon results in one dominant social pathology, the fear of contaminated bodies and resultant neglect of burial rites:

> At first they became ill and died from the unhealthiness of the season and their position; but afterwards the disease was spread merely by attending upon, and coming in contact with, those affected (*curatio ipsa et contactus aegrorum volgabat morbos*); so that those who were seized with it either died neglected and abandoned, or else carried off those who sat by them and those who nursed, having caught the same dread disease. And so every day funerals and death were before the eyes; and lamentations were heard from all sides, day and night. At last, their feelings had become so completely brutalized by being habituated to these miseries, that they not only failed to follow their dead with tears and decent lamentations, but they did not even carry them out and bury them; so that the bodies of the dead lay scattered about (*iacerent strata examina corpora*) exposed to the view of those who were awaiting a similar fate; and thus the dead were the means of destroying the sick, and the sick those who were in health, both by fear and by the filthy state and the foul stench of their bodies. And some, choosing to die by the sword instead, dashed into the outposts of the enemy single-handed (*et ut ferro potius morerentur, quidam inuadebant soli hostium stationes*). The force of the disease, nevertheless, was much greater in the Phoenician camp than in the Roman (*multo tamen uis maior pestis Poenorum castra quam Romana*), for the latter, from having been a long time before in Syracuse, had become more habituated to the climate and the water. Of the army of

[58] Cf. Vallillee (1960, 165), who notes that Silius has transformed Livy's account of the plague, represented as an interruption in combat, into an "impediment to victory."

> the enemy, the Sicilians, as soon as they perceived that diseases had become very common from the unwholesomeness of the situation, dispersed to their respective cities in the neighborhood; but the Carthaginians, who had no place to retire to, perished together with their generals, Hippocrates and Himilco, to a man. Marcellus, on seeing the violence with which the disease was raging, had removed his troops into the city, where their debilitated frames were recruited in houses and shade. Nevertheless many in the Roman army were carried off by this same pestilence (*multi tamen ex Romano exercitu eadem peste absumpti sunt*).
>
> (25.26, translation modified from Gardner Moore 1940)

The presence of the dead and dying among the living deeply unsettles both military *castra*, and Livy indicates a kind of identity between opposing forces in casualties suffered from "the same disease" (*eadem peste*). At the same time, the historian notes that plague was worse in the Carthaginian camp, because Romans had become more accustomed to the climate and water. Drawing on the discrepancy between an ennobling death on the battlefield and the dehumanizing effects of the illness, Livy recognizes that some preferred to die by the sword (*ferrum*) rather than by plague, providing a narrative opportunity that the epic poet will seize on to illustrate a grasp for glory beneficial to the Roman cause. As with his earlier accounts of plague, the historian stresses familiar tropes, the spread of the disease by proximity, failure to bury the dead, the demoralizing effects of watching others die. Yet, because this epidemic occurs far from Rome, and strikes the Carthaginians with greater ferocity, there is less opportunity for reflecting on the Roman body politic or for casting the plague as an agent of discord in the constant negotiations of class privileges that defined the city's early history.[59]

This is the plague that Silius Italicus reworks in his *Punica*, and in doing so he reclaims for pestilence the power to illustrate the effects of an internal crisis and to proffer its remedy. While both authors stress the ubiquity of death and decay during the outbreak, Silius transforms Livy's *commune malum* (25.26.7), a *pestilentia* whose origins lie in atmospheric conditions, into a "hostile disease" and "untimely plague" (*inimica pestis, importuna lues*, 14.582). The redundancy in naming the epidemic allows Silius to combine the Lucretian atmospheric aetiology of plague, as born from "hostile air" (*inimicus aer*,

[59] As I argue above, Chapter 2.

6.1117–20), with Vergil's and Ovid's divinely wrought, punitive *lues* on Crete and Aegina (*Aen*.3.139, *Met*.7.523). The source of divine wrath is hardly explicit (14.616–17; Spaltenstein 1990, 331), though its presence colors the disaster with moral overtones, casting the episode as one to test the character as well as physical stamina of the opposing armies. In the *Punica*, the Romans led by Marcellus have just defeated the Carthaginian fleet off the coast of Syracuse. Using the momentum of such a victory, Marcellus might have been able to take the city (14.580–4), had not plague beset both the Roman and Carthaginian forces. As with Lucan, plague interrupts the momentum of a military siege, but where Lucan's pestilence simply abates with changing climate, adamantly disavowing opportunities for heroic or divine intervention, Silius constructs his plague dramaturgy as a vehicle for illustrating the *virtus* of Marcellus.

Like Livy, Silius notes fear concerning the contaminated corpses of plague victims. Where Livy expands on the nature of this particular social dysfunction and its resultant taboos (leaving corpses unburied), Silius attends to the very ubiquity of death, which serves as a counterweight against processes of differentiation and distinction that can accompany heroic deeds:[60]

succubuit medicina malis. cumulantur acervo
labentum et magno cineres sese aggere tollunt.
passim etiam deserta iacent inhumataque late
corpora, pestiferos tetigisse timentibus artus.
serpit pascendo crescens Acherusia pestis
nec leviore quatit Trinacria moenia luctu
Poenorumque parem castris fert atra laborem.
aequato par exitio et communis ubique
ira deum atque eadem leti versatur imago.
(14.609–17)

The ashes of the fallen are piled up in a heap and raise themselves in a great mound; scattered bodies lie abandoned and unburied far and wide, with men fearing to touch plague-bearing limbs. The infernal disease creeps along, deadly, growing as it feeds, nor does it shake the Trinacrian walls with lighter grief and brings an equal hardship to the camp of the Phoenicians. Equally shared wrath of the gods and the same image of death exist with equal destruction everywhere.

[60] Text is that of Postgate and Summers, printed in Duff (1927).

The accumulation of ashes of the dead, which "raise themselves" up, makes a macabrely ironic return to the *Punica*'s opening lines, where, because of the conflict with Carthage, glory for Aeneas' descendants raises itself to the heavens (*ordior arma, quibus caelo se gloria tollit/ Aeneadum*, 1.1–2). Plague threatens not only to reverse that elevation, but to supplant it with the graphic accumulation of bodies, cut down in decidedly unheroic circumstances. We have observed how Lucretius lent his successors an imagery of corporal accumulation during pestilence, imagery especially useful to Lucan, who transferred the language of bodily accumulation within an epidemic to the realm of the battlefield, as body counts swell in the thick of civil war, defying the poet's commemorative powers.[61] And yet the opposite of corporeal anonymity, the *gloria* of the individual, is also problematic for Silius, as perhaps reflected in his decision to assign *gloria* to the entire Roman race in the opening line of his epic. Critics have drawn attention to the poem's lack of a single protagonist and transformation of "the single epic hero (*virum*) into a Republican multiplicity of heroes (*viros*) who are subordinated to national necessity" (Tipping 2010a, 2). The image of a steadily rising heap of ashes challenges the *Punica*'s focus on the rising glory of those men who made Rome master of the Mediterranean, but plague eventually resets the stage for the emergence of a self-regulating kind of *gloria* in the figure of Marcellus.

Silius' *nec leviore . . . luctu* pointedly diverges from Livy's observation that the Carthaginians experienced greater suffering from the disease (*maior vis*, 25.26.12). For Spaltenstein, such divergence indicates the poet's interest in the tragic notion of equality in the face of disaster (1990, 333). Indeed we have recognized throughout this project the homogenizing effect of plague, its tendency to eradicate distinctions between gender, class, and age, and its impact within the *Punica* extends to nationality as well. Silius' description of the wrath of the gods as afflicting both sides equally with like destruction (*aequato par exitio*) may indicate the influence of Seneca, whose Oedipus laments the ubiquity of the Theban plague: *nec ulla pars immunis exitio vacat, sed omnis aetas pariter et sexus ruit* (*Oed.* 52–3). Even more pertinent to the martial context is Lucan's use of parity to signal the perverted opposition of Roman against Roman on the

[61] See above, p. 203; for Silius' borrowing from Lucretius in his use of *cumulantur*, see Vallillee (1960, 166).

battlefield, parity implicit in his account of two camps under siege from plague and famine at Dyrrachium (see above). Silius pushes back against his predecessors' resistance to identify any figure whose expulsion or promotion can restore difference in a social order collapsing under the weight of its equivalences: he does so by expanding on the role of Marcellus—neither scapegoat nor *devotus*, but a figure whose own distinction prompts a healthy coalescence among the men he leads.

Where Livy's treatment does not credit any single Roman with saving the *castra* (Marcellus merely transfers surviving soldiers into the city, 25.26.15), the dehumanizing prevalence of death in the *Punica*, where afflicted soldiers die like sheep (*in morem pecudum*, 14.631), acts as a foil for Marcellus' leadership:

> nulla tamen Latios fregit vis dura malorum,
> incolumi ductore, viros, cldemque rependit
> unum inter strages tutum caput. ut gravis ergo
> primum letiferos repressit Sirius aestus,
> et minuere avidae mortis contagia pestes,
> ceu, sidente Noto cum se maria alta reponunt,
> propulsa invadit piscator caerula cumba,
> sic tandem ereptam morbis grassantibus armat
> Marcellus pubem, lustratis rite maniplis.
> (14.618–26)

Still no strengthened force of hardships broke the Romans, as long as their leader was unharmed; and a single man's well-being among masses (of dead) compensated for the disaster. Thus as soon as stifling Sirius lifted its deadly waves of heat, and the ravenous plague lessened the infectious spread of death, then, just as, when the high seas grow calm under the subsiding south wind, a fisherman, propelled on his skiff, advances into the sea, just so does Marcellus prepare for arms the soldiers snatched from prowling disease, after the ranks have been duly purified.

In lines 618–20, Silius has deftly collocated a single unharmed leader with both the Latin men (*viros*) he will lead to victory, and the masses of plague victims from whom he is distinguished. Reference to the heaps of dead (*strages*), like the poet's account of accumulating ashes, evokes a tradition that effaces identity in the plague as a counterthrust to the individual's grasp for distinction.[62] Silius—provocatively

[62] See Bruère (2016, 380) on Ovid's influence here. For the language of *strages* to indicate heaps of dead, see also Vergil *G.*3.556.

summoning the body politic metaphor deformed in Lucan's two-headed Rome—allows Marcellus to emerge as one head (*unum caput*) in the heap. Critically, however, Marcellus has not yet been named in the plague narrative and will not be until after a simile likens him to a fisherman heading out to sea when a storm subsides. The simile implies that his leadership is motivated, like a humble *piscator*'s, by necessity rather than desire for individual glory, and as such inspires a community to elevate itself. The comparison is especially striking because its characterization of Marcellus is at odds with his portrayal in other parts of the *Punica*. As Fucecchi has observed, Marcellus' heroism is (outside of Book 14) often marred by impetuosity, haste, and a grasp at *gloria* (2010, 231). He strives for recognition in ways that reflect an "individualistic" and "essentially archaic" outlook (235).[63] Within the context of Book 14, however, Marcellus' flaws as a hero are all but erased, as the siege of Syracuse compels him to operate with restraint and humanity, as an agent of civilized conquest (*vincere servando*; Fucecchi 2010, 236). I would argue that the experience of leading his men through an epidemic is key to Marcellus' somewhat anomalous behavior in Book 14. Silius has revised the literary conventions of his predecessors that use pestilence to disclose the social dysfunction erupting from competition among individuals: Marcellus, observing the workings of contagion and learning from them, takes the helm not as the arrogant winner of *spolia opima* (which he pursues aggressively elsewhere in the poem), but as a lowly fisherman.

Initially invoking but gradually countering the indistinguishable remains of those who experience plague as civil war, Silius' narrative unfolds as a context in which the Roman soldier can earn glory. But as Marcellus' circumspect leadership demonstrates, such honors are only worth winning if they are won by efforts aimed at securing the common good:

> et si fata ferant, iuvat inter proelia ferro
> posse mori; socium miseret, qui sorte pudenda
> in morem pecudum effudere cubilibus atris
> illaudatam animam. tumulos inhonoraque busta
> respiciunt, et vel nullo iacuisse sepulcro
> quam debellari morbis placet. ardua primus

[63] Ahl, Davis, and Pomeroy (1986, 2538) offer a more positive evaluation of Marcellus' heroism and leadership in the poem, though they too emphasize his exceptional humanity during Book 14's siege of Syracuse.

ad muros dux signa rapit. tenuata iacendo
et macie in galeis abscondunt ora, malusque,
ne sit spes hosti, velatur casside pallor.
infundunt rapidum convulsis moenibus agmen
condensique ruunt: tot bellis invia tecta
totque uno introitu capiuntur militis arces.
(14.629–40)

If the fates allow, it is pleasing (for the soldiers) to be able to die in battle by the sword; and he would pity his comrades, who by shameful lot poured forth their lives without praise, on obscure bedding in the manner of beasts. They look back at tombs and graves without honors and it is more pleasing to have fallen without a burial than to be conquered by disease. The leader first hurries the lofty standards up to the walls. In their helmets they hide their faces wasted with sickness, and their unhealthy color is concealed, lest it be a cause for the enemy's hope. They shake the walls and swiftly pour forth a battle line, and tightly packed they rush forth. So many buildings hard to reach in the war and so many citadels are taken by the single advance of the soldiers.

Marcellus' leadership encourages a remarkable brand of distinction that thrives on collective action. As fighting resumes, Roman soldiers pity their comrades who have died like sheep and are denied a glorious death in battle. Thus it is not *gloria* per se that threatens Roman hegemony, but *gloria* achieved in a zero-sum game, in which the success of one *vir* necessarily entails a loss for his rival: at Syracuse all Roman soldiers work to achieve *gloria* and lament those who are not allowed to do the same. Silius nestles the Lucretian (and Thucydidean) phrase comparing plague victims to sheep in close proximity with reminders of praise denied and tombs lacking honors (*illaudatam animam . . . inhonora busta*). Marcellus' leadership is required to prompt the soldiery to decisive action: he is first (*primus*), but not alone. Under his guidance, the Romans unite and storm enemy walls and defenses, scattered and diverse, in a single remarkably uniform blow (*uno introitu*).[64]

By carefully orchestrating the resurrection of the Roman soldiers, who are transformed into a single fighting force, uniformly devoted to a single purpose under the guidance of Marcellus, Silius offers a lesson in managing the pressures of acting as an exceptional individual in the context of a communal crisis. Marcellus' leadership and the quality of his heroism are made clearer not only in contrast with Livy's account of the incident. Lucretius, Vergil, Ovid, and Lucan

64 Cf. Spaltenstein on the rhetorical force of juxtaposing *tot* with *uno* (1990, 334).

have all preceded him in narrating pestilence in hexameters, and yet all forerunners (to varying degrees) make the devastation and triumph of *pestis* something left effectively unchallenged by mortal efforts. One image of the dying warrior (*bellator*) in the *Punica*, borrowed from Vergil's Noric cattle plague in the third *Georgic* (3.478–566) and Ovid's plague of Aegina (*Met.* 7.517–660), has important implications for Silius' articulation of Roman heroism and his effort to present his *pestis* as an opportunity for shaping what Tipping describes as effective leadership through example.[65]

Silius' brief portrait of an *insignis bellator* (14.606–7) alludes to plague-afflicted champion racehorses in the *Georgics* and *Metamorphoses*.[66] After accounting for the physical symptomatology of plague in the Roman *castra*, Silius turns to the discrepancy that defines the formerly proud existence of the distinguished warrior and his present prostration in the face of an *ignavum letum*:

> heu dolor! insignis notis bellator in armis
> ignavo rapitur leto. iactantur in ignem
> dona superba virum, multo Mavorte parata.
> (14.606–8)

What a cause of grief! The warrior distinguished in well-known arms is snatched away by an ignoble death. Proud gifts/trophies of warriors, gained through much fighting, are tossed into the fire.

The image is indebted to Ovid's portrait of a dying champion racehorse:

> acer equus quondam magnaeque in pulvere famae
> degenerat palmas veterumque oblitus honorum
> ad praesepe gemit leto moriturus inerti.
> (*Met.*7.542–4)

The horse once fierce and greatly renowned in the racecourse "disgraces" the victory palm and, forgetful of his old honors, he groans, about to perish by an ignoble death at the stall.

Silius reconfigures the racehorse's *letum iners* as the warrior's *ignavum letum*, following his tendency to use synonyms in adapting Ovidian material (Bruère 2016, 380). An "ignoble death" articulates

[65] Tipping (2010a, 7–8) further argues that exemplarity is, "perhaps the epic hero's principal function in the *Punica*."

[66] As noted above, the flagging war-horse is given a cursory glance in Lucan and Seneca, but no mention is made of past accomplishments cast in the shadow of current malaise.

the plague's power to render former distinctions (redoubled through Silius' collocation of *insignis* with *notis*) meaningless.

Moreover, by recalling the Ovidian image, Silius also evokes Ovid's source, the dying champion *equus* who falls victim to the Noric cattle plague in the third *Georgic*:

> labitur infelix studiorum atque immemor herbae
> victor equus fontisque avertitur et pede terram
> crebra ferit; demissae aures, incertus ibidem
> sudor et ille quidem morituris frigidus.
> (*G.* 3.498–501)

The champion horse, unlucky and unmindful of his races and his fodder, totters and turns away from the fountains, and strikes the earth constantly with his foot; his ears droop, drops of sweat scattered here and there, chilly for those in the grip of death.

For both Vergil and Ovid, there is a pathetic contrast between the former glory of the *equus* and his present malaise. Yet those former glories, especially in the *Georgics,* are also highly problematic, leading to the kind of exultant victories, grievous defeats, and unchecked passions that disrupt the herd (*G.*3.95–122; 209–41). Silius tacitly acknowledges the dangers of distinction in the figure of the *bellator*, whose proud (*superba*) trophies are tossed into the fire. He also, however, presents an alternative model of heroism—that of Marcellus—better accommodated in the civic body. Consistent with his leadership during the plague, if somewhat inconsistent with his depiction elsewhere, Marcellus will issue a critique of unchecked power in victory as he ascertains and laments the plundering and devastation possible in Syracuse (14.665–73). By the end of Book 14, Marcellus' deeds are recognized but also in*corp*orated within a broad swath of exceptional *ductores*: he is one man who illustrates the "ancient customs" of many: *et dabit antiquos ductorum noscere mores* (683).

By allowing Marcellus to illustrate the possibilities of an individual operating effectively to maintain *concordia* in the body politic, Silius does not *ipso facto* promote an overtly sanguine view of the potential for individual achievement in the Principate. Indeed, as those treatments of Scipio Africanus cited above suggest,[67] he has written a belated prequel to the problems of individualism that plague both

[67] See above, p. 222 n. 57.

Lucan's strong-men of the late Republic and the figure of Oedipus in Seneca's drama. However, by offering a novel conclusion to the problem of pestilence at Syracuse, Silius reminds us of the capacity of the plague metaphor, of its power to diagnose and remedy (occasionally, and with varying degrees of optimism) Roman *discordia*. The Latin tradition of narrating pestilence, enacting coalescence within the body politic, has effectively bifurcated the roles played by Roman heroes, who either restore a healthy civic corpus from that coalescence or yield to a drive toward further self-destruction. In so doing, the tradition has equipped plague to address challenges to configuring the body politic across broad temporal, generic, and geographic spectra. In the concluding chapter, we explore the ongoing invocation of Latin pestilence to unveil (in properly apocalyptic fashion) the problems of orienting the individual within his or her community, an orientation constantly challenged by ideological transformations—especially the advent of Christianity—and reformulations of national identity.

7

Relapse

Transmitting Roman Plague in the West

In their study of figurative language, *Metaphors We Live By*, Lakoff and Johnson recognize certain metaphors that pervade life experience to the extent that we use them almost unconsciously; with such metaphors, the vehicle determines how we behave or how we experience the tenor it describes. They offer the example of "argument is war" as one in which war (the vehicle) "structures the actions we perform" (2003, 4) in the experience of an argument (the tenor):

> Our conventional ways of talking about arguments presuppose a metaphor we are hardly ever conscious of. The metaphor is not merely in the words we use—it is in our very concept of argument. The language of argument is not poetic, fanciful, or rhetorical; it is literal. We talk about arguments that way because we conceive of them that way—and we act according to the way we conceive of things. (2003, 5)

In the metaphor describing "civil war" as "plague" the Romans understood the tenor in terms of its vehicle to the extent that plague shaped the way that they thought about and experienced civil war. While according "civil war is plague" the status of a fully-fledged metaphor that the Romans "lived by" would limit its rhetorical effect (and thus does not meet the criteria for those metaphors discussed by Lakoff and Johnson), Lucan's casual transference of the dysfunction associated with the plague at Dyrrachium to the casualties suffered on the battlefield is a clear expression of how thoroughly the conceptual field associated with plague had permeated the experience of civil war for Romans living in the late Republic and early Empire. Strands of civil war discourse threaded throughout accounts of pestilence hindered audiences from thinking of civil war in terms of a more easily remedied condition, like Horace's famous *lippitudo*; instead, they were sensitive to civil war as an interfamilial, contagious catastrophe—one with epoch-changing potential, but without an obvious cure.[1]

The final chapter of this project examines important vectors for the transmission of Roman plague in literary and visual arts, beginning with the early Christian period and proceeding up through the present day. Such an examination, one that identifies sites of reception, as well as the ability of these sites to translate Roman plague topoi into the idioms of their own cultural milieu, is necessarily selective rather than exhaustive. I hope above all to indicate the range of interpretive possibilities available for readers who are sensitive to the conventions developed in the hexameter treatments of Lucretius, Vergil, and Ovid. By concentrating on early Christian literary adaptations, Italian painting in the aftermath of bubonic plague, and finally Anglo-American literary constructions of contagion, we not only get a better understanding of how the plague metaphor allowed Romans at the turn of the first millennium to grapple with internal discord. We can also sift through conventions of narrating pestilence that arise from the norms governing social life in Rome, to isolate those tropes that have persisted because they address relatively constant aspects of the human condition: repeatedly we find that the pressures put on the family, as well as on the individual's relationship with the wider community, emerge as paramount concerns; receptions of Roman plague also speculate on the "clean-slate" potential of an epidemic, either through language of epochal evolution or recognition of expanding governmental control over individual liberties.

If these tropes are no longer used predominantly to address civil war and the transition from one form of government to another, they are quite often used to address internal ideological conflicts or express anxieties surrounding the evolving relationship between the individual and the body politic. I realize that, particularly in light of the

[1] Lakoff and Johnson observe how "a metaphorical concept can keep us from focusing on other aspects of the concept that are inconsistent with that metaphor" (2003, 10). See also Healy (2001, 12–13), who relies on Johnson's *The Body in the Mind* to argue for the way that body and disease metaphors have an especially strong impact on human experiences.

various deconstructive turns taken in cultural criticism at the end of the last century, I skate on thin ice in asserting that there are any qualities that universally define the human condition. Plague narratives, for all their variety, as they chart a process of contagion, are fundamentally concerned with physical and ideological *contactus* among members within any community: that is to say, these accounts reveal bonds between individuals within a collective, whether that collective is an ancient fledgling city on the Tiber or a twenty-first-century superpower or, perhaps more speculatively, but no less compellingly given the number of fictive accounts that address the issue, the species *homo sapiens* under constant threat from the global reach of the next pandemic. While I have made a historicizing argument by circumscribing the generation of certain features of the plague text within the late Roman Republic, it is also true that, at a formal level, plague narratives self-consciously look backward, transhistorically, over the transmission of tropes, augmenting, manipulating, or tiredly rehashing them—as Lucian caustically reminds his readers in the opening epigraph of this study. If the persistence of this transmission does not speak to a "universal" human condition, it does, at the very least grasp at what Martindale has described as "fugitive human communalities across history" (2013, 173).

7.1. ENDELECHIUS AND PAULUS: CHRISTIAN VISIONS OF A NEW JERUSALEM

In her anthology and survey of late twentieth-century approaches to early Christian Latin poets (fourth–sixth centuries CE), Carolinne White addresses the need to recognize innovations among these writers, but also to identify points of continuity between classical Latin authors and their Christian successors (2000, 9; cf. McGill and Pucci 2016, 16). The late-fourth century poet Endelechius straddles innovation and tradition in his Vergilian-inspired *Carmen de mortibus boum*, though he does so largely without the arresting ambivalences of his classical predecessor. Endelechius combines the bucolic setting, dialogic form, and perspectival contrast of Vergil's first *Eclogue* with a reworking of the *Georgic*'s Noric plague. Effectively, the Christian poet has expanded on the *contagia* feared by Meliboeus in the *Eclogue* (1.50), and does so to develop the unenlightened ("pagan") worldview as a foil to the Christian perspective. As Petra Schierl has argued, however, Endelechius does not aim primarily to attack classical tradition using Christian armature,[2] but instead introduces Christian theology as a force of transformation. Thus Vergil's two poems offer recognizable perspectives on death as defining the human condition and a backdrop for Endelechius' dramatization of the changes, especially the assurances of salvation, that Christianity has brought (cf. McGill and Pucci 2016, 21).

Endelechius' *Carmen*, structured in Asclepiadean stanzas,[3] begins as a conversation between the devastated, aptly named Bucolus and his interlocutor Aegon, whose questions prompt Bucolus to narrate the plague's progress among his herd. Tityrus joins the two later, attributing his good fortune, and exemption from the *dira lues* (21), to *Christus*, the *deus* (102) whose beneficence has replaced that of an *otium*-granting *deus* (Octavian) in Vergil's first *Eclogue*. What is striking about Bucolus' account of the plague is the degree to which he personifies his cattle, making overt the familial relationships severed by disease in Vergil's Noricum and expanding on interfamilial tragedies by borrowing and developing elements from other classical writers. In fact, Bucolus' initial reference to the scourge as an Ovidian *dira lues* (*Met.* 7.523) reminds us that Endelechius has marshaled a wider range of plague narratives, a range that facilitates the author's attempt to make plague mean something novel in a Christian context. The poet has, for instance, clearly used a *Georgic* template for modeling the deaths of sibling oxen (cf. *G.*3.515–19), but he also expands on the problematic equality of those afflicted with plague in subsequent classical accounts:

plaustris subdideram fortia corpora
lectorum, studio quo potui, boum;
quis mentis geminae consona tinnulo
concentu crepitacula.

[2] Her approach thus differs from the highly influential study of Schmid (1976), who examines the poem's *Georgic* allusions, but assumes a polemical relationship between Endelechius and his Vergilian models; see Schierl (2016, 242–3), who also provides a good starting point for scholarship examining the conjunction of Christian and classical elements in the poem.

[3] For Endelechius' use of the Asclepiadean meter as a way of distancing his poem from Vergil's bucolic poetry, see Hubbard (1998, 214–15). Green (2004, 23–32) emphasizes the pastoral elements of the *Carmen*, especially those drawn from Vergil's *Eclogues*, but also from Theocritean verse.

aetas consimilis, saetaque concolor;
mansuetudo eadem, robur idem fuit,
et fatum medio nam ruit aggere
par victum parili nece.
(33–40)[4]

I had yoked the strong bodies of chosen oxen to the wagons, as industriously as possible; they were twins in mind and in the same-sounding rattles they made with their ringing (*tinnulo*) (and) harmony (*concentu*). Their age was the same, their bristles the same color; the gentleness the same, so too their strength: for death rushed (upon them) in the middle of their efforts, equally conquered by an equal death.

After a stanza in which Bucolus describes his progress through the soil, he returns to the oxen, recounting in two stanzas how one died just long enough before the other to experience grief over the loss of his partner (45–52). Bucolus conveys his own experience in the fields, as he separates (*disiungo*) the pair after the first has died, leaving behind a *tristis coniunx* (47)—unlike in Vergil's *Georgics*, where, from the relative distance achieved through the didactic frame, readers view a *tristis arator* unyoking (*abiungens*) the sibling *tauri* (3.515–19). In a more dramatic revision of Vergil's portrait, in which the grieving brother's death is only implicit, Bucolus narrates in detail the death of the second *bos*. While Endelechius does not explicitly describe the pair as *fratres*, their equality and sympathetic union (*par victum parili nece*) lays even greater emphasis on the poignancy and privilege of the Roman fraternal bond, recalling how classical writers offered its harmony and stability as a reflection of *concordia* in the Roman body politic.

The parity that defines the experience of the two oxen, however, also retrospectively activates the resonance of civil war coloring the Vergilian tableau of *fraterna mors*, a passage that is itself echoed through later depictions of civil war in Imperial literature.[5] Such equality engages a tradition of writing about internal strife that conveys the horror of having a brother, as *alter* or "second self" (Bannon 1997, 64), become a rival on the battlefield rather than a helpmate.[6] The Christian poet has reversed engineered the

[4] Text is that of Ferdinand Piper (1835).

[5] E.g., Stat. *Theb.* 82–5; see Bannon (1997, 185).

[6] The language of parity is pronounced throughout the poem: the equality of the oxen in death is echoed a few stanzas later by the death of a pregnant cow, in which she and her offspring are "equally" (*pariter*) killed by the plague, so that Bucolus observes "two spirits perish in a single body" (*animas duas/uno in corpore perditas*).

impressive, if disturbing parity that defined Ovid's uniformly loyal Myrmidons as the solution to plague on Aegina, and summons an alternate tradition, one warning that this kind of equality and fraternity in a classical context is especially vulnerable to mutual destruction.

Endelechius' reception of Roman plague tropes is not limited to fraternal expressions of the familial bond. He is equally intent on using the language of classical poets to explore how pestilence exposes contradictions and tensions in the relationships between parents and children. Under the impetus of the reciprocal *pietas* and graphic corporeal entanglement we have observed throughout this project, Endelechius offers a striking image of a mother cow who transmits the disease to her *vitulus*-calf in the very act of nurturing it:

> at parte ex alia, qui vitulus modo
> lascivas saliens texuerat vias,
> ut matrem subiit, mox sibi morbido
> pestem traxit ab ubere.
> mater, tristifico vulnere saucia,
> ut vidit vituli condita lumina;
> mugitus iterans, ac misere gemens,
> lapsa est et voluit mori.
> tunc tamquam metuens, ne sitis aridas
> fauces opprimeret, sic quoque dum iacet,
> admovit moriens ubera mortuo.
> post mortem pietas viget.
> (68–80)

In another part of the field, a calf that recently, while leaping about, had woven playful paths as he went under his mother, soon after contracted the plague in himself from her sickly udder. The mother, hurt by this ill-omened wound, as she saw the eyes of her calf close, letting forth bellows repeatedly and pitiably, collapsed and wished for death. Then, as if fearing that thirst would overcome the calf's dry jaws, she also, while lying there, dying, moved her breast to her dead calf. *Pietas* lives, even after death.

Endelechius recalls the pitiably ironic outcome of family members attempting to succor each other in the context of plague, drawn ultimately from Lucretius' parents and children expiring on each

At the end of the poem, Tityrus and Bucolus make their way equally (*pariter*) along a short path under the assurance of Christ's protection from the plague (125–32).

other outside the walls of Athens,[7] and developed further by Ovid's Aeginetans praying for each other in Jupiter's temple. But Endelechius winnows this tradition in a way that reduces it to the most fundamental source of nurturing within the family, mother's milk: the result is a graphic expression of the bond between parent and child, an expression that (as I argue below) would inform visual depictions of plague in the Renaissance and early Baroque periods. *Pietas* does persist, but its efforts within Bucolus' herd are fatefully misguided.

In concluding his account of plague, Endelechius rounds out the family unit by focusing on a *taurus* ("bull") described as both *vir* and *pater* (81, "husband and father").[8] He too succumbs to death, but not until we glimpse the excessive pride with which he once dominated the herd (*laetus dum sibi met plus nimio placet*, 83), perhaps a nod to the socially disruptive force of claims for supremacy informing plague narratives in Latin epic. With this last vision of the impact of plague on individual lives and identities shaped by familial relationships, the poet, again following the lead of classical authors, turns to the homogenizing and leveling effects of disease, which reduce victims to countless multitudes of falling leaves and snowflakes (85–8). As Schierl notes of the simile (2016, 260), the poet borrows here from Vergil's depiction of souls in *Aeneid* 6 (309–10). For Vergil's souls, however, there is the possibility (delayed in the case of improper burial) of crossing the Styx and either retiring to Elysium or eventually rejoining the stream of human life. For Bucolus' livestock, the simile emphasizes their sheer numbers and directs attention to the emphatically material and deteriorative forms that have littered the landscape. As such, the image borrows equally from Ovid, whose Aeacus likens citizens dying during the Aeginetan plague to rotting fruit and acorns fallen from shaken branches (*Met.*7.584–6).

The possibility of preventing disease, announced by Tityrus soon after he joins the group, buttresses the validity of the new worldview

[7] As Schierl (2016, 249) observes, there is also a hint of Lucretius' famously poignant description of a mother cow in search of her lost calf (Lucr. 2.352–66), as proof that animals (like humans) possess powers of familial recognition. See above (Chapter 4, p. 130) for the scene's relationship to Vergil's plague narrative in the *Georgics*; cf. Green (2004, 28).

[8] Cf. Schierl (2016, 245) on the poet's presentation of "the whole bovine family: a calf, its mother, and the proud father of the herd," as a clear indication of the poem's import for the *condicio humana* (259).

he promotes: to protect the herd, one only needs to renounce "pagan" traditions and acknowledge Christ's divinity (123–8). But Tityrus' injunction also reminds us of the sacrificial economy that operated, or failed to operate properly, in the Latin epic tradition. For the faithful, Christ's death has already solved the problem of plague, with its attendant implications for crisis within the social order, and no further shedding of blood is necessary. Thus, despite Tityrus' strictures against bloodshed on altars of Roman gods (117–20), the poet's rendering of contagion and its impact is not so much anti-sacrificial as post-sacrificial, and sensitive to how authors of the early Principate pondered sacrifice as a solution to destructive rivalries. More broadly speaking, Endelechius' sustained depiction of familial relationships within the community—and of the sacrificial order upon which the stability of such relationships depends—reflects an intense, if highly selective, engagement with poetic tradition: such engagement allows him to manipulate the conventions of the Latin plague narrative most effective for articulating a new understanding of mortality from a Christological perspective.

The plagues that Paul the Deacon (c.720–790 CE) describes in his *Historia Langobardorum*, an account of the Lombard kingdom in Italy up through its conquest by Charlemagne, are less overtly classicizing than Endelechius' *Carmen.*[9] Nevertheless, he too, as a major source in Latin for the so-called plague of Justinian, relies on tropes of pestilence in epic, in order to register the degree of devastation wrought by plague in the Western empire on a social order already compromised by prolonged war and famine. Such conditions would gradually clear a path for Lombard invasions and dominance in the Italian peninsula (Everett 2003, 16–17). Gregory of Tours, who lived through the initial onset of the pandemic, is our most expansive source for the successive waves of bubonic plague that swept through

[9] Though Paul too wrote poems in classical meters (hexameters, elegiacs, Sapphics, etc.) that would be more profitably compared to Endelechius' efforts as a poet. His histories and the intellectual heritage they reflect are discussed at length in Foulke's (1907) introduction to Paul's *History of the Langobards*, xv–xlii. Foulke relies on Mommsen (Neues Archiv., V.) in recognizing the "double marks of classical and national feeling" (xlii) that inform his historical projects. Everett (2003, 12) contextualizes Paul's education (what little we know of it) within a wide range of sources (especially legal and epigraphic) for literacy within Lombard Italy, and recognizes a general antipathy for classical rhetoric among Christian sources (15); he also includes relevant bibliography (esp. 12, n. 47) that addresses Paul's life and classical heritage.

Gaul and Italy during the sixth century (Little 2007, 11–13). Paul, writing about two centuries after Gregory, extends the chronology of the plague and intensifies his focus on Italy. Though not an eye-witness to the outbreaks he describes,[10] he adopts the spectacle-oriented didacticism that we observed as early as Lucretius, who directs readers to imagine visions of physical deterioration in Athens, and in particular the lifeless bodies of family members heaped upon each other outside the city walls (*posses videre*, Lucr. 6.1257; cf. 1268).

In the first of four accounts of plague, Paul remains sensitive to the *pietas*-oriented bonds that structure Roman social life and develops the plague-ravaged landscapes as sites for epochal evolution. After describing the telltale signs of *Yersinia pestis*, Paul addresses the communal response to the disease in Liguria in 565 CE:[11]

> Erant autem ubique luctus, ubique lacrimae. Nam, ut vulgi rumor habebat, fugientes cladem vitare, relinquebantur domus desertae habitatoribus, solis catulis domum servantibus. Peculia sola remanebant in pascuis, nullo adstante pastore. Cerneres pridem villas seu castra repleta agminibus hominum, postero vero die universis fugientibus cuncta esse in summo silentio. Fugiebant filii, cadavera insepulta parentum relinquentes, parentes obliti pietatis viscera natos relinquebant aestuantes. Si quem forte antiqua pietas perstringebat, ut vellet sepelire proximum, restabat ipse insepultus; et dum obsequebatur, perimebatur, dum funeri obsequium praebebat, ipsius funus sine obsequio manebat. Videres seculum in antiquum redactum silentium: nulla vox in rure, nullus pastorum sibilus, nullae insidiae bestiarum in pecudibus, nulla damna in domesticis volucribus. Sata transgressa metendi tempus intacta expectabant messorem; vinea amissis foliis radiantibus uvis inlaesa manebat hieme propinquante. Nocturnis seu diurnis horis personabat tuba bellantium, audiebatur a pluribus quasi murmur exercitus. Nulla erant vestigia commeantium, nullus cernebatur percussor, et tamen visus oculorum superabant cadavera mortorum. Pastoralia loca versa fuerant in sepulturam hominum, et habitacula humana facta fuerant confugia bestiarum. (*Historia Langobardorum* 2.4)

> There was, moreover, grief everywhere, tears everywhere. For as rumor commonly held it that those fleeing would avoid disaster, houses were relinquished, abandoned by their inhabitants, with only pups left to look out for the house. Property (livestock/flocks) remained alone in the

[10] Paul's last account is of plague in Rome in 680; on variations in his account from that in the *Liber Pontificalis*, see Little (2007, 13).

[11] I have used Waitz's text (1876).

> pastures, with no shepherd attending. You would see (*cerneres*) that villas or military camps formerly filled with throngs of men, after everyone had fled together on the following day, were all in the most profound silence. Children fled, leaving behind the unburied corpses of their parents. Parents, forgetful of their *pietas*, abandoned their children who were burning up with fever. If by chance ancient *pietas* bound anyone, so that he wished to give burial to kin, he himself remained unburied; and while he was being dutiful, he approached death; while he furnished burial rites, his own death remained without burial rites. You would see (*videres*) the age driven back to its ancient silence. There was no talk in the countryside, no murmuring of shepherds, no snares of beasts among the flocks, no harm to the domestic fowl. The crops, having exceeded the right time for gathering, awaited a reaper untouched. As winter approached, the vines remained uncut, though their leaves had fallen and grapes were shining. Throughout the hours of night and day, the trumpet of war resounded, and was heard by many as if the murmur of an army. There were no footprints of passersby, nor was any assailant seen; but still the bodies of the dead were an overwhelming sight. Pastoral places had been turned into tombs for men, and places fit for human habitation had become the refuge of beasts.

Paul concludes his account of this particular outbreak by describing its containment within the Italian peninsula and resuming the matter of hostilities between Narses, Justinian's imperial representative, and the Goths, hostilities that ultimately clear the stage for Lombard rule in Italy. While Paul resists acknowledging the outbreak as a turning point for the ascension of the Lombard people, he does stress the plague's confinement to the Romans of Italy, and his account of its dramatic social and environmental impact hints at a conceptual divide between past and future rule. The adjective *antiquus*, used to modify both *pietas* and the primordial *silentium* in which Liguria is enveloped, signals the roles of familial bonds and saecular upheavals as twin pillars of narrating plague in the Latin tradition.[12] And yet his invocation of that tradition as explicitly *antiqua* relegates it to a past, already weakened by Gothic invasions and further atrophied in the plague.

It is worth considering what aspects of "ancient" *pietas* or ancient representations of epochal evolution the historian found so compelling, and why. Paul does not focus with the same intensity as

[12] Cf. similar remarks about grass growing over marketplaces in *Historia Langobardorum* 6.5.

Endelechius on any particular bond between parent and child. In fact, he introduces *pietas* as a compulsion between parents and children that is mostly ineffective, forgotten (*obliti pietatis*) amidst the horrors of disease rapidly spreading. In the rare cases where it binds (*perstringo*) individuals to honor ties of kinship, *pietas* proves as futile for the Ligurians as it had for Lucretius' Romanized Athenians or Ovid's Aeginetans or, in the context of civil war, Lucan's Massilians struggling to bury their own kin, who are rendered unrecognizable on the sea shore after the slaughter of battle. Paul spells out explicitly the certain death from physical proximity that results from *pietas*, rather than (as his predecessors had done) merely lamenting the futility of attempting to bury what was, after all, merely corporeal. *Pietas* is transformed into a harsh zero-sum game, so that a value formerly structured by reciprocity is replaced by one in which reciprocity is inevitably interrupted: if a family member acts dutifully, she will contract the disease, die, and relinquish her only chance for a proper burial.

In contrast to the subtle ironies that he injects in his account of *pietas*, Paul expands with some reverence on the Golden- and Iron-Age inversions that had colored accounts of plague in Latin epic. The plague neutralizes former hostilities between domestic and wild beasts, as observed in Vergil's pastoral Golden Age in the *Eclogues* (4.21–5) and his upending of that age in Noricum (*G.*3.537–47; cf. Ovid *Met.*7.545–6). Moreover, agriculture, an indicator of the Iron Age and its attendant *labores*, ceases altogether; *intacta* crops, in particular, signaling the absence of work, echo Ovid's vision of a Golden Age in which the land, "untouched" (*intacta*, *Met.*1.101), bore all her gifts, although the same sentence in Paul looks back to the former Iron-Age conditions in which the crops were sown (*sata*). Paul's interest in grapes ripe and ready on the vine, moreover, reflects on Vergil's similar fixation on those Golden-Age amenities of the fourth *Eclogue* (4.29, 40). As so often in the traditions of Latin poetry, plague's aberrations locate the infected landscape on a highly tenuous divide between ages. The primordial silence that marks the conditions of prehistory is interrupted by sounds resembling that of the war *tuba*—surely misinterpreted, since no human footprints accompany the sounds of an approaching army, but an effective reminder of the wars against the Goths in Italy that would continue unabated throughout successive epidemics. Of course, like agriculture, war furthers a precipitous decline from the Golden Age in both

Ovidian and Vergilian accounts of saecular evolution (*G.* 1.118–47; cf. 2.532–40; *Met.* 1.97–100, where the *tuba* is explicitly absent).

Crawfurd's early twentieth-century account of pestilence in literature and visual arts contrasts Latin accounts of the pandemic in the Western empire with Greek accounts in the East, primarily those of Procopius and Evagrius: Latin accounts are so intent on "the mental and moral features of the distemper, that they say almost nothing of its physical features" (Crawfurd 1914, 88). Stoclet's (2007) relatively recent examination of Western responses to the plague clarifies the mental and moral features stressed by Crawfurd with a focus on, *inter alia*, omens, portents, and superstition: the plague provided Latin chroniclers of the period ample room for reflection on the efficacy of ancient Roman *superstitio* compared with Christian responses to various outbreaks. Indeed, Paul enriches a subsequent account of pestilence with solar and lunar eclipses as well as the story of the transference of St. Sebastian's remains to the church of St. Peter at Pavia, upon which act the pestilence ceased (*Historia Langobardorum* 6.5).

The responsibility for the details in these treatments by Christian authors does not, however, lie solely on the shoulders of competing pagan vs. Christian worldviews. As I hope to have suggested, such details are partly attributed to the traditions of classical Latin epic:[13] the same account describing the transference of St. Sebastian's remains includes a graphic (faintly Lucretian) depiction of "parents with children and brothers with their sisters" heaped upon one another, on funeral biers.[14] Paul's adaptations of "ancient" tropes, moreover, interprets the most salient and affective elements of the Latin epic tradition for new audiences and transmits them to a culture grappling with the aftermath of its own literal plague. Such audiences were struggling to make sense out of a world whose imperial Roman architecture was crumbling, soon to be replaced in Italy by new governance, as well as by new theological models restructuring

[13] Livy, and especially his depiction of the deserted countryside surrounding plague-stricken Rome in the outbreak of 463 BCE (see above, Chapter 2), may also have influenced Paul here, especially in light of his generic affinity, though the pronounced tropes in *HL* are more easily identified as epic borrowings.

[14] *Historia Langobardum* 6.5: *tantaque fuit multitudo morientium, ut etiam parentes cum filiis atque fratres cum sororibus, bini per feretra positi, apud urbem Romam ad sepulchra ducerentur.*

humankind's relationship with the divine.[15] These models, Christological alternatives largely supplanting ancient Roman religious practices, would similarly guide responses to the second pandemic that struck Europe in the fourteenth century. And evident again within these responses are expressions of the classical past, expressions that would persist in asserting plague's ancient power to address ideological fractures and prompt coalescence among a population.

7.2. VISIONS OF CHAOS, MANIFESTATIONS OF ORDER: PLAGUE ICONOGRAPHY IN THE ITALIAN RENAISSANCE AND BEYOND

7.2.1. Raphael's Plague of Phrygia

The second pandemic to hit the Western world was the Black Death, again *Yersinia pestis* or bubonic plague.[16] It arrived in Europe in 1347 and continued to ravage the continent in successive waves until the last reported outbreak occurred in Marseilles in 1720. Italy's initial experience of plague, perhaps best known from Boccaccio's *Decameron*, was filtered representationally through the lens of antiquity: Boccaccio draws from many tropes explored in this study, and of particular interest is his recognition of familial loyalties and betrayals. While Thucydides clearly influenced his narrative stance as eyewitness to the calamity, the Roman tradition is manifested in his observations that "brothers abandoned brothers, uncles their nephews, sisters their brothers, and in many cases wives deserted their husbands. But even worse, and almost incredible, was the fact that fathers and mothers refused to nurse and assist their own children, as though they did not belong to them."[17] Boccaccio's

[15] The last outbreak of this first pandemic was in 750 CE. For an engaging, if occasionally overreaching argument concerning the plague's impact on the transformation of the Roman Empire and its gradual dissolution into the nation-states that would define Western Europe, see Rosen (2007).

[16] *Yersinia pestis* refers to the bacillus that causes bubonic plague, so called from the painful swellings around the lymph nodes that were a common symptom of the disease. The same bacillus also causes septicemic and pneumonic forms of the disease, less common but with higher mortality rates.

[17] McWilliam's translation (1972, 54)=*Decameron* 27 in Branca's (1992) text.

account of the social pathologies that grip Florence during the outbreak of 1348, combined with a large corpus of plague treatises in Latin and Italian that rely heavily on classical writers and ancient medicine, serve as a textual backdrop to innovative responses to the epidemic in the visual arts—responses that foreground the very tropes that made representations of pestilence so compelling and revelatory in the Rome of the late Republic and early Principate.

By and large these images do not aim to depict the clinical reality of the plague, and thus do not draw on the symptomatology and epidemiology structuring many Roman plague narratives. Mormando's survey of textual sources ranging from medical treatises to personal correspondence to sermons and biblical commentary from the sixteenth through eighteenth centuries distinguishes discourses that aimed at containing the epidemic and treating physical symptoms from those church-mandated *rimedi spirituali* that aimed at healing the soul and assuring laypersons of rewards and punishments in the afterlife (2005, 2–3; 15–28). Most visual arts fell squarely in the camp of the latter, reminding viewers that the cause of plague was god's wrath, hence the coinage of the term "plague" under the belief that epidemic disease, and bubonic plague in particular, was a "blow" from god as punishment for the sins of humankind (cf. Leavy 1992, 4–5). Visual images also promote the role of the church and its representatives as intercessors between god and humankind. From the Roman inheritance, however, we find a preoccupation with the affective bonds that structure the family as well as the power of pestilence to prompt the renewal of a community under specific leadership or according to new models of identity in relation to the state.

The classical Latin inheritance used to frame Renaissance visions of bubonic plague is perhaps best illustrated by an engraving of Marcantonio Raimondi based on a drawing by Raphael. The engraving, referred to as *Il Morbetto* and depicting the episode of pestilence on Crete recounted in *Aeneid* 3, is one of a number of Raphael's images inspired by Vergil's poem and the product of a fruitful collaboration between artist and engraver.[18] Raphael's enthusiasm for antiquity, and especially the architectural ruins of ancient Rome,

[18] Raphael had access to early illuminated manuscripts of Vergil and was inspired by them for his imagery. See also Lord (1984), who speculates that the painter had planned to publish a volume of engravings from the *Aeneid* in its entirety.

was recognized by his earliest biographers and remains the subject of many art historical approaches to the painter's oeuvre.[19] Indeed Raphael's desire to capture ancient images that would convey the prestige and significance of contemporary Rome under Leo X is fully apparent in *Il Morbetto* (Fig. 7.1). [20]

An inscribed herm divides the engraving in two halves: on the right, in the foreground and depicted in the light of day, are afflicted

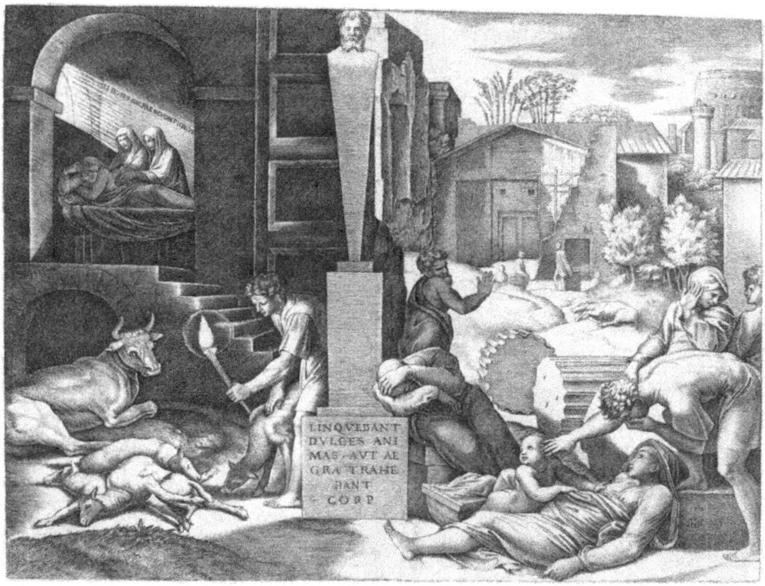
LINQVEBANT
DVLCES ANI
MAS AVT AE
GRA TRAHE
BANT
CORP

Fig. 7.1. Marcantonio Raimondi (after Raphael), *Il Morbetto* (*The Plague of Phrygia*), *c.*1514. National Gallery of Art, Washington, DC, gift of W.G. Russell Allen.

Courtesy of the National Gallery of Art, Washington, DC.

[19] While overseeing a papal building project under Leo X, Raphael helped publish an Italian translation of Vitruvius. For early biographical treatments, cf. *Le Vite* (*c.*1550) of Giorgio Vasari, 1511–74 (cited in Forcellino, 2012, 7–8); Roland Fréart's study of Renaissance painters, including Raphael, emphasizes the influence of Pliny and Quintilian. Fréart's work was translated into English as *An Idea of the Perfection of Painting* by John Evelyn, 1668; Forcellino also notes Raphael's "systematic study of the ancient world" (2012, 177).

[20] On Raphael's collaboration with the Pope in promoting Rome's rebirth through classical imagery, see Farinella (2004, 32).

Trojans in various postures of distress, some of them holding their noses, a gesture originally used to indicate the smell of death, but one that, thanks to the engraving, would become common in depictions of the bubonic plague.[21] Most prominent is the supine form of a woman, dead or near death, with an infant grasping at her breast, while an onlooker, presumably fearing the child will contract the disease, tries to push the infant away from its mother. Receding in the background are various architectural elements, including column drums and an unfinished tower, signs of a city in the making. A mysterious figure stands near an opening in the tower, perhaps a litter bearer removing corpses, and nearby a horse lies dying. This side of the engraving thus corresponds roughly with the plague described in *Aeneid* 3.132–42, and an inscription on the herm from lines 140–1 of the passage confirms as much: *linquebant dulcis animas aut aegra trahebant corp [ora*].

To the left of the herm, chiaroscuro, the play of light and dark that would become characteristic of Italian baroque and mannerist painting, evokes a moonlit evening. In the upper left corner "images" of the Penates are illuminated by light from the window and identified by an inscription drawn from *Aeneid* 3.148 (*effigies sacrae divom Phryg [iique Penatesque*]). They hover over a reclining Aeneas, presumably *in somnis* as Vergil describes him (3.151), and receiving word sent by Apollo that the Trojans should abandon Crete and make their way to Hesperia. Below him, in the left foreground, the artist has depicted a stable scene with a bull or heifer and three lambs lying upon one another. A young man accompanied by a fourth lamb looks over the three bodies with a lit torch. The nighttime setting may indicate that the animals are sleeping,[22] though their bodies appear contorted in a way that suggests death rather than slumber.

As Christine Boeckl has stressed (2000, 95), the engraving reverses the sequence from left to right in Raphael's original drawing, which more faithfully reflects Vergil's sequence of pestilence in the fledgling Pergamum (originally on the left) followed by Aeneas' nocturnal vision (originally on the right). Since viewers tend to read images left to right, the sequence of Raphael's drawing conveys a more hopeful

[21] Boeckl (1991, 121–2); scholars have also suggested that the gesture harkens back to the ancient theory of miasma; see Hipp (2007, 184, esp. n. 25) and Mormando (2005, 9).

[22] See Boeckl (2000, 94); cf. *Aen*.3.147, *nox erat et terris animalia somnus habebat.*

message, juxtaposing "the story of destruction with the promise of rescue" (2000, 94). Why Raimondi chose to execute the design in reverse must remain a subject of speculation,[23] but the effect, along with the addition of the inscription on the herm drawn from the Latin text, draws attention to the morbid nature of the episode. I would also suggest that the new sequence prompts a more comprehensive review of pestilence as depicted throughout Vergil's poetry. Vergil does not mention the effects of the *pestilentia* on livestock in *Aeneid* 3, so the prominence of animal forms is puzzling unless we turn to other Vergilian representations of plague. By turning to *Georgics* 3, we can explain the left foreground of the engraving, in which livestock are afflicted; in the same book the account of Noric plague is preceded by an account of contagion among sheep, perhaps explaining the stable scene, and concludes with the first signs of pestilence among the region's human inhabitants. *Georgic* allusions in the engraving would thus account for a viewing sequence in *Il Morbetto* that conveys the affliction of animals prior to the arrival of pestilence among the human community.

Such a relatively morbid composition, while still reversing the original drawing, does not necessarily eradicate hope from the engraving. The most striking image (or at least most influential, based on its persistent afterlife) is that of the child at the breast of its mother. As Boeckl argues, the fact that the child's head is being averted from its mother's lifeless form suggests hope for survival (2000, 94). The gesture, however, also addresses the plague's tragically ironic impact on the mother's role as primary nurturer and implies that the renewal of the community depends in some instances on the severance of familial bonds.[24] The iconography has an especially pronounced ancient pedigree: most art historians attribute it to Pliny's ecphrasis of a painting by Aristides of Thebes, who had managed to convey the "mind" (*animus*) and "feelings" (*sensus*) of figures he depicted, especially in the image of "the capture of a town, showing an infant creeping to the breast of its mother who is dying of a wound; it is felt that the mother is aware of the child and is afraid

[23] Boeckl suggests that Raimondi published the engraving at a time when fresh waves of the epidemic threatened Italy (2000, 95).

[24] This imagery inverts the common medieval and Renaissance portrayals of the infant Christ nursing at Mary's breast, a theme whose psychological gratification lies partly in its power to restore the fantasy of symbiosis between mother and child; see Adams (1993, 202–8).

that, as her milk is exhausted by death, it may suck blood" (*Nat.* 35.98).[25] Pliny's discussion of Greek painting helped shape the ideals of Renaissance art, and we know that Leonardo at least owned and consulted his copy of the *Natural History*.[26] The text no doubt played some role in promoting the image of an infant attempting to nurse from its lifeless mother, albeit it the context of war rather than pestilence.[27] It is also possible, however, that the tradition of Latin plague narratives, with their sustained emphasis on often self-destructive familial entanglements, primed the canvas for the transference of this particular configuring of mother and child from a setting of war to one of rampant contagion.

The impact of Raphael's image was somewhat delayed, but increased dramatically after it was quoted for the first time in Nicolas Poussin's *Plague of Ashdod* (1630), a painting with a similarly ancient (although biblical) subject matter that would have created a comforting temporal distance between the viewer and the catastrophe depicted (Hipp 2007, 195). By the early seventeenth century the figural group of mother and child had also worked its way into literary discourses, as reflected in a French moralizing treatise on responses to bubonic plague; the author, Etienne Binet, condemns how the disease "separates father from his son and the mother from the infant at her breast; and even before killing people, it first kills charity and friendship" (from Binet's *Remèdes souverains contre la peste et la mort soudaine* [1628], cited in Hipp 2007, 208). The composition of mother separated from child serves as a reminder of the plague's power to corrode familial bonds, and how the corrosion of such bonds can permeate relationships within the wider community. In Poussin's painting, as in Raphael's image, a glimmer of hope is afforded as a man leans over the mother and child directing the

[25] *Oppido capto ad matris morientis ex volnere mammam adrepens infans, intellegiturque sentire mater et timere, ne emortuo lacte sanguinem lambat.*

[26] On Leonardo's use of Pliny, see Adams (1993, 26); for the importance of Pliny's ecphrasis and evaluation of Aristides' painting on the ideals of Renaissance art, see Summers (1989, 17–18); for Pliny's description as the primary source of inspiration for Raphael's drawing, see also Hipp (2007, 182), Mormando et al. (2005, 187, cat. 5), and Blunt (1967, 94).

[27] Ghirlandaio's *Massacre of the Innocents*, which includes a scene likely inspired by Pliny's description, precedes Raphael's drawing (Blunt 1967, 94; Boeckl 2000, 94), though Raphael is the first known artist to use the iconography in the context of plague.

child's head away from her breast, a gesture indicating the possibility of salvation.

It is worth noting that between the time of *Il Morbetto*'s circulation and Poussin's painting Endelechius' *Carmen de mortibus boum* had been rediscovered and published (1590) by the French lawyer and scholar Pierre Pithou.[28] The poem's circulation of highly Vergilian (if also highly Christianized) plague imagery may have prompted audiences to review the implications of Raimondi's Vergilian engraving and perhaps even informed new depictions of the mother and suckling infant motif, such as that in Poussin's painting: Endelechius' bitter-sweet affirmation of the familial bond expressed by the mother cow and her nursing *vitulus*—despite its ultimately destructive implications—confirms the endurance of *pietas* in the face of pestilence: *post mortem pietas viget* (80). The fear experienced by the mothers in both Pliny's and Endelechius' descriptions is minimized in the compositions of Poussin and Raphael, of course, since she appears dead or nearly dead. Our attention is drawn to the possibility of the child's survival, despite the mother's demise, and the role of the community in that salvation. This redirection may imply a more hopeful reading of the potential for recovery than its classical models, while at the same time using pestilence to question what relationships within the family unit and between the family and the wider community are required to shore up the social order and optimize its functioning.

7.2.2. A Tale of Two Cities: Coppola's Visions of Naples after the Plague of 1656

After Poussin's *Plague at Ashdod*, the mother and child motif recurs in countless paintings of plague, executed by a wide range of talents and contextualized in both sacred and secular settings.[29] In the late

[28] For the publication of Pithou's edition, see Schierl (2016, 241 n. 4).

[29] See especially paintings by Caroselli (after Poussin), Crespi, Sweerts, Tiepolo, and Mignard, nos. 1, 2, 6, 7, and 25 in Mormando et al. (2005). Other notable variations on the motif include, in the San Bartolomeo all' Isola, Antonio Carracci's (*c*.1612) painting of *St. Charles Borromeo Giving Communion to a Plague Victim* (where the mother and child are the only dead figures, placed in the foreground; in the background another plague victim receives final sacraments); in Chiesa di San Rocco, Tintoretto's *St. Roch Heals the Plague Stricken*; in the Scuola di San Rocco, Zanchi's

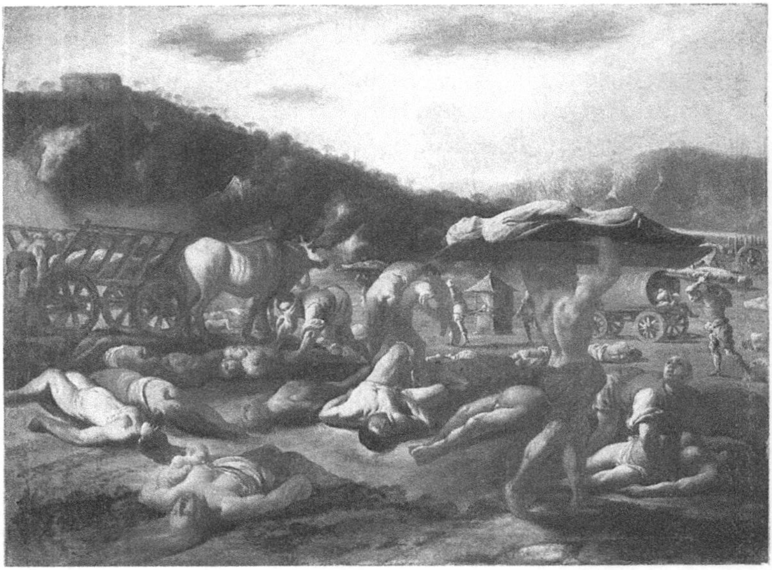

Fig. 7.2. Carlo Coppola, *The Pestilence of 1656 in Naples*, after 1656. Princeton University Art Museum, Caroline G. Mather Fund.
Photo: Princeton University Art Museum/Art Resource.

seventeenth century, Carlo Coppola painted two representations of the outbreak in Naples in 1656: on one canvas (Fig. 7.2) bodies are scattered on the earth in contorted positions at various stages of decomposition, indicated by flesh tones graduating from grey to pink. While a few living figures hoist shrouded corpses above their shoulders, most of the bodies are nude, exposed in a context removed from civic space, which at first glance might be mistaken for a battlefield.[30] Left of center, and pushed prominently to the foreground, lies the figure of a woman, eyes shut and mouth agape, with a living child nursing at her lifeless breast. While Coppola's image clearly quotes similar configurations in Raphael and Poussin, the artist here suppresses the element of hope implicit in the works of

(1666) *Virgin Appearing to Plague Victims*; in Chiesa di Sant' Anna dei Lombardi (Naples), Francesco di Maria's (1688) *The Communion of the Plague Victims*.

[30] See cat. 26 in Mormando et al. (2005, 229) for Coppola's experience in battle and its possible impact on his images of plague.

his predecessors: the living figures in the scene are so distracted with their own grief or with removal of the dead that they do not attempt to remove the child from its dead mother.

The mother and child are the only explicit reference to the familial bond, though they may be complemented by figures in the right lower corner, where a young man clings to the ashen figure of a woman, perhaps his mother or wife. The desperation in his eyes signals his fear of relinquishing the body to those charged with filling up the death carts. The mortality and chaos that dominate the bottom half of the canvas are met with sloping hills and a cloudy sky in the upper portion, a disinterested nature refusing to answer the call for sympathy. Coppola's "journalistic" approach to depicting pestilence here suggests an unscripted and erratic response to the calamity that has befallen Naples, by most accounts the worst the city had suffered, a response valuable for its bleak realism in contrast to more positive images of divine intercession (Mormando et al. 2005, 229).

Coppola's second painting (Fig. 7.3), of a market square in Naples during the same outbreak, is similarly framed by a disinterested natural world, this time more sinister as Mt. Vesuvius rises in the background. The square itself, filled with miniature, almost indistinguishable human figures, consumes the canvas. This space, however, is definitively civic. The geometry of the piazza imposes order upon its citizens: as Clifton observes, the buildings are arranged with striking regularity, and "even the supposedly frantic figures are carefully arranged in rows parallel to the bottom edge of the canvas" (2005, 115). Human forms drawn in industrious ranks that dispose of bodies answer the call of officials, slightly larger figures whose authority is marked by dress, gesture, or positioning on horseback. We glimpse the conventional horrors of plague: futile appeals to heaven, crowding of fountains, a scattering of corpses. But these horrors are contained and offered for the viewer's surveillance.[31] A woman near the fountain exposes her buboes to a man nearby. A handful of death carts enter and exit the square, while a few figures in quarantined buildings throw themselves from upper story windows. The operations used to meet the catastrophe reveal a community interacting, enduring punishment for violating

[31] For an antecedent to Coppola's approach, see Clifton, who examines Garguilo's painting of the Largo del Mercatello, in which the use of space, geometry, and distance works similarly to contain the threatening aspects of plague (2005, 113).

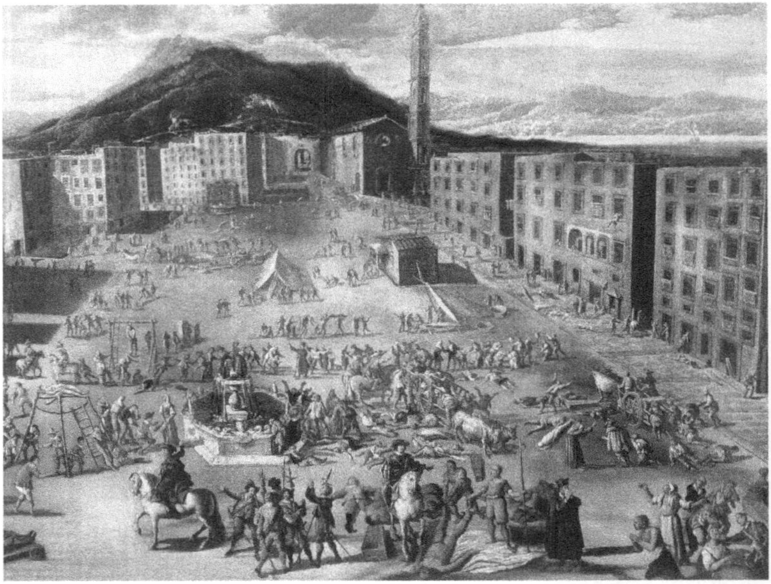

Fig. 7.3. Carlo Coppola, *Piazza del Mercato during the Plague of 1656*, *c.*1660. Museo di S. Martino, Naples.

Photo by DeAgostini/Getty Images. DEA/A. DAGLI ORTI.

quarantine, and complying with the dictates of authority. Bureaucracy is forged; life, for some, will go on.

While the two paintings present starkly divergent images of how contagious disease impacts human life, their observations of that impact should be viewed as complementary rather than antithetical, together narrating the collapse of the social order and its subsequent restructuring, described by Foucault as two dreams: one is a dream of utter lawlessness and the other is that moment "when political power is exercised to the full" (2003, 47). As demonstrated in Chapter 5, these two dreams of plague are anticipated by Ovid's before and after snapshots of Aegina, first in the throes of disease and then in the wake of recovery, in which healthy, serviceable Myrmidon bodies are distributed throughout the kingdom. Viewers may find comfort in the containment Coppola offers in his rendering of the Piazza, confirming a critical function of both visual and textual representations of disease as articulated by Sander Gilman: "our examination of the image of the sufferer provides us with rigid structures for our definition of the boundaries of disease, boundaries that are reified by the very limits inherent in the work of art" (1988, 2). Within that consolation, however, there is also revelation—revelation of pestilence as an opportunity for the expansion of governmental oversight and intrusion within the population. If Naples was not left with a slate quite so clean as Ovid's Aegina, mortality rates and upheaval in the social order had given secular and ecclesiastical authorities enough of a new order to justify their power over and production of a civic body for whose well-being they were increasingly responsible.[32]

The stringent order that Coppola gestures toward in his painting would, in fact, be exercised more fully in Rome, which experienced an outbreak of plague just after Naples in 1656, but with a remarkably lower mortality rate.[33] As Gentilcore observes, "Rome became a city of boundaries" (2016, 157). While there were some minority groups targeted for expulsion (mendicants, vagrants, prostitutes), the city's Congregation of Health worked fastidiously to control the movement of people and goods, not only through quarantine, but also through pesthouses, health status reporting, licensing for remedies, prohibitions on public gatherings, and restrictions on the departure of physicians, surgeons, and barbers (Gentilcore 2016, 156–7). Cohn (2010, 7–8) assigns the growing state and church authority to the success of mandates from the health boards in Italy, beginning in the wake of earlier outbreaks during the sixteenth century: "The mobilization of massive resources to combat plague in 1575–8 and the successful encouragement of clergy and health workers to remain at their posts . . . fueled the growth of the new Counter-Reformation Church and secular states alike."[34] While spiritual remedies would continue to offer an answer to god's wrath as manifested in plague, earthly measures emerged to manage populations, giving birth to a "biopolitics" centered on the state's need to justify and defend its

[32] Clifton stresses ecclesiastical law over secular, noting that the initial response to plague was one of "re-affirmation of the stringency of the Rule and devotion to celestial advocates" (2005, 109). Literary sources also reflect, however, a sharp reversion to more indulgent habits after the plague had abated.

[33] About 40 percent of Naples' population died in the outbreak of 1656, reducing the population from about 400,000 in 1655 to about 240,000 after the plague abated. Rome's population by contrast was reduced by about 20,000. See Gentilcore (2016, 157–8).

[34] For Cohn, such success "led to the glorification of individual rulers and instructed on the need and value of subjects to obey, thereby boosting absolutist authority at the end of the sixteenth century into the next" (2010, 8).

oversight as it reshaped the relationship between the individual and the body politic (Foucault 1997, 73; cf. Wald 2012, 114).[35]

7.3. A NEW ORDER FOR *HOMO SAPIENS?* FROM BIOPOLITICS TO BIOENGINEERING IN ANGLO-AMERICAN FICTION

If visual images of seventeenth-century Italy hint at the opportunities for exercising authority that accompany the disaster of bubonic plague, Defoe's *Journal of the Plague Year* gives full voice to the efforts of London magistrates to manage an infected population.[36] The fictive account, while based on the pestilence that struck London in 1665, was published in 1722, with some concern for the possibility of the plague's return after Marseilles experienced an outbreak in 1720. The author meticulously records measures established by the "Lord Mayor and Aldermen" to ensure public safety and order (*JPY* 38–47; 90–2) and to restrict manufacture and trade (90–2).[37] While he views the efficacy of quarantine procedures with some skepticism, Defoe's narrator "H.F." mostly applauds London's officials and citizens for respecting the rule of law. Through constant reflection on the movement of individuals throughout the larger London community, the *Journal* exposes tension between the desire for self-preservation and interest in the overall "public good" (Leavy 1992, 33–4): this tension in turn fuels progress

[35] In his course on "Security, Territory, and Population" (1997, 67), Foucault describes a shift from a nation's imperative to manage territories to national concerns with managing populations. In "The Birth of Biopolitics" (1997, 73–9), he stresses that such population management was answered by a "Liberalism" that regularly questioned the need for governmental regulation. For Foucault's particular use of the term "biopolitics," see Chapter 5, p. 180 n. 43. Wald's (2012) study explores how twenty-first-century contagion narratives, especially those written after the bombing of the World Trade Towers, explore vulnerabilities within the biopolitical mechanisms of the US.

[36] On the flourishing of plague discourses, from physicians' treatises to narrative poems, in England in the sixteenth and seventeenth centuries, as a response to repeated outbreaks of bubonic plague, see Healy (2001, 54–64), who demonstrates a consistent reliance on both classical and Old Testament sources for representations of disease and its physical and social impact.

[37] References to Defoe's *Journal of the Plague Year* are indicated with the abbreviation *JPY* and taken from the 2001 Modern Library edition, with introduction by Jason Goodwin.

toward articulating what we might consider a contemporary and highly alienated sense of self, if only by creating a foil, a self that feels the constant pull of civic and familial duty.[38]

Barbara Fass Leavy has argued that plague texts from different historical contexts are united by their attention to "the psychological and moral issues concerning what constitutes human beings as a group and what individuates its members," and by their tendency to confront readers with the threat of estrangement (1992, 11). A broad range of Anglo-American plague narratives, from Defoe's eighteenth-century *Journal* to Margaret Atwood's twenty-first century *MaddAddam* trilogy again draw from the traditions of the Latin plague narrative by invoking the family in order to reflect on the autonomy of the self. And, as in Roman plague texts, imagery of the Golden Age and epochal evolution, in many cases enhanced through the language of dissolution and bodily decay, allow these writers to frame the question of the individual's relationship to the larger community as one whose answers shed light on the ideal conditions of human existence. To ponder the question more dramatically, what features, if any, of *homo sapiens* should survive a sweep of contagion that could wipe the slate clean?

While Defoe is by no means consumed with the question of familial obligations—H.F. is a bachelor and mentions only a brother who leaves London with his family (*JPY* 10–11)—his examination of kinship in the outbreak glances at the traditions of Latin epic. He returns constantly to the plight of afflicted and quarantined families: H.F. converses with a man who, with some consternation, avoids his stricken family (*JPY* 102); so too does "self Preservation" appear "to be the first Law . . . for the Children ran away from their Parents, as they languished in the utmost distress: And in some places . . . Parents did the like to their children" (*JPY* 110); more succinctly, he observes that "Families" were "made even a terror to themselves" (*JPY* 168). Defoe, however, also observes citizens guided by a more compassionate impulse, recalling the efforts of family members to attend to each other in Ovid's Aegina, Seneca's Thebes, and more recently,

[38] See Leavy (1992, 7): "[S]uch alienation, however, had not (in Defoe's London) become virtually synonymous with the human condition. Civic duty, a very important concept in the *Journal*, . . . supplies a grounds for moral action in 1722 London . . . The view of selfhood that modern criticism takes for granted is the very one that the *Journal* struggles against."

Endelechius' pastoral landscape. The narrator expounds at length on the dynamics of birth and motherhood, citing many instances of infected women who gave birth to children "half born or born but not parted from the mother" (*JPY* 111) as well as mothers who, while nursing, "has poison'd, that is, infected the Infant with [their] Milk, even before they knew they were infected themselves; nay, and the Infant has dy'd in such a case before the Mother" (*JPY* 113). From there H.F. invokes the increasingly familiar visual motif of "living Infants being found sucking the Breasts of the Mothers" (*JPY* 113).

Again we confront the paradox of familial solidarity—the bedrock of the social contract—rendered a source of contamination and threat to both personal autonomy and communal stability. Eventually, writers and filmmakers will question whether joining the ranks of the infected is such a threat after all, and allow the trope to expose new possibilities for (post) human identity, but these will emerge in the midst of contagion that is not, as with the bubonic plague, often fatal; such recent, fictive contagions tend to be transformative rather than deadly.[39] The fear that lingered from London's very real experience of pestilence would not be alleviated by prospects of joining the ranks of the infected. With the closure of the *Journal*, in fact, comes the restoration of the old social contract, where individuals can once again commune with each other, an outcome that ensures approval of the London bureaucrats who have managed to maintain a semblance of order.[40] H.F. has only half-reluctantly witnessed the dissolution of hierarchy within the city as demonstrated through the operations at the death pits, where "bodies [were] shot into the pit promiscuously" (*JPY* 60), and where there was "no difference made, but poor and rich went together" (*JPY* 61). But readers can rest assured that, with some individual liberties conceded (cf. Leavy 1992, 33), the law has navigated Londoners through the worst of the crisis. The otherworldly, "profound Silence" (*JPY* 100) that cloaked the streets early in the plague will be lifted by commerce and the exchange of friendly greetings (*JPY* 233).

[39] See below (pp. 269–70) for examples of this type of contagion narrative. Wald (2012, 112–14) discusses species evolution as a preoccupation of many bio-terror narratives, and argues that such preoccupation is grounded in fears concerning the long-term biological impact of contagious diseases on humankind.

[40] See David Steel on how bureaucratic routines in the *Journal* quantify and control the plague (1981, 103).

Defoe had a remarkable impact on the traditions of plague writing, most notably on Camus, who uses an epigraph taken from *Robinson Crusoe* to open his own *La Peste*.[41] A more immediate successor to the Englishman's preoccupation with human subjectivity and human survival amidst the impending collapse of civilization is found in Mary Shelley's *The Last Man*.[42] In her temporally stratified approach to inscribing a plague of the future (2073–2100 CE) from the vantage of early nineteenth-century England, Shelley turns to Roman oracular power to speculate on how pestilence impacts the human subject and her relationship with the larger community—whether that community is defined as a body politic (England) or the vestiges of the human race. In her author's introduction, "Shelley" cites the leaves of Vergil's Sibyl at Cumae as the source of the fragmented prophecies she has reassembled as testimony for the future envisioned in *The Last Man*:[43]

> Scattered and unconnected as they were, I have been obliged to add links and model the work into a consistent form. But the main substance rests on the truths contained in these poetic rhapsodies, and the divine intuition which the Cumaean damsel obtained from heaven. I have often wondered at the subject of her verses, and at the English dress of the Latin poet. (*LM* 4)[44]

The introduction to the testimony of the "last man," structured as a kind of katabasis in which the author and her companion make their way down into the Sibyl's cave, overtly conjures Vergil's Aeneas (*LM* 3), whose access to the afterlife reveals the culmination of

[41] "It is as reasonable to represent one kind of imprisonment by another, as it is to represent anything that really exists by that which exists not." The epigraph signals (*inter alia*) the allegorical import of the plague in Oran that is the subject of Camus' novel. For the influence of Defoe's plague narratives (*Due Preparations for the Plague, as well for Soul as Body* in addition to the *Journal*) on Camus, see especially Steel (1981, esp. 91–5) and Cooke (2009, 16–43).

[42] On the lukewarm reception of the novel, which handles a theme already treated in verse by Byron and Thomas Campbell, see Paley (1993) and Thomas (2000). Ridicule was garnered largely from the notion that "lastness" was fundamentally un-representable.

[43] The gender of the introduction's author is perhaps intentionally ambiguous, though many readers equate the authorial voice with Shelley herself; see esp. Mellor (1993, xxiv–xxv); cf. Eberle-Sinatra (2000, 101–2).

[44] References to passages in Shelley's novel are taken from Luke's (1993) edition and abbreviated *LM*.

Rome's future under Augustan rule.[45] Shelly's novel, while doggedly eschatological in speculating on possibilities for a renewed, if Christianized Golden Age (Paley 1993, 116–18), will find no such reassurances in the future that Lionel Verney, the narrator and titular hero, records. It is one contention of this book that Shelley and the many interpreters of the Western plague narrative have chosen the "Latin poet"—and Latin epic in particular—as a source for understanding plague's expurgatory power, its power to wash away old ways of being in the world and speculate on new templates for human relationships. These same imaginatively constructed, communally experienced disasters also, however, articulate a hesitant wavering between a clean slate and those relics of the past that pestilence leaves behind, fragments, like the Sibyl's leaves, worth piecing together as a memorial to what went before, in the face of incipient change. Her novel's use of the prophetic mode grants Shelley a vatic stance, not too distant from Vergil's Noric seer, seizing on plague's power to explore and in some cases challenge the conditions that determine the individual's relationship to the body politic.[46]

The mythologies of Rome's founding also frame the internal testimony of the "last man." Lionel Verney devotes much of his account to his childhood spent "as uncouth a savage as the wolf-bred founder of Rome" (*LM* 9) and his gradual enculturation among the English aristocracy. By the novel's closure, Verney arrives in Rome pondering its relics and perusing its libraries (*LM* 335–9), reflecting self-consciously on his former identity as a Romulus figure, where his "robber and shepherd propensities, similar to those of [the city's] founder, were of advantage to its sole inhabitant" (*LM* 338). Verney's final observations of Rome as the crowning achievement of human civilization and his concerted engagement with Latin literature brings his journey full circle (Thomas 2000, 31).

[45] For Shelley's use of the Sibyl and the episode from Book 6 of the *Aeneid*, which she records having read in 1824, see Goldsmith (1993, 277–80), who argues that the Sibyl, as mouthpiece of the god Apollo, underscores the constraints of patriarchy encountered by the author.

[46] Gender is one condition determining the relationship between individual and community that Shelley's novel interrogates, though much of the topic, aside from its intersections with familial identities, remains beyond the scope of this discussion, which I have limited to focus on echoes of Roman pestilence treated in earlier sections of this book. Goldsmith (1993, 261–313) and Mellor (1993, x–xviii) address the novel's treatment of gender within the family, and the ways in which that treatment may have been informed by Shelley's own marital and parental experiences.

Within the circle and engaging the traditions of Latin epic that explicitly colored pestilence with shades of internal *discordia*, a specter of civil war haunts England throughout Verney's account of his maturity and well into his record of the plague's encroachment. In particular, Verney befriends England's former crown prince, Adrian, a relationship formalized as brotherhood through marriage. While Adrian expresses strong support for the country's new republican constitution, others among the English aristocracy are less sanguine about the change in governance, including the ambitious Raymond, another of Verney's "brothers," again through marriage. Raymond sets his designs initially on restoration of the monarchy, but eventually wins election as Lord Protector, England's highest office under its new constitution. Despite the novel's futuristic setting, Verney makes references to Roman civil war and revolution (*LM* 241), as well as the political revolutions in France and America (*LM* 39). His understanding of these events guides his observations on the strife that plagues England (*LM* 30). Verney views England as constantly "on the eve of civil war" (*LM* 34), a threat not entirely dissipated until after the plague has made its way into Western Europe and invaded England's shores—and even then the "contagion of rebellion" (*LM* 293) will threaten the motley crew of emigrant survivors as they travel throughout Europe (e.g., *LM* 274–5).[47]

Civil war comes closest to erupting when Irish refugees, fleeing pestilence in their own territory, enter England in hopes of finding succor, but find hostility instead. Adrian manages to quell the discord, as he invokes English troops to recall that, "these are your brothers, commit not fratricide; soon the plague will not leave one for you to glut your revenge upon" (*LM* 219). Indeed it is through brotherhood that the narrator gives such civil discord a specifically Roman inflection. And, as with hostilities between the English and Irish, Verney stages contention for the Protectorship—fought after Raymond's death between Adrian and himself—as wrangling between brothers. Ultimately Verney, who stood for the position primarily to spare the perennially poor health of his brother-in-law, concedes to Adrian and is told to return to the care of his family ("Return to Windsor then, my brother," *LM* 185).

[47] Verney further tightens the association between plague and civil war through his observance that the latter diverts English attention from the former (*LM* 161; cf. 163).

In fact, Adrian's status as a bachelor positions him in the novel as explicitly suited for assuming leadership of England during the plague. As with Defoe's narrator H.F., a lack of certain familial entanglements (marriage or paternity) liberates him from the affective bonds that complicate behaviors during an atmosphere of contagion, a freedom reflected in the improved health that he assumes in tending to others stricken with disease (*LM* 187).[48] In contrast, Verney feels the constant pull of his wife, Idris, and their two children; the desire to protect them shapes his attitude toward interacting with the larger community (*LM* 179, 188), though compassion for those outside the familial unit ultimately guides his moral compass (*LM* 188). As Mellor notes, Shelley betrays a certain cynicism about family life and the constancy of "domestic affections" (1993, xvii), as human folly and the plague play equal roles in eradicating Verney's kin. At the same time, the narrator observes that, even amidst an atmosphere of self-preservation and licentiousness, the crisis of plague and looming mortality "drew closer the ties of kindred and friendship" (*LM* 197). If Shelley's novel enacts the "drama of self and other" described by Stephanson, it recognizes a fundamental human impulse towards companionship as much as toward alienation and autonomy. From a Girardian perspective, the mimetic rivalries reflected in representations of plague as a trope for internal strife ironically culminate in the supreme autonomy of Verney ("I alone . . . I alone . . . ," *LM* 326), our narrator who wishes for nothing more than companionship. Conscious of the tension between the human drive for distinction and the ambiguous comforts of group identity and continuity (*LM* 167), Verney is, in the end, granted only the cold-comfort of unfettered individuality.

As Sterrenburg has demonstrated, Shelley's "anatomy of failed revolutions" (1978, 345) in *The Last Man* responds to body politic metaphors articulated in such thinkers as Godwin, Wollstonecraft, and Burke, who contemplate disease in the civic corpus as either

[48] A similar convention governs Michael Crichton's sci-fi plague thriller, *The Andromeda Strain* (1969). Dr. Mark Hall, as the only unmarried male working with a team of scientists to study an extraterrestrial pathogen that has annihilated a small southwestern town, is solely authorized to disarm the research facility's nuclear self-destruct mechanism (to be triggered in the event of the pathogen's escape from the containment lab). The so-called "odd man" hypothesis, emphasized in later screen (1971) and televisual (2008) adaptations of the book, relies on assumptions concerning the emotional detachment of men who are not linked by familial ties.

necessary, restorative, or detrimental—but ultimately able to be remedied (Burke, for instance, advocates a kind of conceptual quarantine). But while the author clearly engages the political philosophy of her near contemporaries, she also relies on the Roman writers who have figured pestilence as indicative of civil war partly because of its irremediable status. Moreover, the tendency of Latin epic to foreground the familial bonds that are frequently the casualties of internal strife grants Shelley's novel a deeper meditation on the relationship between the individual and the various members of the body politic with whom she must engage.[49] It is with pronounced cynicism, however, that such bonds are depicted in the novel (Mellor 1993, xvi): in so far as the template for the body politic lay in domestic life, the gendered inequalities that structured the family would for Shelley continue to infect the wider community.

As a backdrop to humankind's largely self-destructive tendencies, Shelley posits nature, a force identified equally with plague's destruction and the earth's relentless capacity for renewal. Such a polarity finds a conceptual ancestry in Lucretius' bracketing of his excursus on Epicurean principles between generative Venus and deteriorative *pestilitas*, both of which are conceptually fused with *natura*. Shelley also relies on Lucretius' epic successors, especially the hexameters of Vergil, who had used the flourishing of nature to evoke a morally inflected Golden Age—one that spoke of civilization's utter dismantling with an eye to possibilities of renewal. For Shelley, nature, along with its Golden-Age bounty, is no longer a source of moral authority, but instead a source of indifference,[50] offering up harvests left uncultivated as a foil to and painful reminder of humanity's wretched condition (*LM* 305): "all plenty and yet alas! All poverty, painted in wondrous hues and fantastic groupings this land of beauty" (*LM* 313; cf. 198–9). Shelley does not so much dwell on Golden-Age neutralization

[49] Scholars have often viewed representations of and challenges to the apocalypse, such as that issued in Shelley's novel, as attempts to generate an apolitical discourse (e.g., Northrop Frye's view of formal apocalypse as absolute freedom from circumstance and a means of liberating its human participants from history; 1957, 117–19; cf. Goldsmith 1993, 9). As Goldsmith argues, however, any speculation on the circumstances that attend human life beyond history is undeniably entangled in the historical and political moment that has produced such speculation (Goldsmith 1993, esp. 11–24).

[50] Cf. Mellor (1993, xvii), who emphasizes how Shelley resists Romantic tendencies to idealize nature in *The Last Man*.

of hostilities as she does indicate the gradual reduction of "man's" stature in relation to the animal world.[51]

While "a vague picture of perpetual spring, fragrant groves, and sparkling streams" (*LM* 279) inspires Verney and his fellow survivors to head for Versailles, what they find there is ultimately useless. Golden-Age conditions outside of Versailles merely blunt the impulse to endure:

> At first I likened it to a colony, which borne over far seas, struck root for the first time in a new country. But where was the bustle and industry characteristic of such an assemblage; the rudely constructed dwelling, which was to suffice till a more commodious mansion could be built; the marking out of fields; the attempt at cultivation; the eager curiosity to discover unknown animals and herbs; the excursions for the sake of exploring the country? Our habitations were palaces—our food was already stored in granaries—there was no need of labour, no inquisitiveness, no restless desire to get on. (*LM* 279)

Here Shelley invokes Vergil's emphasis on *labor* as an ambiguous by-product of humanity's fall from a Golden-Age existence, while contextualizing such conditions in a failed foundation narrative, one that summons Aeneas' failed attempt at founding a colony in Crete. But where Vergil allows Aeneas to depart from Crete "with a few Trojans left behind," found an empire and perhaps, through Augustus (*Aen.* 6.791–7), a new Golden Age in Rome, Shelley resists the enticements of an *aurea aetas* as well as ideologies that would view plague's expurgating power as a means to achieving that end. Her narrator, in any case, in so far as his testimony overwhelmingly concerns familial bonds broken by departure, abandonment, and death, remains fixated on the ones left behind.

As Paley has stressed (1993, 115–16), various Christian "millennial" predictions of renewed paradise are voiced throughout the novel only to be discredited, in particular, the astronomer Merrival's prophecy that a "universal spring will be produced and the earth become a paradise" (*LM* 158). Verney's account of his final meal before entering Rome, of arbutus berries and chestnuts consumed under the shade of an ilex tree (*LM* 333), underscores the earth's restoration of the very Golden-Age offerings denied by Dodona in Vergil's *Georgic*

[51] This is especially evident in Verney's increasingly uncivilized condition after he survives the shipwreck that drowns his last surviving companions, Adrian and Clara; cf. *LM* 329, 331.

Iron Age (1.147–9) and enjoyed by humans in Ovid's Golden one (*Met.* 1.101-12). And yet, over and against a tradition that pondered the renewal of a Golden Age (however modified) in the wake of civil war, Shelley's overtures to epochal evolution conjure apocalypse without revelation (cf. Paley 1993). As the title suggests, and as many critics have found problematic, there is no afterward, only endlessly deferred finality (Thomas 2000, 23; Wright 2000, 145). In this respect, the novel finds closer kinship with the plagues that conclude Lucretius' *De Rerum Natura* and Vergil's third *Georgic* than those remedied by the recovery of the hive in *Georgics* 4 or the repopulation of Aegina in Ovid's ant-born race of Myrmidons.

Shelly's novel advertises an interest in humanity's pre- and postlapsarian orientation through its introductory epigraph, drawn from Milton's *Paradise Lost*: "Let no man seek/ Henceforth to be foretold what shall befall/ Him or his children" (11.770–2). The lines, spoken by Adam after he has learned of the near eradication of humankind through the Flood, explicitly censure efforts to know the future (Paley 1993, 114–15). Margaret Atwood takes up precisely this strand of eschatological thinking in her trilogy on the near eradication of the human race through a genetically engineered virus: *Oryx and Crake* (2003), *The Year of the Flood* (2009), and *MaddAddam* (2013). The biblical injunction against certain forms of knowledge is most resonant in the second installment, which largely concerns a cult resistant to technological progress known as God's Gardeners. The series, however, consistently fixates on human efforts to master knowledge of nature through bio-engineering—whose crowning achievement is the virus JUVE (Jetspeed Ultra Virus Extraordinary), designed by the character referred to as Crake, which nearly obliterates the human species in a "waterless Flood." The world before the Flood is imaginatively dystopic in its experimentation with life forms created to support a jarringly imbalanced economic structure. Equal to Atwood's interest in speculating on the darker side of human ingenuity (for which of course she is also indebted to Shelley) is a concern with the power of contagious disease to enact dissolution at both the individual and communal levels and, in that process, to speculate on what—if anything—is worth salvaging. To address this concern, she engages the Roman tropes of pestilence that we have explored throughout this project.

Crake's motive for designing the JUVE virus is what he understands as the fundamentally flawed condition of humanity, one born from "king-of-the-castle hard-wiring" and perpetuated by property acquisition, marriage bonds, and familial lineage (*Oryx and Crake*, 305).[52] Within a sealed-off compound dubbed "Paradice" he engineers the species of Crakers, physically flawless creatures with enhanced immune systems, to replace *homo sapiens*; Crakers have no propensity for ownership or the erotic attachments that lead to marital and kinship bonds. In fact, most of the human protagonists of the trilogy, whose pre-plague existence is revealed in recurring flashbacks, have no familial attachments, except those that have been seriously, often tragically compromised. That is to say, the intensely problematic familial relationships within Atwood's doomed dystopia provide a reasonable defense for Crake's plan, though one compelling feature of the narrative is its interest in how, in the absence of traditional family structures, characters form new, often salutary quasi-familial bonds.

The virus is unleashed through the efforts of Oryx, Crake's lover, and his unwitting friend Jimmy (also Oryx's lover), renamed "Snowman" by the end of the first novel and that novel's primary focalizer. A skeletal symptomatology and epidemiology emerge at *Oryx and Crake*'s conclusion, followed by equally elusive references to JUVE's outbreak in the successor novels, from different narrative perspectives.[53] Despite (perhaps because of) Atwood's short shrift of the usual plague dramaturgy, bodily dissolution functions as virtually the only symptom of disease. News commentators in *Oryx and Crake* identify the virus as a "rogue hemorrhagic" (*OAC* 325). From there, in *The Year of the Flood*, symptomatology remains alarmingly imprecise: Ren, an exotic dancer who once lived with God's Gardeners and whose perspective shapes much of the novel, describes victims as "just sort of melting" (283).[54] Ren's account of her experience alternates with that of Toby, who recognizes a similar dissolution (*YOTF* 322) and describes the afflicted as "clot(s) on legs" (*YOTF* 323). So too minor characters in the tale make reference to

[52] References are to the 2003 Doubleday edition of the novel, abbreviated hereafter as *OAC*.

[53] Ursula K. Le Guin, in her largely positive review of *The Year of the Flood*, remarks that "failure to describe the nature of the illness and the days of its worse virulence leaves the epidemic an abstraction, novelistically weightless" (https://www.theguardian.com/books/2009/aug/29/margaret-atwood-year-of-flood).

[54] References to *The Year of the Flood* are taken from the Doubleday 2009 edition and abbreviated hereafter as *YOTF*.

victims who "kind of melted" (*YOTF* 334) or were transformed into "pink porridge" (*YOTF* 354). The very lack of specificity, while medically frustrating, serves the same purpose as does the liquefaction of livestock in the streamlined symptomatology of Vergil's cattle plague: by emphasizing dissolution, both accounts foreground the role that a deadly pestilence plays in orchestrating the collapse of body as body politic. Readers only need to know that this virus initiates the dismantling of human life, and a rapidly operating "rogue hemorrhagic" efficiently conveys the end result.

In order to transfer the implications of the melting human form to the larger social order in which such forms are embedded, Atwood relies on a general atmosphere of decay, where characters constantly confront putrid odors and deteriorating bodies (e.g., *YOTF* 325, 328, 339, 378). She also uses a language of epochal evolution, especially in *The Year of the Flood*, which intermittently looks back to Eden, humankind's fall from paradise, and the possibility of Eden's restoration after the Flood. The novel opens with a kind of primordial silence observed by Toby, who has survived the ravages of the JUVE virus, alone as far as she can tell. More often, the hymns and sermons of the Gardeners, the latter of which are spoken by the aptly named leader, Adam One, clarify the epoch-changing implications of the disaster. The first hymn (*YOTF* 14) speaks of a time when, "Adam first had that breath of life / All in that golden peace," peace shared with god and other species. Midway through the novel Adam One accounts for the fall of man, which began with lapsed vegetarianism and culminated in "sexual twitching" and "the anxious contemplation of the vanished past and distant future" (*YOTF* 188). By *The Year of the Flood*'s conclusion, however, Adam One upholds the prospect that the waterless Flood has both destroyed and cleansed, and perhaps set the stage for a new Eden (*YOTF* 345).

While Ren and Toby often eye such prospects skeptically, their own movements throughout the post-Flood landscape locate them in the symbolic economy of the Latin Golden Age. Toby in particular is entrusted with the care of the Gardeners' beehive, after her mentor, Pilar, has died. She develops a sympathetic, virtually symbiotic relationship with the bees, which protect her when she is attacked by a violent former employer. At the same time, the hive's collective nature is stressed ("all the bees of the hive are one bee," *YOTF* 99) as well as their golden status (*YOTF* 258), positioning them as both an ideal and a foil for human existence. Atwood's speculations on the fallen human condition are not without a wry sense of humor: among more perverse instantiations of a literalized Golden Age are the liobams, a lion–sheep splice commissioned by a religious sect hoping to force the return of the Peaceable Kingdom. The creatures, in which lions and lambs literally co-exist, prove to be dangerous predators, "not strictly vegetarian" beasts with golden fur (350–1) and a deceptively cute countenance (94–5).[55] Equally perverse, if less harmful, are the Mo'Hair sheep, genetically engineered to grow pink, purple, and green fleece (238), reminiscent of the self-dyeing flocks in Vergil's fourth *Eclogue* (4.41–5)—and equally designed as a human luxury.[56]

For all its pretensions of a new order to follow in the wake of the Flood, the conclusion of the trilogy is highly ambiguous in its evaluation of humanity, as such. For the essentially docile Crakers, nearly every gesture is directed towards the good of their species, even sexual reproduction, which is experienced collectively when a female Craker goes into heat, and thus prevents recognition of paternity, or any other kinship bonds. At the conclusion of *MaddAddam*, however, Crakers have mated with humans, anticipating a hybrid offspring in which the more desirable traits of humans and Crakers might combine (*MA* 377).[57] While Atwood only glances at what those traits might be, it is surely telling that one Craker, named Blackbeard, develops an individual voice in learning to read and write, and eventually memorialize in literature the deaths of the human companions who were dear to him. We also observe in the species the equally human power of art and the persistence of symbolic representation: the Crakers dream and have an affinity for song, inherited

[55] Biblical tradition is also relevant (cf. Isaiah 11:6, "The calf and the young lion will grow up together . . . "), especially given the (quasi) Judeo-Christian orientation of the sect that produces these creatures. Atwood's deft handling of Judeo-Christian and classical tropes and the cross-contamination between them in the West make it difficult to assign priority to either influence here. For speculation on the Semitic roots of Roman Golden Age imagery, see Newman (1998, 228–9).

[56] As such Atwood revises the paradox of luxury without human artifice implicit in Vergil. As Coleman observes, "The paradox of the Golden Age is that man, now free from his obsession with luxury, is surrounded by it and does not need to transgress nature's bounds to obtain it" (1977, 143). Atwood's sheep indeed remove the need for human intervention in the dyeing process, but only because humans have already intervened in realms of creation that were formerly subject to nature or divinity.

[57] References to *MaddAddam* are taken from the 2013 Doubleday edition (abbreviated *MA*).

from human hard wiring that Crake "couldn't manage to wipe out" (*OAC* 352).[58]

Thus the brave new world emerging, for all its egalitarian momentum, is perhaps bound to falter in the pitfalls of a mutually dependent relationship between artistic production and individual expression. In imagining the potential of human-Craker hybrids, the author may be picking at more problematic threads frequently sewn into human affiliations. With some awareness of his name but still awkwardly referring to himself in the third person, young Blackbeard notes after his own first mating that, "he is more happy than anyone," because during the process the female Craker being inseminated chose the flower he had offered her (*MA* 380). Atwood's backward reach has harnessed Roman images of collective crises and used them to pose basic questions about the capacity of humans to co-exist: in subtle counterpoint to the largely beneficent role of bees who attend the Gardeners and subtend their system of values, Jimmy, at *Oryx and Crake*'s conclusion, reflects more caustically on the nature of ants: "He checks the inside of his hat, flicks out an ant. Can a single ant be said to be alive, in any meaningful sense of the word, or does it only have relevance in terms of its anthill? An old conundrum of Crake's" (*OAC* 372). Indeed, Ovid, in the context of an ancient political order that was marketing itself as a new age, had already posed a similar question.

7.4. EPILOGUE

The Craker–human hybrids anticipated at the end of Atwood's trilogy allow the novelist to consider the possibilities of post-human subjectivity and the role that an epidemic might play in its accomplishment. As observed above, this has been the concern of a good number of contagion narratives since the mid-twentieth century. The vampire virus that afflicts humans in Richard Matheson's *I Am*

[58] For a relatively realistic novel that tracks the endurance of artistic expression among survivors in a post-plague world, see Emily St. John Mandel's *Station Eleven* (2014). Shelley's *The Last Man* is also concerned with the value of the arts in a fallen world, though she is perhaps more cynical than either successor concerning their redemptive or restorative value.

Legend (1954, repr. 1995) ends with a realization by the novel's protagonist that his species is obsolete: those beings infected with the virus are the new normal, but they can control its more sinister compulsions (cf. Wald 2012, 112–13). Similarly, in *The Girl with All the Gifts* (M.R. Carey, 2014) most of humanity is wiped out by an epidemic, in this case a brain-colonizing fungus that transforms victims into zombie-like cannibals; but a few survivors, children of infected individuals who have an ability to control the fungus' debilitating symptoms, are by the end of the book building a New Jerusalem and have a questionably benign authority over the earth's remaining human occupants.[59] Another recent entry in this body of literature is Joe Hill's *The Fireman* (2016), in which a virus either causes its victims to combust or allows the afflicted to share in a kind of beatific group-think, experienced as unparalleled bliss, but eradicating autonomy and individuality in the process. Unsurprisingly perhaps, bees are invoked as a model for group experiences throughout the novel (e.g., 345, 475).[60]

At the same time, another strain of narrative has replicated, one that asserts human identity in the face of an unequivocally undesirable model of subjectivity. George Romero's creation of the infectious zombie, or "undead," opened up a new vista for representations of contagious disease on screen. Within its trenchant observations of social dysfunction, the persistence of racism in particular, *Night of the Living Dead* (1968) observes the spread of contagion from the perspective of Ben (Duane Jones), an apparently unattached African-American man. The living individuals who attempt to escape disease and survive with him enter the film's diegesis bound to each other by familial or erotic attachments. Frictions are generated among survivors primarily over indecision concerning how to treat infected loved ones. For instance, the nearly catatonic woman Barbra (Judith O'Dea)

[59] As testimony to the author's engagement with Greco-Roman tradition, it is worth noting that the novel was developed from a short story entitled, "Iphigenia in Aulis," and a classical heritage informs the Pandora-like central protagonist Melanie, the girl "with all the gifts" who offers both hope and devastation to the human race.

[60] Greg Bear's (1985) *Blood Music* offers a similar approach in so far as it suggests the power of a pandemic to dissolve subjectivity as genetically modified bacteria colonize human bodies and gradually envelope nearly all of human life in North America. Human consciousness is thus replaced with microbial consciousness, whose dialogue with human survivors in Europe, transmitted through a transcript on a computer monitor, dramatizes familiar tensions: "What you think of as INDIVIDUAL may be spread across the *totality *" (163).

responds first with uncertainty and then with fatal vulnerability to her infected brother, Johnny.

It is, however, the fate of the Cooper family that most effectively challenges our notions of human identity and the relationships we rely on to support that identity. Near the end of the film, it becomes apparent that Karen (Kyra Schon), the young daughter of Helen (Marilyn Eastman) and Harry Cooper (Karl Hardman), has been bitten and is coming down with the vaguely defined zombie disease. The survivors agree that it would be prudent to relegate the child in the basement; but her parents refuse to leave Karen alone there and cannot register that their daughter is becoming something very dangerous (Fig. 7.4). The familial crisis is perhaps predictable,[61] but its

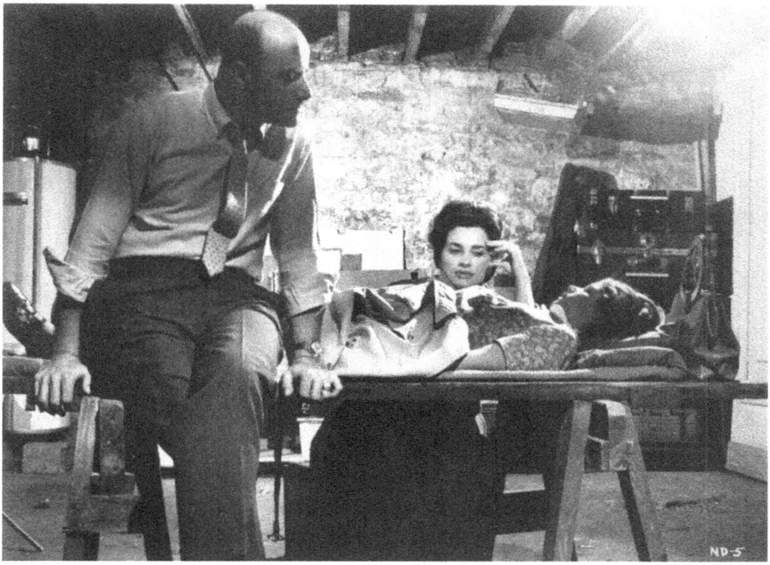

Fig. 7.4. The Coopers (Marilyn Eastman and Karl Hardman) attend to their sick daughter, Karen (Kyra Schon), in *Night of the Living Dead* (George Romero, 1968). Image Ten.

[61] That predictability is partly due to hindsight, since the infection of loved ones becomes a persistent source of dramatic tension in the genre. Romero continued to produce and direct influential examples of the zombie/contagion film until 2009's *Survival of the Dead*. Among his critically acclaimed successors are *28 Days Later* (Boyle 2003) and *28 Weeks Later* (Fresnadillo 2009), the latter of which is especially

predictability is matched by equal poignancy and eventually horror over images of Karen biting her father in the arm and then brutally murdering her mother with a trowel.[62]

Amplifying the resonance of the Coopers' familial tragedy, the contemporary series *Fear the Walking Dead* (2015–present, a satellite of the more well-known *The Walking Dead*) focuses intently on the fate of an uneasily blended family living in Los Angeles during the outbreak of the zombie virus: the series not only reveals how familial relationships condition our response to contagion, but also frequently dramatizes the dysfunction of contemporary American family life. Moral dilemmas faced by the series' central protagonist, Madison Clark (Kim Dickens), and her children are framed increasingly by how their decisions will affect the family unit, a unit that had been plagued by significant disruption prior to the outbreak (e.g., suicide, divorce, drug addiction). As Jeremiah Otto (Dayton Callie), the patriarch and founder of a survivalist compound introduced in Season 3, quips: "Nothing heals a family like a purpose."[63] While Madison outwardly expresses a desire to integrate her family within the compound community, she also tells her son Nick that she is prepared to kill: "I'll bring our family together, take what we need, and stop anyone who gets in our way" (Episode 3.2).

Both horrific and questionably salutary consequences of such parental devotion must be situated in a long history of narratives that find

focused on loyalty and betrayal within the family. While the zombie/contagion film has been a largely Anglo-American phenomenon, the past few decades have observed noteworthy contributions to the genre by French (e.g., *La Horde* [Rocher 2009]), Spanish (e.g., *REC* [Balaguero and Plaza 2007]), German (e.g., *Virus Undead* [Wolff 2008]), and Korean directors (e.g., *Train to Busan* [=*Busanhaeng*, Sang-ho Yeon 2016]).

62 In his essay using the zombie to determine whether personal identity is determined more by psychological or bodily continuity, Larkin uses Karen's fate and audience reactions to it to defend the position that "persons are most fundamentally corporeal objects" (2006, 15). That is to say, audiences would not react with horror to the scene unless they assumed continuity between Karen before she becomes infected and Karen after she attacks her parents. In his study of the impact of *NOTLD* on popular culture, Flint notes that Mr. Cooper is branded a coward in the film primarily for his desire to protect his family (2009, 76).

63 It is worth noting that Mr. Otto must deal with his own familial burdens—divorce, alcoholism, and two sons with competing ideas about the moral climate and future of the compound. Evoking Girard's mimetic doubles, the "better" brother Jake tells his sibling Troy after interrupting a mission for fuel that Troy was charged with: "Why do you think Dad sent you here? Cast out the one to protect the many" (Episode 3.1).

their origins among the casualties of plague in Latin literature: as I have emphasized throughout this project, contagion materializes and makes visible those social interactions that are most dear and familiar even as it destroys them. As devastating as contagious diseases can be, that heightened visibility has proven invaluable in determining what unites or fractures the social order. And it is largely to Roman writers, as they imagine the causes and effects of disease as a means of reflecting on their own morbid *res publica*, that we are indebted for enhancing that visibility. In assuring readers that "you would be able to see" the bodies of family members entangled in death and by igniting brawls over funeral pyres, Lucretius directed us to the power of an epidemic to exacerbate and eradicate (at least temporarily) the rivalries and loyalties that enervated the body politic of the late Republic: it is a power that Vergil and Ovid capitalized on and channeled into their own visions of suffering and renewal after Actium, visions that we have been marveling at ever since.

Bibliography

Adams, Laurie S. 1993. *Art and Psychoanalysis*. New York.

Ahl, Frederick. 1976. *Lucan: An Introduction*. Ithaca.

Ahl, Frederick. 2008. *Two Faces of Oedipus: Sophocles'* Oedipus Tyrannus *and Seneca's* Oedipus. Ithaca and London.

Ahl, Frederick with Davis, M.A. and Pomeroy, A. 1986. "Silius Italicus." *ANRW* 32.4 II: 2493–561.

Albini, Umberto. 1995. "La storia di Edipo in Seneca." *RFIC* 123: 428–32.

Anderson, William S. 1963. "Multiple Change in the *Metamorphoses*." *TAPA* 94: 1–27.

Anderson, William S., ed. 1972. *Ovid's Metamorphoses: Books 6–10*. Norman, OK.

Armstrong, Rebecca. 2002. "Crete in the *Aeneid*: Recurring Trauma and Alternative Fate." *CQ* 52.1: 321–40.

Artaud, Antonin. 1958. *The Theater and Its Double*. Trans. by Mary Richards. New York.

Artaud, Antonin. 1964 (reissue of 1938). *Le théâtre et son double*. Paris.

Atkinson, J.E. 1981. "Seneca and his Oedipus." *Akroterion* 26.1/2: 22–9.

Atwood, Margaret. 2003. *Oryx and Crake*. New York and London.

Atwood, Margaret. 2009. *The Year of the Flood*. New York and London.

Atwood, Margaret. 2013. *MaddAddam*. New York and London.

Augoustakis, Antony. 2010. "Silius Italicus, a Flavian Poet." In A. Augoustakis, ed., *Brill's Companion to Silius Italicus*, 1–23. Leiden and Boston.

Bailey, Cyril. 1947. *Titi Lucreti Cari de Rerum Natura Libri Sex. Volume 3: Commentary, Books IV–VI*. Oxford.

Baker, Geoffrey. 2003. "Nietzsche, Artaud, and Tragic Politics." *Comparative Literature* 55.1: 1–23.

Bandera, Cesáreo. 1981. "Sacrificial Levels in Virgil's *Aeneid*." *Arethusa* 14: 217–39.

Bannon, Cynthia J. 1997. *The Brothers of Romulus: Fraternal* Pietas *in Roman Law, Literature, and Society*. Princeton.

Barchiesi, Alessandro. 1997a. "Endgames: Ovid's *Metamorphoses* 15 and *Fasti* 6." In D.H. Roberts, F. Dunn, and D. Fowler, eds., *Classical Closure: Reading the End in Greek and Latin Literature*, 181–208. Princeton.

Barchiesi, Alessandro. 1997b. *The Poet and the Prince: Ovid and Augustan Discourse*. Berkeley.

Barchiesi, Alessandro. 2017. "Colonial Readings in Virgilian Geopoetics: The Trojans at Buthrotum." In V. Rimell and M. Asper, eds., *Imagining Empire: Political Space in Hellenistic and Roman Literature*, 151–66. Heidelberg.

Bartsch, Shadi. 1997. *Ideology in Cold Blood: A Reading of Lucan's Civil War*. Cambridge, MA.

Bear, Greg. 1985 (reprint 2006, SFBC). *Blood Music*. Westminster, MD.

Berger, James. 1999. *After the End: Representations of Post-Apocalypse*. Minneapolis, MI.

Bettini, M. 1983. "L'arcobaleno, l'incesto e l' enigma: a proposito dell' *Oedipus* di Seneca." *Dioniso* 54: 137–53.

Bignone, E. 1945. *Storia della letteratura latina*. Vol. 2. Florence.

Bishop, J.D. 1978. "Seneca's *Oedipus*: Opposition Literature." *CJ* 73: 289–302.

Blunt, Anthony. 1967. *Nicolas Poussin: The A.W. Mellon Lectures in the Fine Arts*. Bollingen Series XXXV.7. New York.

Bockemueller, F., ed. and comm. 1873. *Lucretius. De Rerum Natura*. Stade.

Bodel, John. 1995. "Chronology and Succession 2: Notes on Some Consular Lists on Stone." *Zeitschrift für Papyrologie und Epigraphik* 105: 279–96.

Bodel, John. 2000. "Dealing with the Dead: Undertakers, Executioners and Potter's Fields in Ancient Rome." In V.M. Hope and E. Marshall, eds., *Death and Disease in the Ancient City*, 128–51. London and New York.

Boeckl, Christine M. 1991. "A New Reading of Nicolas Poussin's 'The Miracle of the Ark in the Temple of Dagon'." *Artibus et Historiae* 12.24: 119–145.

Boeckl, Christine M. 2000. *Images of Plague and Pestilence: Iconography and Iconology*. Kirksville, MO.

Bömer, Franz P. 1976. *P. Ovidius Naso, Metamorphosen: Kommentar. Vol. 3*. Wissentschaftliche Kommentare zu griechischen und lateinischen Schriftstellern. Heidelberg.

Boyle, A.J., ed. 2011. *Seneca: Oedipus*. Oxford.

Bradley, Mark with Stow, K., eds. 2016. *Rome, Pollution, and Propriety: Dirt, Disease and Hygiene in the Eternal City from Antiquity to Modernity*. Cambridge.

Branca, Vittore, ed. 1992. *Giovanni Boccaccio: Decameron*. Turin.

Braund, S.H., trans. 1992. *Lucan: Civil War*. Oxford.

Bright, D.F. 1971. "The Plague and the Structure of *De Rerum Natura*." *Latomus* 30: 607–32.

Bruère, R.T. 2016. "*Color Ovidianus* in Silius' *Punica*." In A. Augoustakis, ed., *Flavian Epic. Oxford Readings in Classical Studies*, 345–87. Oxford.

Busch, Austin. 2007. "*Versane Natura Est*? Natural and Linguistic Instability in the Extispicium and Self-Blinding of Seneca's *Oedipus*." *CJ* 102.3: 225–67.

Cabisius, Gail. 1985. "Social Metaphor and the Atomic Cycle in Lucretius." *CJ* 80.2: 109–20.

Camus, Albert. 2001. *The Plague*. Trans. by Robin Buss (orig. publication as *La Peste*, 1947). New York.

Carnes, Jeffery. 1995. "Why Should I mention Aiakos? Myth and Politics in Pindar's 'Nemean' 8, Part 1." *Quaderni Urbinati di Cultura Classica*. N.S. 51.3: 7–48.

Cary, Earnest, trans. 1914. *Dio's Roman History, Vol. VI*. Cambridge, MA.

Casali, Sergio. 2011. "The *Bellum Civile* as an Anti-*Aeneid*." In P. Asso, ed., *Brill's Companion to Lucan*, 82–109. Leiden and Boston.

Claridge, Amanda. 1998. *Oxford Archaeological Guides: Rome*. Oxford.

Clay, Diskin. 1983. *Lucretius and Epicurus*. Ithaca and London.

Clifton, James. 2005. "Art and Plague in Naples." In F. Mormando, G.A. Bailey, and P.M. Jones, eds., *Hope and Healing: Painting in Italy in a Time of Plague 1500–1800*, 97–117. Worcester Art Museum.

Cohn, S.K., Jr. 2010. *Cultures of Plague: Medical Thinking at the End of the Renaissance*. Oxford.

Coleman, Robert, ed. 1977. *Vergil: Eclogues*. Cambridge.

Commager, H.S., Jr. 1957. "Lucretius' Interpretation of the Plague." *Harvard Studies in Classical Philology* 62: 105–18.

Conte, G.B. 2001. "Aristaeus, Orpheus, and the *Georgics*: Once Again." In S. Spence, ed., *Poets and Critics Read Vergil*, 44–63. New Haven, CT.

Cooke, Jennifer. 2009. *Legacies of Plague in Literature and Film*. Basingstoke.

Craik, E.M. 2001. "Thucydides on the Plague: Physiology of Flux and Fixation." *CQ* 51.1: 102–8.

Crawfurd, Raymond. 1914. *Plague and Pestilence in Literature and Art*. Oxford.

Csillag, Pál. 1976. *The Augustan Laws on Family Relations*. Budapest.

Davis, Cynthia. 2002. "Contagion as Metaphor." *American Literary History* 14.4: 828–836.

Dawe, R.D., ed. 1982. *Sophocles: Oedipus Rex*. Cambridge.

Defoe, Daniel. 2001. *A Journal of the Plague Year*. Mineola, NY.

Delcuve, Jules. 1936. "*Dira Lues* (Ovide, *Metam*. VII, 523)." *Les études classiques* 5: 200–8.

Derrida, J. 2004. *Dissemination*. Trans. by B. Johnson. London and New York.

DeVeau, F.J., ed. and comm. 1935. *The Bucolics of Vergil*. New York and Oxford.

Duckworth, G.E. 1952. *The Nature of Roman Comedy: A Study in Popular Entertainment*. Princeton.

Duff, J.D., ed. and trans. 1927. *Punica, Volume 2, Books 9–17*. Cambridge, MA.

Duff, J.D., ed. and trans. 1928. *Lucan: The Civil War (Pharsalia)*. Cambridge, MA.

Dutoit, E. 1948. "Tite-Live s'est-il intéressé à la medicine?" *MH* 5: 116–23.

Eberle-Sinatra, Michael. 2000. "Gender, Authorship and Male Domination: Mary Shelley's Limited Freedom in *Frankenstein* and *The Last Man*." In

M. Eberle-Sinatra, ed., *Mary Shelley's Fictions: From* Frankenstein *to* Falkner, 95–108. Basingstoke and London.

Evans, Rhiannon. 2008. *Utopia Antiqua: Readings of the Golden Age and Decline at Rome*. New York and London.

Evelyn-White, H.G., trans. 1977. *Hesiod: The Homeric Hymns and Homerica* (reprint of 1914). Cambridge, MA.

Everett, Nicholas. 2003. *Literacy in Lombard Italy, c.568–774*. Cambridge.

Eyben, Emiel. 1993. *Restless Youth in Ancient Rome*. Trans. by P. Daly. London.

Fairclough, H.R. 1999. *Virgil: Eclogues, Georgics, Aeneid 1–6*. Revised by G.P. Goold. Cambridge, MA.

Fantham, Elaine, ed. 1992. *Lucan: De Bello Civili, Book II*. Cambridge.

Fantham, Elaine. 2013. *Roman Literary Culture: From Plautus to Macrobius*, second ed. Baltimore.

Farinella, Vincenzo. 2004. *Raphael. Gallery of the Arts 4*. Trans. by Susan Wise. Milan.

Farrell, Joseph. 1991. *Vergil's* Georgics *and the Traditions of Ancient Epic*. Oxford.

Fear, Trevor. 2005. "Propertian Closure: The Elegiac Inscription of the Liminal Male and Ideological Contestation in Augustan Rome." In R. Ancona and E. Greene, eds., *Gendered Dynamics in Latin Love Poetry*, 13–40. Baltimore.

Feeney, Denis. 1991. *The Gods in Epic: Poets and Critics of the Classical Tradition*. Oxford.

Feeney, Denis. 2004. "Interpreting Sacrificial Ritual in Roman Poetry: Disciplines and their Models." In A. Barchiesi, J. Rüpke, and S. Stephens, eds., *Rituals in Ink: A Conference on Religion and Literary Production in Ancient Rome*, 1–22. Munich.

Feeney, Denis. 2007. *Caesar's Calendar: Ancient Time and the Beginnings of History*. Berkeley.

Feldherr, Andrew. 1997. "Livy's Revolution: Civic Identity and the Creation of the *Res Publica*." In T. Habinek and A. Schiesaro, eds., *The Roman Cultural Revolution*, 136–57. Cambridge.

Feldherr, Andrew. 1998. *Spectacle and Society in Livy's History*. Berkeley.

Ferry, David, trans. 2005. *The Georgics of Virgil*. New York.

Flemming, Rebecca. 2009. "Pliny and the Pathologies of Empire." *PLLS* 14: 19–42.

Flint, David. 2009. *Zombie Holocaust: How the Living Dead Devoured Pop Culture*. London.

Forcellino, Antonio. 2012. *Raphael: A Passionate Life*. Trans. by Lucinda Byatt. Cambridge and Malden, MA.

Foster, Jonathan. 1988. "The End of the Third *Georgic*." *Proceedings of the Virgil Society* 19: 32–45.

Foucault, Michel. 1975. *Surveiller et punir: Naissance de le prison*. Paris.

Foucault, Michel. 1995. *Discipline & Punish: The Birth of the Prison*. Trans. by Alan Sheridan. New York.

Foucault, Michel. 1997. *Ethics: Subjectivity and Truth. The Essential Works of Michel Foucault, vol. 1*. Trans. by Robert Hurley et al. New York.

Foucault, Michel. 1999. *Les anormaux: Cours au Collège de France (1974–1975)*. Paris.

Foucault, Michel. 2003. *Abnormal. Lectures at the Collège de France, 1974–1975*. Trans. by G. Burchell. Paris.

Foulke, W.D., trans. 1907. *History of the Langobards by Paul the Deacon*. Philadelphia.

Fowler, D.P. 1988. "Review of *Lucretius and the Late Republic*, by J.D. Minyard." *JRS* 78: 215.

Fowler, D.P. 1989. "Lucretius and Politics." In M. Griffin and J. Barnes, eds., *Philosophia Togata: Essays on Philosophy and Roman Society*, 120–50. Oxford.

Fowler, D.P. 1997. "Second Thoughts on Closure." In D.H. Roberts, F. Dunn, and D. Fowler, eds., *Classical Closure: Reading the End in Greek and Latin Literature*, 3–22. Princeton.

Fowler, D.P. 2000. "The Didactic Plot." In M. Depew and D. Obbink, eds., *Matrices of Genre: Authors, Canons, and Society*, 205–19. Cambridge, MA.

Fowler, Peta. 1997. "Lucretian Conclusions." In D.H. Roberts, F. Dunn, and D. Fowler, eds., *Classical Closure: Reading the End in Greek and Latin Literature*, 112–38. Princeton.

Frank, Marica. 1995. "The Rhetorical Use of Family Terms in Seneca's *Oedipus* and *Phoenissae*." *Phoenix* 49.2: 121–30.

Fucecchi, Marco. 2010. "The Shield and the Sword: Q. Fabius Maximus and M. Claudius Marcellus as Models of Heroism in Silius' *Punica*." In A. Augoustakis, ed., *Brill's Companion to Silius Italicus*, 219–39. Leiden and Boston.

Gale, Monica. 1991. "Man and Beast in Lucretius and the *Georgics*." *CQ* 41.2: 414–26.

Gale, Monica. 1994. *Myth and Poetry in Lucretius*. Cambridge.

Gale, Monica. 2000. *Vergil on the Nature of Things*: The Georgics, *Lucretius and the Didactic Tradition*. Cambridge.

Gale, Monica, ed. 2009. *Lucretius: De Rerum Natura V*. Oxford.

Gale, Monica. 2013. "Piety, Labour, and Justice in Lucretius and Hesiod." In D. Lehoux, A.D. Morrison, and A. Sharrock, eds., *Lucretius: Poetry, Philosophy, Science*, 25–50. Oxford.

Galinsky, G.K. 1975. *Ovid's* Metamorphoses: *An Introduction to the Basic Aspects*. Oxford.

Galinsky, G.K. 1981. "Augustus' Legislation on Morals and Marriage." *Philologus* 125: 126–44.

Galinsky, G.K. 1996. *Augustan Culture: An Interpretive Introduction.* Princeton.
Galinsky, G.K., ed. 2014. *Memoria Romana: Memory in Rome and Rome in Memory.* Supplements to the Memoirs of the American Academy in Rome, 10. Ann Arbor, MI.
Gardner, Hunter. 2013. *Gendering Time in Augustan Love Elegy.* Oxford.
Gardner, Hunter. 2014. "Bees, Ants, and the Body Politic: Vergil's Noric Plague and Ovid's Origin of the Myrmidons." *Vergilius* 60: 3–31.
Gardner Moore, Frank. 1940. *Livy: History of Rome, Books 23–25.* Cambridge, MA.
Garrett, Laurie. 1994. *The Coming Plague: Newly Emerging Diseases in a World out of Balance.* New York.
Gentilcore, David. 2016. "Purging Filth: Plague and Responses to it in Rome, 1656–7." In M. Bradley with K. Stow, eds., *Rome, Pollution, and Propriety: Dirt, Disease and Hygiene in the Eternal City from Antiquity to Modernity,* 153–68. Cambridge.
Gigante, M. and Dorandi, T. 1980. "Anassarco e Epicuro 'Sul regno.'" In F. Romano, ed., *Democrito e l'atomismo antico,* Siculorum Gymnasium 33, 479–97. Catania.
Girard, René. 1974. "The Plague in Myth and Literature." *Texas Studies in Literature and Language* 15.5: 833–50.
Girard, René. 1977. *Violence and the Sacred.* Trans. by P. Gregory. Baltimore and London.
Girard, René. 1986. *The Scapegoat.* Trans. by Y. Freccero. Baltimore.
Gilliam, J.F. 1961. "The Plague under Marcus Aurelius." *AJP* 82.3: 225–51.
Gilman, Sander L. 1988. *Disease and Representation: Images of Illness from Madness to AIDS.* Ithaca and London.
Godwin, John, ed. 1991. *Lucretius: De Rerum Natura VI.* Warminster, UK.
Goldsmith, Steven. 1993. *Unbuilding Jerusalem: Apocalypse and Romantic Representation.* Ithaca and London.
Gomel, Elana. 2000. "The Plague of Utopias: Pestilence and the Apocalyptic Body." *Twentieth Century Literature* 46.4: 405–33.
Green, Roger. 2004. "Refinement and Reappraisal in Vergilian Pastoral." In R. Rees, ed., *Romane Memento: Vergil in the Fourth Century,* 17–32. London.
Greenough, J.B., ed. 1988. *Livy. Books I and II.* New Rochelle, NY.
Griffin, Jasper. 1979. "The Fourth 'Georgic', Virgil, and Rome." *Greece and Rome* 26.1: 61–80.
Grimm, Jürgen. 1965. *Die literarische Darstellung der Pest in der Antike und in Romania.* Munich.
Gruen, Erich S. 1992. *Cultural and National Identity in Republican Rome.* Ithaca and London.
Habinek, Thomas. 1990. "Sacrifice, Society, and Vergil's Ox-born Bees." In M. Griffith and D. Mastronarde, eds., *Cabinet of the Muses: Essays on*

Classical and Comparative Literature in Honor of Thomas G. Rosenmeyer, 209–24. Atlanta.

Habinek, Thomas. 1998. *The Politics of Latin Literature: Writing, Identity, and Empire in Ancient Rome*. Princeton.

Hardie, Philip. 1993. *The Epic Successors of Virgil*. Cambridge.

Harper, Kyle. 2017. *The Fate of Rome: Climate, Disease, and the End of an Empire*. Princeton.

Harrison, E.L. 1979. "The Noric Plague in Vergil's Third Georgic." *Papers of the Liverpool Latin Seminar* 2: 1–65.

Hawkins, Julia N. 2019. *Therapoetics after Actium: Narrative, Medicine, and Authority in Augustan Epic*. Baltimore.

Hays, J.H. 1998. *The Burdens of Disease: Epidemics and Human Response in Western History*. New Brunswick, NJ.

Healy, Margaret. 2001. *Fictions of Disease in Early Modern England: Bodies, Plagues, and Politics*. Basingstoke.

Heinze, Richard. 1993. *Virgil's Epic Technique*. Trans. by H. Harvey, D. Harvey, and F. Robertson. Berkeley.

Hellegouarc'h, J. 1963. *Le vocabulaire latin des relations et des parties politiques sous la république*. Paris.

Henderson, John. 1998. *Fighting for Rome: Poets and Caesars, History, and Civil War*. Cambridge.

Herrmann, L. 1931. "Le Quatrième Livre des Géorgiques et les Abeilles d' Actium." *REA* 33: 219–24.

Heyworth, S.J. and Morwood, J.H.W., eds. 2017. *A Commentary on Vergil: Aeneid 3*. Oxford.

Hill, D.E., ed., trans., and comm. 2000. *Ovid: Metamorphoses XIII–XV*, and indexes. Warminster, UK.

Hinds, Stephen. 1998. *Allusion and Intertext: Dynamics of Appropriation in Roman Poetry*. Cambridge.

Hinds, Stephen. 2011. "Seneca's Ovidian *Loci*." *SIFC* 9: 5–63.

Hipp, Elisabeth. 2007. "Poussin's The Plague at Ashdod: A Work of Art in Multiple Contexts." In F. Mormando and T. Worcester, eds., *Piety and the Plague: From Byzantium to the Baroque*, 177–223. Kirksville, MO.

Holmes, Brooke. 2010. *The Symptom and the Subject: The Emergence of the Physical Body in Ancient Greece*. Princeton.

Hope, V.M. and Marshall, E., eds., 2000. *Death and Disease in the Ancient City*. London and New York.

Horsfall, Nicholas, ed. 2006. *Virgil, Aeneid 3, A Commentary*. Leiden and Boston.

Hubbard, T.K. 1998. *The Pipes of Pan: Intertextuality and Literary Filiation in the Pastoral Tradition from Theocritus to Milton*. Ann Arbor, MI.

Hutchinson, G.O. 2001. "The Date of *De Rerum Natura*." *CQ* 51.1: 150–62.

Jackson, Ralph. 1988. *Doctors and Diseases in the Roman Empire*. London.

Jakobi, R. 1988. *Der Einfluss Ovids auf den Tragiker Seneca*. Berlin and New York.

Jal, Paul. 1963. *La guerre civile à Rome: Étude littéraire et morale*. Paris.

Janan, Micaela. 2001. *The Politics of Desire: Propertius IV*. Berkeley.

Jannarone, Kimberly. 2010. *Artaud and his Doubles*. Ann Arbor, MI.

Jermyn, L.A.S. 1947. *The Singing Farmer: A Translation of Virgil's* Georgics. Oxford.

Johnson, W.R. 1987. *Momentary Monsters: Lucan and his Heroes*. Ithaca and London.

Johnston, Patricia. 1980. *Vergil's Agricultural Golden Age: A Study of the* Georgics. Leiden and Boston.

Jones, W.H.S. 1923. *Hippocrates. Volume II*. Cambridge, MA.

Kelly, R.T. 1980. "The Last Line of the *De Rerum Natura*." *Latomus* 39: 95–7.

Kennedy, Duncan F. 1993. *The Arts of Love: Five Studies in the Discourses of Roman Love Elegy*. Cambridge.

Kenney, E.J. 1977. *Lucretius. Greece & Rome, New Surveys in the Classics 11*. Oxford.

Keyser, Paul T. 2010. "Science." In A. Barchiesi and W. Scheidel, eds., *The Oxford Handbook of Roman Studies*, 859–81. Oxford.

Kilburn, K., trans. 1913. *Lucian, Volume 3*. Cambridge, MA.

Knox, B.M.W. 1956. "The Date of the *Oedipus Tyrannus* of Sophocles." *AJP* 77: 133–47.

Kosak, Jennifer Clarke. 2000. "*Polis Nosousa*: Greek ideas about the city and disease in the fifth century BC." In V.M. Hope and E. Marshall, eds., *Death and Disease in the Ancient City*, 35–54. London and New York.

Kristeva, Julia. 1982. *Powers of Horror: An Essay in Abjection*. Trans. by Leon Roudiez. New York.

Lakoff, George and Johnson, Mark. 2003. *Metaphors We Live By*. Chicago.

La Penna, A. 1988. "Brevi considerazioni sulla divinizzazione degli eroi e sul canone degli eroi divinizzati." In D. Porte and J.-P. Neraudeau, eds., *Hommages à Henri Le Bonniec: Res Sacrae, Collection Latomus* 201, 275–87. Brussels.

Larkin, W.S. 2006. "*Res Corporealis*: Persons, Bodies, and Zombies." In R. Greene and K.S. Mohammad, eds., *Zombies, Vampires, and Philosophy: New Life for the Undead*, 15–26. Chicago and La Salle, IL.

Leavy, Barbara Fass. 1992. *To Blight with Plague: Studies in a Literary Theme*. New York.

Lee, M.O. 1979. *Fathers and Sons in Virgil's* Aeneid: *Tum Genitor Natum*. Albany, NY.

Lewis, C. Day. 1963. *The Georgics of Virgil*. London.

Liebeschuetz, W. 1965. "Beast and Man in the Third Book of Virgil's *Georgics*." *G&R* 12: 68–72.

Lintott, Andrew. 1990. "Electoral Bribery in the Roman Republic." *JRS* 80: 1–16.

Little, L.K., ed. 2007. *Plague and the End of Antiquity: The Pandemic of 541–750*. Cambridge.

Littlewood, C.A.J. 2004. *Self-representation and Illusion in Senecan Tragedy*. Oxford.

Littman, R.J. and Littman, M.L. 1973. "Galen and the Antonine Plague." *AJP* 94.3: 243–55.

Lloyd, R.B. 1957. "*Aeneid* III and the Aeneas Legend." *AJP* 78: 382–400.

Lombardo, Stanley, trans. 2010. *Ovid: Metamorphoses*. Indianapolis, IN.

Longrigg, James. 1995. "Epidemic, ideas and classical Athenian society." In T. Ranger and P. Slack, eds., *Epidemics and Ideas: Essays on the Historical Perception of Pestilence*, 21–44. Cambridge.

Lord, Carla. 1984. "Raphael, Marcantonio Raimondi, and Virgil." *Source: Notes in the History of Art* 3.4: 81–92.

Luce, T.J. 1977. *Livy: The Composition of his History*. Princeton.

Luke, H. J., ed. 1993. *The Last Man by Mary Shelley*. Lincoln and London.

Mack, Sara. 1978. *Patterns of Time in Vergil*. Hamden, CT.

Magnusson, Bruce and Zalloua, Zahi. 2012. "Introduction: The Hydra of Contagion." In B. Magnusson and Z. Zalloua, eds., *Contagion: Health, Fear, Sovereignty*, 3–24. Vancouver.

Manson, Michel. 1975. "La *Pietas* et le sentiment de l' enfance à Rome d'après les monnaies." *RBN* 121: 21–80.

Marks, Raymond. 2010. "Silius and Lucan." In A. Augoustakis, ed. *Brill's Companion to Silius Italicus*, 127–53. Leiden and Boston.

Marks, Raymond. 2016. "*Per vulnera regnum*: Self-destruction, Self-sacrifice, and *Devotio* in Silius' *Punica* 4–10." In A. Augoustakis, ed., *Flavian Epic. Oxford Readings in Classical Studies*, 408–33. Oxford.

Martindale, Charles. 1993. *Redeeming the Text: Latin Poetry and the Hermeneutics of Reception*. Cambridge.

Martindale, Charles. 2013. "Reception: a new humanism? Receptivity, pedagogy, the transhistorical." *Classical Receptions Journal* 5.2: 169–83.

Masters, Jamie. 1992. *Poetry and Civil War in Lucan's* Bellum Civile. Cambridge.

McConnell, Sean. 2012. "Lucretius and Civil Strife." *Phoenix* 66.1: 97–121.

McGill, Scott and Pucci, J. 2016. "Introduction." In S. McGill and J. Pucci, eds., *Classics Renewed: Reception and Innovation in the Latin Poetry of Late Antiquity*, 13–23. Heidelberg.

McGuire, Donald T. 1997. *Acts of Silence: Civil War, Tyranny, and Suicide in the Flavian Epics*. Hildesheim.

McWilliam, G.H., trans. 1972. *Giovanni Boccaccio: The Decameron*. London.

Mebane, Julia. 2016. "Pompey's Head and the Body Politic in Lucan's *De bello civili*." *TAPA* 146.1: 191–215.

Mellor, A.K. 1993. "Introduction." In H.J. Luke, ed., *The Last Man by Mary Shelley*, vii–xxvi. Lincoln and London.

Mezzanotte, Alessandro. 2016. "Echoes of the Contemporary World in Silius Italicus." In A. Augoustakis, ed., *Flavian Epic. Oxford Readings in Classical Studies*, 434–57. Oxford.

Miles, Gary. 1980. *Vergil's* Georgics: *A New Interpretation*. Berkeley.

Miles, Gary. 1995. *Livy: Reconstructing Early Rome*. Ithaca.

Miller, F.J., trans. 1921. *Ovid 3: Metamorphoses 1–8*. Cambridge, MA.

Miller, John F. 2009. *Apollo, Augustus, and the Poets*. Cambridge.

Miller, P.A. 2004. *Subjecting Verses: Latin Love Elegy and the Emergence of the Real*. Princeton.

Milnor, Kristina. 2005. *Gender, Domesticity, and the Age of Augustus: Inventing Private Life*. Oxford.

Minadeo, R. 1965. "The Formal Design of the *De Rerum Natura*" *Arion* 4: 444–61.

Mineo, Bernard. 2015a. "Livy's Political and Moral Values and the Principate." In B. Mineo, ed., *A Companion to Livy*, 125–38. Chichester, UK.

Mineo, Bernard. 2015b. "Livy's Historical Philosophy." In B. Mineo, ed., *A Companion to Livy*, 139–52. Chichester, UK.

Minyard, J.D. 1985. *Lucretius and the Late Republic: An Essay in Roman Intellectual History* (Mnemosyne, Supp. XC). Leiden.

Mitchell-Boyask, Robin. 2008. *Plague and the Athenian Imagination: Drama, History, and the Cult of Asclepius*. Cambridge.

Moi, Toril. 1985. *Sexual/Textual Politics: Feminist Literary Theory*. London and New York.

Morgan, Llewelyn. 1999. *Patterns of Redemption in Virgil's* Georgics. Cambridge.

Morley, N. 2007. "Civil War and Succession Crisis in Roman Beekeeping." *Historia* 56: 462–70.

Mormando, Franco, Bailey, G.A. and Jones, P.M., eds. (=Mormando et al.). 2005. *Hope and Healing: Painting in Italy in a Time of Plague 1500–1800*. Worcester Art Museum.

Mormando, Franco. 2005. "Introduction: Response to the Plague in Early Modern Italy: What the Primary Sources, Printed and Painted, Reveal." In F. Mormando, G.A. Bailey and P.M Jones, eds., *Hope and Healing: Painting in Italy in a Time of Plague 1500–1800*, 1–44. Worcester Art Museum.

Morrison, A.D. 2013. "*Nil igitur mors est ad nos*? Iphianassa, the Athenian Plague, and Epicurean Views of Death." In D. Lehoux, A.D. Morrison, and A. Sharrock, eds., *Lucretius: Poetry, Philosophy, Science*, 211–32. Oxford.

Müller, Gerhard. 2007. "The Conclusions of the Six Books of Lucretius." In M. Gale, ed., *Oxford Readings in Lucretius*, 234–54. Oxford.

Myers, K. Sara. 1994. *Ovid's Causes: Cosmogony and Aetiology in the* Metamophoses. Ann Arbor, MI.

Mynors, R.A.B., ed. 1990. *Virgil: Georgics*. Oxford.

Nadeau, Yvan. 1984. "The Lover and the Statesman." In T. Woodman and D. West, eds., *Poetry and Politics in the Age of Augustus*, 59–82. Cambridge.

Nappa, Christopher. 2005. *Reading After Actium: Vergil's* Georgics, *Octavian, and Rome*. Ann Arbor, MI.

Narducci, Emanuelle. 1979. *La provvidenza crudele: Lucano e la distruzione dei miti augustei*. Pisa.

Nelson, Stephanie. 1998. *God and the Land: The Metaphysics of Farming in Hesiod and Vergil*. Oxford.

Newman, J.K. 1967. *The Concept of* Vates *in Augustan Poetry, Collection Latomus*, vol. 89. Brussels.

Newman, J.K. 1998. "*Saturno Rege*. Themes of the Golden Age in Tibullus and other Augustan Poets." In A. E. Radke, ed., *Candide Iudex: Beiträge zur augusteischen Dichtung. Festschrift für Walter Wimmel zum 75*, 225–46. Stuttgart.

Nichols, James H. 1976. *Epicurean Political Philosophy: The* De Rerum Natura *of Lucretius*. Ithaca and London.

Nugent, S.G. 1994. "Mater Matters: The Female in Lucretius' *De Rerum Natura*." *Colby Quarterly* 30: 179–205.

Nutton, Vivian. 1983. "The Seeds of Disease: An Explanation of Contagion and Infection from the Greeks to the Renaissance." *Medical History* 27: 1–34.

Nutton, Vivian. 2000. "Medical Thoughts on Urban Pollution." In V.M. Hope and E. Marshall, eds., *Death and Disease in the Ancient City*, 65–73. London and New York.

Oakley, S.P. 1998. *A Commentary on Livy Books VI–X*. Vol. 2, books VII–VIII. Oxford.

Oakley, S.P. 2015. "Reading Livy's Book 5." In B. Mineo, ed., *A Companion to Livy*, 230–42. Chichester, UK.

Ogilvie, R.M. 1970. *A Commentary on Livy Books 1–5*. Oxford.

Ogilvie, R.M., ed. 1974. *Titi Livi: Ab Urbe Condita. Libri I–V*. Oxford.

O'Hara, James. 2007. *Inconsistency in Roman Epic: Studies in Catullus, Lucretius, Vergil, Ovid and Lucan*. Cambridge.

Otis, Brooks. 1995 (reprint of 1964). *Virgil: A Study in Civilized Poetry*. Norman, OK.

Padel, Ruth. 1992. *In and Out of the Mind: Greek Images of the Tragic Self*. Princeton.

Paley, M.D. 1993. "The Last Man: Apocalypse without Millennium." In A. Fisch, A. Mellor, and E. Schor, eds., *The Other Mary Shelley: Beyond* Frankenstein, 107–23. Oxford.

Parry, Adam. 1969. "The Language of Thucydides' Description of the Plague." *BICS* 16: 106–18.

Pelling, Christopher. 2010. "'Learning From That Violent Schoolmaster': Thucydidean Intertextuality and Some Greek Views of Roman Civil War." In B. Breed, C. Damon, A. Rossi, eds., *Citizens of Discord: Rome and its Civil Wars*, 105–18. Oxford.

Perkell, Christine. 1978. "A Reading of Vergil's Fourth Georgic." *Phoenix* 32.3: 211–21.

Perkell, Christine. 1989. *The Poet's Truth: A Study of the Poet in Virgil's* Georgics. Berkeley.

Perkell, Christine. 2002. "The Golden Age and Its Contradictions in the Poetry of Vergil." *Vergilius* 48: 3–39.

Piper, Ferdinand, ed. 1835. *Titi Flavii Clementis Alexandrini Hymnus in Christum Salvatorem. Severi Sancti Endelechii, Rhetoris et Poetae Christiani, Carmen Bucolicum De Mortibus Boum.* Gottingen.

Pomeroy, Arthur. 2010. "To Silius through Livy and His Predecessors." In A. Augoustakis, ed., *Brill's Companion to Silius Italicus*, 27–45. Boston and Leiden.

Pomeroy, Arthur. 2016. "Silius' Rome: The Rewriting of Vergil's Vision." In A. Augoustakis, ed., *Flavian Epic. Oxford Readings in Classical Studies*, 321–44. Oxford.

Pope, Michael. 2016. "Sweating with Blood and Civil Conflict in *De Rerum Natura*." *CJ* 112.1: 41–55.

Porter, Roy and Rousseau, G.S. 1998. *Gout: The Patrician Malady*. New Haven, CT.

Preston, Richard. 1995. *The Hot Zone*. New York.

Prince, Meredith. 2011. "Ties that (Un)bind: Fathers, Daughters, and *Pietas* in Ovid's *Metamorphoses*." *Syllecta Classica* 22: 39–68.

Putnam, Michael. 1979. *Virgil's Poem of the Earth: Studies in the* Georgics. Princeton.

Quint, David. 1993. *Epic and Empire: Politics and Generic Form from Vergil to Milton*. Princeton.

Rand, E.K. 1925. *Ovid and His Influence*. Boston.

Ransmayr, Christoph. 1990. *The Last World*. Trans. by J. Woods. London.

Rho, Piero. 1966. *Antologia Lucreziana. Serie Latina, Vol. XXXVI*. Milan.

Ricoeur, Paul. 1984. *Time and Narrative*, 3 Vols. Trans. by K. Blamey and D. Pellaver. Chicago.

Roche, Paul. 2009. *Lucan:* De Bello Civili, *Book 1*. Oxford.

Rosen, William. 2007. *Justinian's Flea: Plague, Empire, and the Birth of Europe*. New York.

Ross, D.O. 1987. *Virgil's Elements: Physics and Poetry in the* Georgics. Princeton.

Rouse, W.H.D. and Smith, M.F., trans. 1992. *Lucretius: De Rerum Natura*. Cambridge, MA.

Rusten, J.S., ed. 1989. *Thucydides: The Peloponnesian War, Book II*. Cambridge.

Saller, R.P. 1994. *Patriarchy, Property, and Death in the Roman Family*. Cambridge.

Saylor, C.F. 1978. "*Belli Spes Inproba*: The Theme of Walls in Lucan, *Pharsalia* VI." *TAPA* 108: 243–57.

Scheid, John. 2015. "Livy and Religion." In B. Mineo, ed., *A Companion to Livy*, 78–89. Chichester, UK.

Scheidel, Walter. 2003. "Germs for Rome." In C. Edwards and G.Woolf, eds., *Rome the Cosmopolis*, 158–76. Cambridge.

Schierl, Petra. 2016. "A Preacher in Arcadia? Reconsidering Tityrus Christianus." In S. McGill and J. Pucci, eds., *Classics Renewed: Reception and Innovation in the Latin Poetry of Late Antiquity*, 241–64. Heidelberg.

Schmid, W. 1976. "Tityrus Christianus: Probleme religiöser Hirtendichtung an der Wende vom vierten zum fünften Jahrhundert." In K. Garber, ed., *Europäische Bukolik und Georgik*, 44–121. Darmstadt.

Schrijvers, P.H. 1970. *Horror ac Divina Voluptas: Études sur la poétique et la poésie de Lucrèce*. Amsterdam.

Sedley, David. 1998. *Lucretius and the Transformation of Greek Wisdom*. Cambridge.

Segal, Charles. 1969. "Myth and Philosophy in the *Metamorphoses*: Ovid's Augustanism and the Augustan Conclusion of Book XV." *AJP* 90.3: 257–92.

Segal, Charles. 1988. *Orpheus: The Myth of the Poet*. Baltimore.

Segal, Charles. 1990. *Lucretius on Death and Anxiety: Poetry and Philosophy in* De Rerum Natura. Princeton.

Severy, Beth. 2003. *Augustus and the Family at the Birth of the Roman Empire*. London.

Sklenář, R. 2003. *A Taste for Nothingness: A Study of* Virtus *and Related Themes in Lucan's* Bellum Civile. Ann Arbor, MI.

Slaney, Helen. 2009. "Liminal's Kosky's Hughes's Artaud's Seneca's *Oedipus*." *New Voices in Classical Reception Studies* 4: 52–69.

Solodow, Joseph. 1988. *The World of Ovid's* Metamorphoses. Chapel Hill, NC.

Sontag, Susan. 1988. *Illness as Metaphor* and *AIDS and Its Metaphors*. New York.

Spaltenstein, François. 1990. *Commentaire des Punica de Silius Italicus (livres 9 à 17)*. Geneva.

Steel, David. 1981. "Plague Writing: From Boccaccio to Camus." *Journal of European Studies* II: 88–110.

Stephanson, Raymond. 1987. "The Plague Narratives of Defoe and Camus." *Modern Language Quarterly* 48: 224–41.

Stoclet, Alain J. 2007. "*Consilia humana, ops divina, superstitio*: Seeking Succor and Solace in Times of Plague, with Particular Reference to Gaul in the Early Middle Ages." In L.K. Little, ed., *Plague and the End of Antiquity: The Pandemic of 541–750*, 135–49. Cambridge.

Stoddard, Kate. 1996. "Thucydides, Lucretius, and the End of the *De Rerum Natura*." *Maia* 48.2: 102–28.

Summers, David. 1989. "*ARIA II*: The Union of the Image and Artist as an Aesthetic Ideal in Renaissance Art." *Artibus et Historiae* 10.20: 15–31.

Thibodeau, Philip. 2011. *Playing the Farmer: Representations of Rural Life in Vergil's* Georgics. Berkeley.

Thomas, Richard. 1982. *Lands and Peoples in Roman Poetry: The Ethnographical Tradition*. Cambridge.

Thomas, Richard, ed. 1988. *Virgil: Georgics III–IV*. Cambridge.

Thomas, Richard. 1991. "The 'Sacrifice' at the End of the *Georgics*, Aristaeus, and Vergilian Closure." *Classical Philology* 86.3: 211–18.

Thomas, Sophie. 2000. "The Ends of the Fragment, the Problem of the Preface: Proliferation and Finality in *The Last Man*." In M. Eberle-Sinatra, ed., *Mary Shelley's Fictions: From* Frankenstein *to* Falkner, 22–38. Basingstoke and London.

Thompson, Lynette and Bruère, R.T. 2010. "Lucan's Use of Vergilian Reminiscence." In C. Tesoriero, ed. (with F. Muecke and T. Neal), *Oxford Readings in Classical Studies: Lucan*, 107–48. Oxford.

Tipping, Ben. 2010a. *Exemplary Epic: Silius Italicus'* Punica. Oxford.

Tipping, Ben. 2010b. "Virtue and Narrative in Silius Italicus' *Punica*." In A. Augoustakis, ed., *Brill's Companion to Silius Italicus*, 193–218. Leiden and Boston.

Tissol, Garth. 1997. *The Face of Nature: Wit, Narrative, and Cosmic Origins in Ovid's* Metamorphoses. Princeton.

Tracy, Jonathan. 2011. "Internal Evidence for the Completeness of the *Bellum Civile*." In P. Asso, ed., *Brill's Companion to Lucan*, 33–56. Leiden and Boston.

Trinacty, Christopher. 2014. *Senecan Tragedy and the Reception of Augustan Poetry*. Oxford.

Turner, B.S. 1984. *The Body and Society: Explorations in Social Theory*. London and New Delhi.

Vallillee, Gerald. 1960. *The Plague in Lucretius and Later Latin Poets*. Dissertation, University of Chicago.

Van Noorden, Helen. 2015. *Playing Hesiod: "The Myth of the Races" in Classical Antiquity*. Cambridge.

Vasaly, Ann. 2015. "The Composition of the *Ab Urbe Condita*: The Case of the First Pentad." In B. Mineo, ed., *A Companion to Livy*, 217–29. Chichester.

Versnel, H.S. 1981. "Self-Sacrifice, Compensation and the Anonymous Gods." In J. Rudhardt and O. Reverdin, eds., *Le sacrifice dans l'antiquité*. 135–85. Geneva.

Volk, Katharina. 2010. "Lucretius' Prayer for Peace and the Date of *De Rerum Natura*." *CQ* 60: 127–31.

Von Glinski, Marie Louise. 2012. *Simile and Identity in Ovid's* Metamorphoses. Cambridge.

Wald, Pricilla. 2008. *Contagion: Cultures, Carriers, and the Outbreak Narrative*. Durham, NC.

Wald, Pricilla. 2012. "Hybridity in the Biohorror Narrative or What We Can Learn from Monsters." In B. Magnusson and Z. Zalloua, eds., *Contagion: Health, Fear, Sovereignty*, 99–122. Vancouver.

Wallace-Hadrill, Andrew. 1985. "Propaganda and Dissent? Augustan Moral Legislation and the Love-Poets." *Klio* 67: 180–184.

Walsh, P.G. 1961. *Livy: His Historical Aims and Methods*. Cambridge.

Wasik, Bill and Murphy, Monica. 2012. *Rabid: A Cultural History of the World's Most Diabolical Virus*. New York.

Waszink, J.H. 1948. "Varro, Livy, and Tertullian on the History of the Roman Dramatic Art." *Vigiliae Christianae* 2: 224–42.

Warmington, E.H. 1940. *Remains of Old Latin, vol. 1: Ennius and Caecilius*. Cambridge, MA.

Wazer, Caroline. 2016. "Between Public Health and Popular Medicine: Senatorial and Popular Responses to Epidemic Disease in the Roman Republic." In W.V. Harris, ed., *Popular Medicine in Greco-Roman Antiquity*, 126–46. Leiden and Boston.

Welch, Tara S. 2005. *The Elegiac Cityscape: Propertius and the Meaning of Roman Monuments*. Columbus, OH.

West, David. 1979. "Two Plagues: Virgil, *Georgics* 3.478–566 and Lucretius 6.1090–1286." In D. West and T. Woodman, eds., *Creative Imitation and Latin Literature*, 71–88. Cambridge.

White, Carolinne. 2000. *Early Christian Latin Poets: The Early Church Fathers*. London and New York.

Wilkinson, L.P., trans. 1982. *Virgil: The Georgics*. London.

Williams, Gareth. 2009. "Apollo, Aesculapius, and the Poetics of Illness in Ovid's *Metamorphoses*." *PLLS* 14: 63–92.

Williams, R.D., ed. 1962. *Aeneidos: Liber Tertius*. Oxford.

Wills, Jeffrey. 1996. *Repetition in Latin Poetry: Figures of Allusion*. Oxford.

Woodman, A.J. 1988. *Rhetoric and Classical Historiography*. London and Sydney.

Woodman, A.J. 2009. "Community Health: Metaphors in Latin Historiography." *PLLS* 14: 43–61.

Wright, J.M. 2000. "'Little England': Anxieties of Space in Mary Shelley's *The Last Man*." In M. Eberle-Sinatra, ed., *Mary Shelley's Fictions: From* Frankenstein *to* Falkner, 129–49. Basingstoke and London.

Yavetz, Z. 1984. "The *Res Gestae* and Augustus' Public Image." In F. Millar and E. Segal, eds., *Caesar Augustus: Seven Aspects*, 1–36. Oxford.

Zanker, Paul. 1990. *The Power of Images in the Age of Augustus*. Trans. by Alan Shapiro. Ann Arbor, MI.

Index Locorum

Index

Lightning Source UK Ltd.
Milton Keynes UK
UKHW021828101221
395293UK00002B/281

9 780198 796428